Praise for *Spastic Hemiplegia—Unilateral Cerebral Palsy*

"Wow! This book is the most amazing and comprehensive source of information available for persons with unilateral CP and their families I have ever seen, and it should be required reading for any professionals who care for them. I was frankly astounded by the breadth of information here. Not only did I learn several things I had not known before, but I also am not able to think of anything the authors may have missed. Perhaps even more notable is that the information is understandable and digestible to all audiences and presented in a very caring and respectful manner that does not minimize the inherent challenges of having CP while also highlighting the limitless possibilities. The story of Ally and all the voices of those with CP and their families add tremendously to the content and the overall tone of the book. The lifespan perspective is to be applauded as well."

DIANE DAMIANO, Senior Investigator and Chief, Neurorehabilitation and Biomechanics Research Section, National Institutes of Health; Past-President Clinical Gait and Movement Analysis Society; Past President American Academy of Cerebral Palsy and Developmental Medicine, US

"I found this book to be an exceptional resource. It not only provides a thorough exploration of the unique challenges faced by those of us living with CP but also brings these experiences to life through personal stories and insights. This blend of practical advice and real-life experiences makes it an essential guide for anyone looking to empower themselves or support others in the CP community."

EMMA LIVINGSTONE, Founder and CEO, UP–The Adult Cerebral Palsy Movement; Adult with spastic hemiplegia, UK

"This publication provides a comprehensive review of medical team decision-making and addresses important aspects of surgical and clinical care. Perhaps most importantly, it includes an emphasis on community connection and provides personal experiences from individuals with CP and their families to learn from. Interested individuals, families, and clinicians will benefit from this effort."

JUSTIN RAMSEY, Associate Medical Director, Movement Clinic and Cerebral Palsy Program, Bethany Children's Health Center; Volunteer Clinical Associate Professor of Neurology, University of Oklahoma; Adult with spastic hemiplegia, US

T0325445

"In a world where it is so hard for parents of children with cerebral palsy to navigate conversations in health care systems, this book gets my highest recommendation: it is useful for parents. In particular, the explanations of concepts that they will hear doctors and therapists refer to, the importance of mental health considerations, and the perspective of other parents make this a uniquely practical resource. An unexpected and wonderful addition is the stories from adults with cerebral palsy—unvarnished and honest—which shed light on their experiences while also offering hope for a positive future for our children and patients."

NATHALIE MAITRE, Professor of Pediatrics in Neonatology, Neonatologist at Children's, and Director of Early Development and Cerebral Palsy Research, Emory University School of Medicine; Mother of son with hemiplegia, US

"How refreshing to read a book that is as relevant to doctors and health professionals as it is to people with cerebral palsy and their families. Learning from real-life experiences like those of Ally and her family, shared with openness and vulnerability, make the book compelling. Their story, interwoven throughout the text, provides valuable insights, and the photographs add depth. This book strikes a balance between being informative and respectful toward health care professionals and people with lived experience, written in language that can facilitate open communication to achieve the best outcome for the child and their family. There is a refreshing emphasis on shared decision-making and multidisciplinary care, as well as family- and person-centered care. A highlight is the information on transition to adulthood and living as an adult with cerebral palsy. It felt like a genuine conversation, addressing the person with CP directly: informative, respectful, and heartwarming. This book just wants to do the right thing by families. It is a generous resource of other sources of knowledge and help. I recommend this book to both health professionals and to families living with cerebral palsy."

NADIA BADAWI, CP Alliance Chair of Cerebral Palsy Research, University of Sydney; Medical Director and Co-Head, Grace Centre for Newborn Intensive Care, The Children's Hospital at Westmead, Australia

"As someone with right spastic hemiplegia, I was amazed by how much of the information was relevant to my memories of childhood therapy appointments and doctor visits. I deeply enjoyed reading the testimonies of those with CP, and I felt recognized inside their stories. From small things like official medical terminology to detailed explanations on why I was receiving certain treatments as a child, this book helped me not only recontextualize my own experiences but also prepared me to be a better medical advocate for myself moving into adulthood."

EMMALYNNE SHUMARD, Student; Adult with spastic hemiplegia, US

"*This book is a comprehensive distillation of current medical knowledge and best practice to guide all involved with children, families, and individuals with unilateral cerebral palsy. The delivery is straightforward, organized, and well informed. Individuals with hemiplegia and their parents will be drawn to this one source that focuses on the specifics of the condition. What makes this stand out is the 'humanistic holistic' approach to daily life, which is pertinent to quality of life. Especially noteworthy is the emphasis on activity, sports, and the discussion on how to participate at the community as well as Paralympic level. This book is a unique contribution.*"

DEBORAH GAEBLER-SPIRA, Director Emeritus Cerebral Palsy Program, Shirley Ryan AbilityLab; Professor Emeritus of Pediatrics and Physical Medicine and Rehabilitation, Northwestern Feinberg School of Medicine; Past President, American Academy for Cerebral Palsy and Developmental Medicine, US

"*Spastic Hemiplegia—Unilateral Cerebral Palsy is an essential read for anyone with an interest, either professional or personal, in understanding the condition. It successfully distills a huge volume of research into an accessible text that vitally provides a lifespan perspective. It provides parents with a much-needed toolkit to be their child's advocate. It also equips parents with knowledge to pass on to their child, empowering them to become their own advocate in the future. One of the book's standout features is the inclusion of personal stories. I found myself searching for the personal narrative in each chapter, wanting to understand Eimear's and Ally's perspectives, which brings the robust evidence-based content to life. The book beautifully illustrates what is often said, that each experience of cerebral palsy is unique. The diversity of personal experiences highlights the varied paths to diagnosis, management, and support, as well as both the unique and shared strengths and challenges faced by those living with spastic hemiplegia. This book is a valuable resource that successfully merges scientific evidence with lived experiences, making it a compelling and informative read.*"

JENNIFER RYAN, Director, Cerebral Palsy Lifespan Health and Well-being (CP-Life) Research Centre, Royal College of Surgeons in Ireland

"*Spastic Hemiplegia is a perfect primer for parents wanting more information about their child's condition, allied health care professionals interested in gaining more evidence-based information about the care of children with spastic hemiplegia, and for the layperson who knows someone with hemiplegia and is looking to understand the condition better. It is rare to find a book that weaves the patient experience into the content as nicely as has been done in this book. The authors have done a fine job of providing evidence-based information in a patient and family-centered fashion—a must-read for all!*"

BENJAMIN SHORE, Director, Cerebral Palsy and Spasticity Center, Boston Children's Hospital; Associate Professor of Orthopedic Surgery, Harvard Medical School, US

In these days when information is so prolific, misinformation seems to rule. It is no different in the world of cerebral palsy. Sadly, I have seen the wheel being reinvented over and over—erroneous treatment recommendations and overdosed surgeries, proposed and performed by low-volume clinicians and surgeons. Underwhelming treatment outcomes often go unrecognized. Parents and patients seeking comprehensive information on hemiplegia will find in this book clear explanations and sound information on diagnosis, prognosis, treatment strategies, and expected outcomes. I hope that all parents and patients have access to this wonderful work.

PAULO SELBER, Attending Orthopedic Surgeon, Hospital for Special Surgery; Professor of Orthopedic Surgery, Weill Cornell Medical College, US

Being suddenly immersed in a world of medical terminology, professional opinion, and service provision is surely overwhelming. This book centralizes children, families, and adults and provides a wealth of information on living with CP spastic hemiplegia throughout the life course. It has an excellent blend of medical and scientific information, practical application, and real-life excerpts. It is carefully written with clear but thorough explanations. This book is a must-read, not only for parents of children and adults with spastic hemiplegia but for the professionals working with them.

MICHELLE SPIRTOS, Associate Professor and Head of Discipline of Occupational Therapy, School of Medicine, Trinity College Dublin, Ireland

It has been an absolute pleasure to read Spastic Hemiplegia—Unilateral Cerebral Palsy. *The book communicates cutting-edge knowledge about the causes, development, and treatment of cerebral palsy in clear and accessible language. The perspectives of people with CP and their families are thoughtfully integrated. Even the most complex aspects are presented in a way that is easy to understand. I highly recommend this book to families, health care professionals, and researchers studying various aspects of cerebral palsy.*

EVA PONTÉN, Consultant Orthopaedic and Hand Surgeon, Karolinska University Hospital; Associate Professor, Karolinska Institutet, Sweden

SPASTIC HEMIPLEGIA UNILATERAL CEREBRAL PALSY

SPASTIC HEMIPLEGIA
Unilateral Cerebral Palsy

Understanding and
managing the condition
across the lifespan:
A practical guide for families

Marcie Ward, MD
Lily Collison, MA, MSc
Eimear Gabbett, Parent

Edited by
Elizabeth R. Boyer, PhD
Tom F. Novacheck, MD
GILLETTE CHILDREN'S

Gillette Children's Healthcare Press
200 University Avenue East
St Paul, MN 55101
www.GilletteChildrensHealthcarePress.org
HealthcarePress@gillettechildrens.com

ISBN 978-1-952181-13-9 (paperback)
ISBN 978-1-952181-14-6 (e-book)
LIBRARY OF CONGRESS CONTROL NUMBER 2024941673

COPYEDITING BY Ruth Wilson
ORIGINAL ILLUSTRATIONS BY Olwyn Roche
COVER AND INTERIOR DESIGN BY Jazmin Welch
PROOFREADING BY Ruth Wilson
INDEX BY Audrey McClellan

Printed by Hobbs the Printers Ltd, Totton, Hampshire, UK

For information about distribution or special discounts for bulk purchases, please contact:
Mac Keith Press
2nd Floor, Rankin Building
139-143 Bermondsey Street
London, SE1 3UW
www.mackeith.co.uk
admin@mackeith.co.uk

To individuals and families whose lives are affected by these conditions, to professionals who serve our community, and to all clinicians and researchers who push the knowledge base forward, we hope the books in this Healthcare Series serve you very well.

Gillette Children's acknowledges a grant from the Cerebral Palsy Foundation for the writing of this book.

All proceeds from the books in this series at Gillette Children's go to research.

Contents

Authors and Editors xv

Series Foreword by Dr. Tom F. Novacheck xvii

Series Introduction xix

1 CEREBRAL PALSY 1

    1.1   Introduction 3

    1.2   The nervous system 9

    1.3   Causes, risk factors, and prevalence 14

    1.4   Diagnosis 21

    1.5   Function 25

    1.6   Classification based on predominant motor type and topography 30

    1.7   Classification based on functional ability 39

    1.8   The International Classification of Functioning, Disability and Health 55

    Key points Chapter 1 59

2 SPASTIC HEMIPLEGIA 61

    2.1   Introduction 63

    2.2   The brain injury 73

    2.3   Growth 77

    2.4   Bones, joints, muscles, and movements 80
            WITH ARIANA PETERSON, OTR/L, AND JEAN STOUT, PT, MS, PhDc

    2.5   Typical hand function and typical walking 90

    2.6   Primary problems 95

    2.7   Secondary problems 104

    2.8   Tertiary problems 123

    2.9   Motor function in individuals with spastic hemiplegia 125

    2.10 Associated problems 132

    Key points Chapter 2 139

3   MANAGEMENT AND TREATMENT
    OF SPASTIC HEMIPLEGIA TO AGE 20 141

    3.1   Introduction 143
    3.2   What does best practice look like? 145
    3.3   Overall management philosophy 153
    3.4   Therapies 158
          WITH SUSAN ELLERBUSCH TOAVS, MS, CCC, CANDICE JOHNSON, OTD, OTR/L,
          AND AMY SCHULZ, PT, NCS
    3.5   The home program 181
          WITH CANDICE JOHNSON, OTD, OTR/L, AND AMY SCHULZ, PT, NCS
    3.6   Assistive technology 196
          WITH CANDICE JOHNSON, OTD, OTR/L, KAITLIN LEWIS, CTRS,
          KATHRYN PIMENTEL, MPO, CPO, AND AMY SCHULZ, PT, NCS
    3.7   Tone reduction 218
    3.8   Orthopedic surgery 229
          WITH TOM F. NOVACHECK, MD, JEAN STOUT, PT, MS, PhDc,
          AND ANN VAN HEEST, MD, FAOA
    3.9   Managing associated problems 243
    3.10 Alternative and complementary treatments 248
    3.11 Community integration, education, independence,
          and transition 251
          WITH TORI BAHR, MD
    Key points Chapter 3 266

4   THE ADULT WITH SPASTIC HEMIPLEGIA 267

    4.1   Introduction 269
    4.2   Aging in the typical population 274
    4.3   Aging with spastic hemiplegia 278
    4.4   Management and treatment of spastic hemiplegia
          in adulthood 290
          WITH JILL GETTINGS, MD, CANDICE JOHNSON, OTD, OTR/L,
          AND LEE SCHUH, MD
    Key points Chapter 4 301

5   LIVING WITH SPASTIC HEMIPLEGIA 303

6   FURTHER READING AND RESEARCH 331
    WITH ELIZABETH R. BOYER, PhD

Acknowledgments 341

APPENDICES (ONLINE)

Appendix 1: Measurement tools

Appendix 2: Scoliosis management

Appendix 3: Positioning

Appendix 4: Exercise and physical activity

Appendix 5: Selective dorsal rhizotomy

Appendix 6: Gait analysis

Appendix 7: Rehabilitation after single-event multilevel surgery

Appendix 8: Epilepsy management

Glossary 343

References 348

Index 371

Authors and Editors

Marcie Ward, MD, Pediatric Rehabilitation Medicine Physician, Gillette Children's

Lily Collison, MA, MSc, Program Director, Gillette Children's Healthcare Press

Eimear Gabbett, Parent

Elizabeth R. Boyer, PhD, Clinical Scientist, Gillette Children's

Tom F. Novacheck, MD, Medical Director of Integrated Care Services, Gillette Children's; Professor of Orthopedics, University of Minnesota; and Past President, American Academy for Cerebral Palsy and Developmental Medicine

Series Foreword

You hold in your hands one book in the Gillette Children's Healthcare Series. This series was inspired by multiple factors.

It started with Lily Collison writing the first book in the series, *Spastic Diplegia–Bilateral Cerebral Palsy*. Lily has a background in medical science and is the parent of a now adult son who has spastic diplegia. Lily was convincing at the time about the value of such a book, and with the publication of that book in 2020, Gillette Children's became one of the first children's hospitals in the world to set up its own publishing arm—Gillette Children's Healthcare Press. *Spastic Diplegia–Bilateral Cerebral Palsy* received very positive reviews from both families and professionals and achieved strong sales. Unsolicited requests came in from diverse organizations across the globe for translation rights, and feedback from families told us there was a demand for books relevant to other conditions.

We listened.

We were convinced of the value of expanding from one book into a series to reflect Gillette Children's strong commitment to worldwide education. In 2021, Lily joined the press as Program Director, and very quickly, Gillette Children's formed teams to write the Healthcare Series. The series includes, in order of publication:

- *Craniosynostosis*
- *Idiopathic Scoliosis*
- *Spastic Hemiplegia—Unilateral Cerebral Palsy*
- *Spastic Quadriplegia—Bilateral Cerebral Palsy*
- *Spastic Diplegia—Bilateral Cerebral Palsy, second edition*
- *Epilepsy*
- *Spina Bifida*
- *Osteogenesis Imperfecta*
- *Scoliosis—Congenital, Neuromuscular, Syndromic, and Other Causes*

The books address each condition detailing both the medical and human story.

Mac Keith Press, long-time publisher of books on disability and the journal *Developmental Medicine and Child Neurology,* is co-publishing this series with Gillette Children's Healthcare Press.

Families and professionals working well together is key to best management of any condition. The parent is the expert of their child while the professional is the expert of the condition. These books underscore the importance of that family and professional partnership. For each title in the series, medical professionals at Gillette Children's have led the writing, and families contributed the lived experience.

These books have been written in the United States with an international lens and citing international research. However, there isn't always strong evidence to create consensus in medicine, so others may take a different view.

We hope you find the book you hold in your hands to be of great value. We collectively strive to optimize outcomes for children, adolescents, and adults living with these childhood-acquired and largely lifelong conditions.

Dr. Tom F. Novacheck

Series Introduction

The Healthcare Series seeks to optimize outcomes for those who live with childhood-acquired physical and/or neurological conditions. The conditions addressed in this series of books are complex and often have many associated challenges. Although the books focus on the biomedical aspects of each condition, we endeavor to address each condition as holistically as possible. Since the majority of people with these conditions have them for life, the life course is addressed including transition and aging issues.

Who are these books for?

These books are written for an international audience. They are primarily written for parents of young children, but also for adolescents and adults who have the condition. They are written for members of multidisciplinary teams and researchers. Finally, they are written for others, including extended family members, teachers, and students taking courses in the fields of medicine, allied health care, and education.

A worldview

The books in the series focus on evidence-based best practice, which we acknowledge is not available everywhere. It is mostly available in high-income countries (at least in urban areas, though even there, not always), but many families live away from centers of good care.

We also acknowledge that the majority of people with disabilities live in low- and middle-income countries. Improving the lives of all those with disabilities across the globe is an important goal. Developing scalable, affordable interventions is a crucial step toward achieving this. Nonetheless, the best interventions will fail if we do not first address the social determinants of health—the economic, social, and environmental conditions in which people live that shape their overall health and well-being.

No family reading these books should ever feel they have failed their child. We all struggle to do our best for our children within the limitations of our various resources and situations. Indeed, the advocacy role these books may play may help families and professionals lobby in unison for best care.

International Classification of Functioning, Disability and Health

The writing of the series of books has been informed by the International Classification of Functioning, Disability and Health (ICF).[1] The framework explains the impact of a health condition at different levels and how those levels are interconnected. It tells us to look at the full picture—to look at the person with a disability in their life situation.

The framework shows that every human being can experience a decrease in health and thereby experience some disability. It is not something that happens only to a minority of people. The ICF thus "mainstreams" disability and recognizes it as a widespread human experience.

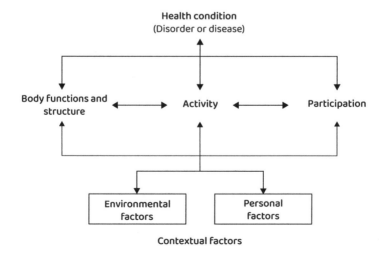

International Classification of Functioning, Disability and Health (ICF). Reproduced with kind permission from WHO.

In health care, there has been a shift away from focusing almost exclusively on correcting issues that cause the individual's functional problems to focusing also on the individual's activity and participation. These books embrace maximizing participation for all people living with disability.

The family

For simplicity, throughout the series we refer to "parents" and "children"; we acknowledge, however, that family structures vary. "Parent" is used as a generic term that includes grandparents, relatives, and carers (caregivers) who are raising a child. Throughout the series, we refer to male and female as the biologic sex assigned at birth. We acknowledge that this does not equate to gender identity or sexual orientation, and we respect the individuality of each person. Throughout the series we have included both "person with disability" and "disabled person," recognizing that both terms are used.

Caring for a child with a disability can be challenging and overwhelming. Having a strong social support system in place can make a difference. For the parent, balancing the needs of the child with a disability with the needs of siblings—while also meeting employment demands, nurturing a relationship with a significant other, and caring for aging parents—can sometimes feel like an enormous juggling act. Siblings may feel neglected or overlooked because of the increased attention given to the disabled child. It is crucial for parents to allocate time and resources to ensure that siblings feel valued and included in the family dynamics. Engaging siblings in the care and support of the disabled child can help foster a sense of unity and empathy within the family.

A particular challenge for a child and adolescent who has a disability, and their parent, is balancing school attendance (for both academic and social purposes) with clinical appointments and surgery. Appointments outside of school hours are encouraged. School is important because the cognitive and social abilities developed there help maximize employment opportunities when employment is a realistic goal. Indeed, technology has eliminated barriers and created opportunities that did not exist even 10 years ago.

Parents also need to find a way to prioritize self-care. Neglecting their own well-being can have detrimental effects on their mental and physical health. Think of the safety advice on an airplane: you are told that you must put on your own oxygen mask before putting on your child's. It's the same when caring for a child with a disability; parents need to take care of themselves in order to effectively care for their child *and* family. Friends, support groups, or mental health professionals can provide an outlet for parents to express their emotions, gain valuable insights, and find solace in knowing that they are not alone in their journey.

For those of you reading this book who have the condition, we hope this book gives you insights into its many nuances and complexities, acknowledges you as an expert in your own care, and provides a road map and framework for you to advocate for your needs.

Last words

This series of books seeks to be an invaluable educational resource. All proceeds from the series at Gillette Children's go to research.

Chapter 1

Cerebral palsy

Section 1.1 Introduction 3

Section 1.2 The nervous system 9

Section 1.3 Causes, risk factors, and prevalence 14

Section 1.4 Diagnosis 21

Section 1.5 Function 25

Section 1.6 Classification based on predominant motor type
and topography 30

Section 1.7 Classification based on functional ability 39

Section 1.8 The International Classification of Functioning,
Disability and Health 55

Key points Chapter 1 59

Introduction

So be sure when you step.
Step with care and great tact
and remember that Life's
a Great Balancing Act ...
And will you succeed?
Yes! You will, indeed!
(98 and ¾ percent guaranteed.)
Kid, you'll move mountains!
Dr. Seuss

To fully understand hemiplegia, it is worth first having an understanding of the umbrella term "cerebral palsy" (CP). "Cerebral" refers to a specific part of the brain (the cerebrum) and "palsy" literally means paralysis (cerebrum paralysis). Although paralysis describes something different from the typical features of CP, it is the origin of the term "palsy."

CP was first described in 1861 by an English doctor, William Little, and for many years it was known as "Little's disease." Over the years there has been much discussion of the definition of CP, and different definitions have been adopted and later discarded. Following is the most recently adopted definition, published in 2007:

> *Cerebral palsy describes a group of permanent disorders of the development of movement and posture, causing activity limitation, that are attributed to non-progressive disturbances that occurred in the developing fetal or infant brain. The motor disorders of cerebral palsy are often accompanied by disturbances of sensation, perception, cognition, communication, behaviour, by epilepsy and by secondary musculoskeletal problems.[2]*

In other words, CP is a *group* of conditions caused by an injury to the developing brain, which can result in a variety of motor and other problems that affect how the child functions. Because the injury occurs in a *developing brain and growing child*, problems often change over time, even though the brain injury itself is unchanging. Table 1.1.1 explains the terms used in the definition of CP above, in order.

Table 1.1.1 Explanation of terms in definition of CP

TERMS	EXPLANATION
Cerebral	"Cerebral" refers to the cerebrum, one of the major areas of the brain responsible for the control of movement.
Palsy	"Palsy" means paralysis, that is, an inability to activate muscles by the nervous system, though paralysis by pure definition is not a feature of CP.
Group	CP is not a single condition, unlike conditions such as type 1 diabetes. Rather, CP is a group of conditions. The location, timing, and type of brain injury vary, as do the resulting effects.
Permanent	The brain injury remains for life; CP is a permanent, lifelong condition.
Disorders	A disorder is a disruption in the usual orderly process. To meet the definition of CP, the disorder must cause activity limitation.
Posture	Posture is the way a person holds their body when, for example, standing, sitting, or moving.

Cont'd.

TERMS	EXPLANATION
Activity limitation	An activity is the execution of a task or action by an individual. Activity limitations are difficulties an individual may have in doing activities. Walking with difficulty is an example.
Nonprogressive	The brain injury does not worsen, but its effects can develop or evolve over time.
Developing fetal or infant brain	The brain of a fetus or infant has not finished developing all its neural connections and is therefore immature. An injury to an immature brain is different from an injury to a mature brain.
Motor disorders	Motor disorders are conditions affecting the ability to move and the quality of those movements.
Sensation	"Sensation" refers to the physical feeling or perception arising from something that happens to or that comes in contact with the body.
Perception	Perception is the ability to incorporate and interpret sensory and/or cognitive information.
Cognition	"Cognition" means the mental action or process of acquiring knowledge and understanding through thought, experience, and the senses.
Communication	Communication is the imparting or exchanging of information.
Behavior	"Behavior" refers to the way a person acts or conducts themselves.
Epilepsy	Epilepsy is a neurological disorder in which brain electrical activity becomes abnormal, causing seizures or periods of unusual behavior, sensations, and sometimes loss of awareness.
Secondary musculoskeletal problems	"Musculoskeletal" refers to both the muscles and the skeleton (i.e., the muscles, bones, joints, and their related structures). Musculoskeletal problems appear with time and growth and are therefore termed "secondary problems." They develop as a consequence of the brain injury. People with CP may develop a variety of musculoskeletal problems, such as bone torsion (twist), or muscle contracture (a limitation of range of motion of a joint).

Adapted from Rosenbaum and colleagues.[2]

CP is the most common cause of physical disability in children.[3] It is acquired during pregnancy, birth, or in early childhood, and it is a life-long condition. There is currently no cure, nor is one imminent, but good management and treatment (addressed in Chapter 3) can help alleviate some or many of the effects of the brain injury.

When the brain injury occurs is important. The consequences of a brain injury to a fetus developing in the uterus are generally different from those of a brain injury sustained at birth, which in turn are different from those of a brain injury acquired during infancy. The European and Australian Cerebral Palsy Registers use two years of age as the cutoff for applying the diagnosis of CP.[4,5] A brain injury occurring after two years of age is called an "acquired brain injury." This two-year cutoff is applied because of the differences in brain maturity relative to when the brain injury occurs.

Although the development of movement and posture is affected in individuals with CP, as seen above, other body systems can also be affected.

How to read this book

To help you navigate the information in this book, it has been organized so that you can read it from beginning to end or, alternatively, dip into different sections and chapters independently. Because much of the information builds on previous sections and chapters, it is best to first read the book in its entirety to get an overall sense of the condition. After that, you can return to the parts that are relevant to you, knowing that you can ignore other sections or revisit them if and when they do become relevant.

This chapter addresses the overall condition of CP. Chapter 2 addresses hemiplegia, and Chapter 3 covers the management of treatment of hemiplegia to age 20. Chapter 4 looks at hemiplegia in adulthood.

Throughout Chapters 1 to 4, medical information is interspersed with personal lived experience. Orange boxes are used to highlight the personal story. Chapter 5 is devoted to vignettes from individuals and families around the globe. Chapter 6 provides further reading and research.

At the back of the book, you'll find a glossary of key terms.

A companion website for this book is available at www.GilletteChildrens HealthcarePress.org. This website contains some useful web resources and appendices. A QR code to access **Useful web resources** is included below.

It may be helpful to discuss any questions you may have from reading this book with your medical professional.

Ally was born prematurely in Limerick, Ireland, on May 2011, at 25 weeks gestation and weighed 2 lb. The early birth was due to cervical insufficiency and a premature rupture of my membranes[*] with consequent loss of amniotic fluid. I had been in hospital for five days prior to delivery, and because I developed an infection, I had an emergency cesarean section. Following delivery, it was nearly 24 hours before I got to meet Ally in her tiny red hat, in an incubator, and with lots of tubes and machines attached to her. I just could not believe that any baby could be so small; she literally was the size of a soda can with tiny arms and legs.

---

[*] Cervical insufficiency is a condition where the cervix, the lower part of the uterus, is unable to maintain tight closure during pregnancy, resulting in possible loss of the pregnancy or preterm birth. Premature rupture of membranes occurs when the amniotic sac surrounding and protecting the fetus in the uterus breaks before labor starts, resulting in possible preterm birth and the risk of infection.

Ally was intubated with full life support,[*] and the clear message we got from the doctors and nurses was how critical the next 24 hours would be. The risk of brain bleeds, breathing issues, and infection was significant, and this would really determine whether Ally would survive.

At the time, this did not mean a lot to me. I did not research or delve into the implications or what it would mean in the future. Instead, I wanted to focus on what I could do to help her there and then, which for me was the immediate focus of generating breast milk and having skin-to-skin contact.

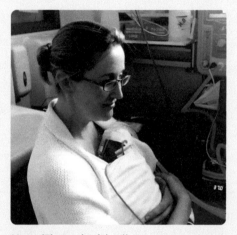

Mom (Eimear) with Ally.

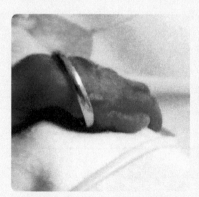
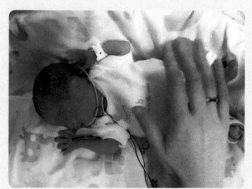

Ally's hand in her dad's wedding ring.

* Life support for a newborn infant typically involves providing mechanical ventilation (a tube down the throat to help with breathing) and other interventions to support vital functions.

The nervous system

The Brain—is wider than the Sky
Emily Dickinson

CP results from an injury to the developing fetal or young child's brain, or a difference in how the fetal brain forms. A basic understanding of the nervous system is useful to help understand the effects of the brain injury. This section briefly explains the main components of the nervous system.

The nervous system is composed of the:

- Central nervous system (CNS)—the brain and spinal cord.
- Peripheral nervous system (PNS)—a large network of nerves that carry messages between the CNS and the rest of the body. The autonomic nervous system is part of the PNS; it controls involuntary functions of the brain and body, such as breathing, heart rate, and digestion.

See Figure 1.2.1.

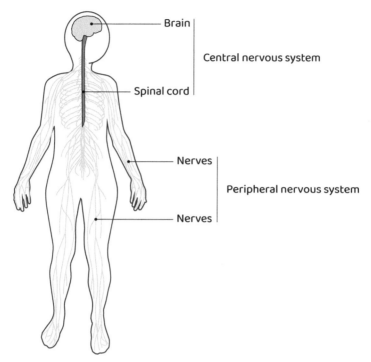

Figure 1.2.1 The nervous system.

Nerve cells

The nerve cell (also known as "neuron" or "neurone") is the basic unit of the nervous system. Nerve cells carry information between the CNS and the rest of the body as electrical impulses. There are three types of nerve cells:

- Motor nerve cells, which take information from the CNS to a muscle or gland
- Sensory nerve cells, which do the opposite, taking messages from the rest of the body to the CNS
- Interneurons (also known as "relay neurons"), which carry information between nerve cells

Figure 1.2.2 shows a typical nerve cell. Note the cell body and axon. Information enters the nerve cell through the dendrites and cell body, and exits via the axonal endings. The cell bodies form the gray matter of the brain, and the axons form the white matter, or the communication tracts.

The whitish color of the white matter is due to the fatty substance, called "myelin," that covers the axons; this insulates and speeds up the transmission of electrical impulses. Nerve cells receive, interpret, and transfer messages as electrical impulses. These electrical impulses form the brain's electrical activity, which can be measured and recorded on an electroencephalogram (EEG).

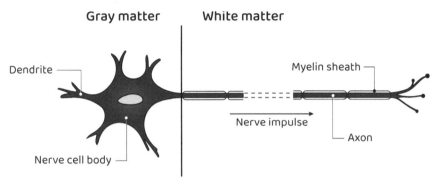

Figure 1.2.2 Nerve cell. Adapted with permission from *The Identification and Treatment of Gait Problems in Cerebral Palsy*, 2nd edition, edited by James Gage et al. (2009). Mac Keith Press.

Brain structure and functions

The brain is housed inside the cranium, a bony covering that protects the brain from external injury. Together, the cranium and the bones that protect the face make up the skull.

The brain is divided into several distinct parts that serve important functions. See Figure 1.2.3.

The *cerebrum* is the front and upper part of the brain. The cerebral cortex (the outer layer, the surface of the brain) is the gray matter where the cell bodies of the nerve cells are found. The cerebral cortex has a large surface area and, due to its folds, it appears wrinkled. Different regions of the cerebral cortex have different functions.

The *cerebellum* is located at the back of the brain, under the cerebrum, and helps with maintaining balance and posture, coordination, and fine motor movements.

The *brain stem* is the bottom part of the brain that connects the cerebrum to the *spinal cord*. It also serves as a relay station for messages between different parts of the body and the cerebral cortex. Many functions responsible for survival are located here (e.g., breathing and heart rate).

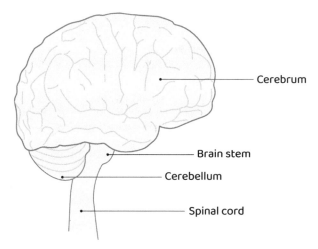

Cerebrum

Brain stem

Cerebellum

Spinal cord

Figure 1.2.3 Parts of the brain.

The cerebrum is divided in two halves, referred to as hemispheres (see Figure 1.2.4). In general, the right half controls the left side of the body, and the left half controls the right side of the body. Therefore, damage on the right side of the cerebrum will impact the left side of the body and vice versa. Communication between the two halves occurs in the corpus callosum, located in the center of the cerebrum.

The *basal ganglia* and *thalamus* are located in the middle of the cerebrum, deep beneath the cerebral cortex. The basal ganglia are important in the control of movement, including motor learning and planning. The thalamus is sometimes referred to as a relay station—it relays various sensory information (e.g., sight, sound, touch) to the cerebral cortex from the rest of the body.

Cerebrospinal fluid is found within the brain and around the spinal cord. It is produced within channels in the brain, called "ventricles." Cerebrospinal fluid helps protect the brain and spinal cord from injury.

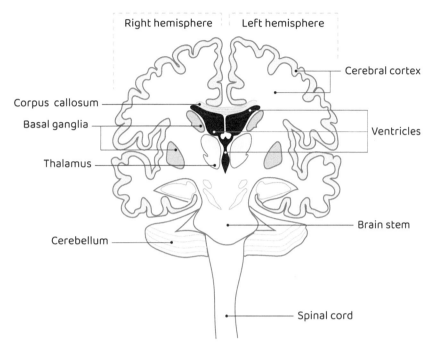

Figure 1.2.4 Vertical cross-section of the brain.

Causes, risk factors, and prevalence

The little reed, bending to the force of the wind,
soon stood upright again when the storm had passed over.

Aesop

The US Centers for Disease Control and Prevention (CDC) defines "cause" as:

> *A factor (characteristic, behavior, event, etc.) that directly influences the occurrence of disease. A reduction of the factor in the population should lead to a reduction in the occurrence of disease.*

It defines "risk factor" as:

> *An aspect of personal behavior or lifestyle, an environmental exposure, or an inborn or inherited characteristic that is associated with an increased occurrence of disease or other health-related event or condition.*[6]

Causes thus have a stronger relationship with CP than do risk factors. A significant stroke in the infant's brain, for example, is a cause of CP.

Preterm birth (i.e., less than 37 weeks gestation) is a risk factor but not a cause of CP—in other words, not every preterm infant is found to have CP. There are many possible causes of brain injury, including events during fetal development, pregnancy, birth, or early infant life. Much is known about the causes and risk factors for CP, but more remains unknown.

Causes

Data from Australia shows that 94 percent of children with CP had a brain injury in the prenatal or perinatal periods (i.e., during pregnancy and up to the first 28 days after birth), while only 6 percent had a recognized postnatal brain injury (acquired more than 28 days after birth and before two years of age).[4] Seventy to 80 percent of CP cases are associated with prenatal factors, and birth asphyxia (lack of oxygen during birth) plays a relatively minor role.[7]

There are many causes of brain injury, including:

- **Hypoxia-ischemia:** from hypoxia, which is a deficiency of oxygen, and ischemia, which is reduced blood flow to the brain. Hypoxia-ischemia is a combination of both terms.
- **Hemorrhage:** bleeding in the brain, also termed a "cerebral vascular accident" (CVA) or a stroke.
- **Infection**
- **Abnormalities in brain development**[7]

A decrease in oxygen and insufficient blood supply to the brain have different effects in preterm infants compared with term infants due to the different stages of their brain development. As noted in section 1.2, the nerve cell bodies form the gray matter while axons form the white matter or the communication tracts. It has been found that white matter injuries predominate in infants born preterm, whereas gray matter injuries are more common in infants born at term.[7]

Approximately 90 percent of cases of CP result from healthy brain tissue becoming damaged rather than from abnormalities in brain development.[3] The cause of CP in an individual child is very often unknown.[8,9]

Risk factors

Infants who are born preterm (earlier than 37 weeks) or who have low birth weight have a higher risk of CP.[10] Twins and other multiple-birth siblings are at particular risk because they tend to be born early and at lower birth weights. Australian data shows that:[4]

- Forty-three percent of children with CP were born preterm compared to 9 percent in the typical population.
- Forty-three percent of children with CP were born with low birth weight (under 2,500 grams, or 5.5 lb) compared to 7 percent in the typical population.
- The prevalence of children with CP was higher for twin than singleton births. This is why single embryo transfer in assisted reproductive technology (ART)* is strongly encouraged.[11,12]

In addition to the above, other risk factors for CP include the following (not an exhaustive list):[7]

- Prior to conception:
  - Young or advanced maternal age
  - A history of stillbirth or multiple miscarriages
  - Low socioeconomic status
  - Genetic factors
- During pregnancy:
  - Male sex: Males account for a greater proportion of individuals with CP than females. Australia data shows that 58 percent of those with CP were male.[4]
  - TORCH complex: TORCH is an acronym used to refer to a group of infections that can affect a developing fetus or a newborn: **T**oxoplasmosis (caused by a parasite), **O**ther infections, **R**ubella (also known as German measles), **C**ytomegalovirus, and **H**erpes simplex virus.
  - Maternal thyroid disorder.

---

* A broad term encompassing various fertility treatments, including in vitro fertilization, intrauterine insemination, and egg freezing.

- o Pre-eclampsia (high blood pressure that can pose serious risks to both mother and fetus if left untreated).
  - o Placenta problems (e.g., placenta previa, placenta abruption).[*]
- Around the time of birth and during the neonatal (newborn) period:
  - o An acute hypoxic event (lack of oxygen) during birth
  - o Meconium aspiration[†]
  - o Seizures
  - o Low blood sugar

Some risk factors are declining, but others are increasing. Although any one risk factor may cause CP, if that factor is severe enough, it is more often caused by the combination of multiple risk factors.[13] Although preterm birth is a large risk factor for CP, it's the causal pathways that have led to it, or the consequences of it, that may cause the CP, rather than the preterm birth itself.

Mutations or changes in the genes involved in brain development or function (either inherited or *de novo*, which is a change in a gene that appears for the first time in a child but is not present in either parent) can increase susceptibility to CP. These genetic risk factors may affect the severity of symptoms, the specific type of CP, or the likelihood of associated conditions. Genetic risk factors may interact with other risk factors, highlighting the complex interplay between multiple risk factors in determining the development of the condition.

In low- and middle-income countries, causes and risk factors differ. In these countries, few preterm infants survive. Birth asphyxia is more common due to complications during labor or delivery. Also more common is Rhesus incompatibility (a mismatch in the Rhesus blood group system between the mother and the fetus). As well, a higher proportion of postnatally acquired CP is associated with infections such as meningitis, septicemia, and malaria.[7]

---

[*] "Placenta previa" means the placenta partially or fully covers the cervix. It can lead to bleeding and complications during birth. "Placenta abruption" means the placenta detaches from the uterus before the infant is born, with potentially life-threatening risks for both the mother and infant. It requires immediate medical attention.

[†] When a newborn breathes in a mixture of amniotic fluid (fluid that was surrounding the fetus in the uterus) and stool during or shortly after birth, potentially causing respiratory issues.

Prevalence

The prevalence of a condition is how many people in a defined population have the condition at a specific point in time. Prevalence can vary geographically and change over time because of medical advances and social and economic development.

Having an understanding of prevalence, along with causes and risk factors, can help with prevention of CP. A systematic review[*] of interventions for prevention and treatment of CP reported that effective prenatal interventions include corticosteroids and magnesium sulfate; effective neonatal (newborn) interventions include caffeine (methylxanthine) and hypothermia.[†14]

CP registers[‡] are essential for tracking and analyzing the prevalence and trends of CP in populations. They provide researchers and health care providers with critical data on the incidence, types, severity, and outcomes of CP, which can lead to improved health care policies and practices. It would be very helpful if, once a child is diagnosed with CP, parents would give consent to have their child added to a CP register. Many countries maintain CP registers. There are two major networks of registers: the Surveillance of Cerebral Palsy in Europe (SCPE, established in 1998) and the Australian Cerebral Palsy Register (ACPR, established in 2007). A newer network of registers was established in 2018: the Global Low- and Middle-Income Countries CP Register (GLM CPR). There is no single national CP register in the US. There, instead, CP data is often collected and maintained by various state or regional programs, research facilities, or health care centers.

The current CP birth prevalence in high-income countries is declining and is now 1.6 per 1,000 live births (data 1995 to 2014).[5] However, in the US, prevalence was found to be higher at 2.9 per 1,000 eight-year-olds (2010 data)[15] and 3.2 per 1,000 3- to 17-year-olds (2009–2016 data).[16]

Current CP birth prevalence is also higher in low- and middle-income countries.[5] The prevalence in rural Bangladesh was reported as 3.4

---

[*] A systematic review summarizes the results of a number of scientific studies.

[†] The controlled cooling of a newborn's body temperature.[20]

[‡] Confidential databases that store important data about individuals with CP.

per 1,000 children, and the majority had potentially preventable risk factors.[17] For example, only 30 percent of mothers received regular prenatal care.[17]

The most recent report from the Australian Cerebral Palsy Register shows a decrease in both prevalence and severity of CP between 1997 and 2016.[4] The decrease in prevalence was from 2.4 to 1.5 per 1,000 live births, a decrease of almost 40 percent. The decrease in severity was evidenced by a decrease in the proportion of children with greater functional mobility challenges, and in the proportion of children with epilepsy or intellectual impairment. This is encouraging because it suggests that with the application of resources, prevalence and severity may be able to be reduced in other countries.

Unfortunately, funding for CP research is very low. Although the reported prevalence of CP is double that of Down syndrome,[18] funding awarded for CP research in 2023 ($30 million) was significantly lower than for Down syndrome research ($133 million).[19]

And so the journey began. Ally did great for the first few days and all the signs were good: she was accepting my milk, she was free from infection, she was breathing room air without the addition of oxygen, and she did not appear to have had a brain bleed. The nurses and doctors were sending messages that things were looking positive.

On day three, we met our first setback when, unfortunately, her liver was punctured when a central line* was being inserted. This left her so unwell that they really did not think she would survive, and we christened her on day five. Ally, however, is a fighter, and despite that setback, plus two bouts of sepsis,† breathing issues due to underdeveloped lungs, and feeding issues, she fought her way through a three-month intensive care stay. We eventually brought her home at the beginning of September weighing a hefty (as far as we were concerned) 5 lb.

---

* A central line is a catheter placed into a large blood vessel to administer medications and fluids.

† Sepsis is a serious condition; it is the body's response to infection in the blood or other tissues. It can lead to organ failure, shock and death.

At this stage, despite numerous brain ultrasounds while Ally was in hospital, there was no evidence that she had had a brain bleed or hypoxic[*] event. I had no clue that Ally had cerebral palsy; as far as I was concerned, with the exception of prematurity and a tiny stature, she had no major challenges. The first few months were so intense with feeding I didn't notice anything significant with Ally, but on reflection she did not move her right side as much and there probably was some tone present. The doctors did not inform or educate me on the high likelihood that Ally might have CP. With hindsight, I would urge parents who have premature babies or a difficult birth to be very aware of any unusual signs or developmental delays and to ask questions and try to secure an early brain MRI as knowledge is power, and at least if you have an early diagnosis you can begin interventions as early as possible.

Early detection is of paramount importance, as the earlier you can intervene the better the outcome.

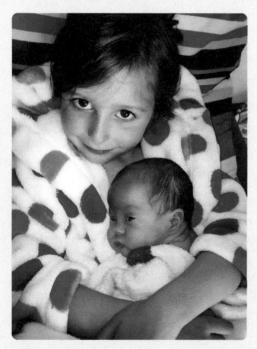

Milly (sister) with Ally.

---

[*] "Hypoxic" means lack of oxygen.

1.4

Diagnosis

Acceptance is knowing that grief is a raging river.
And you have to get into it. Because when you do,
it carries you to the next place. It eventually
takes you to open land, somewhere where it
will turn out OK in the end.

Simone George

There is no single test to confirm CP, unlike other conditions such as type 1 diabetes, which is confirmed through a simple blood test for glucose, or Down syndrome, which is confirmed through a genetic test. Recall that CP is not a single condition; rather, it is a group of conditions. The location, timing, and type of brain injury vary, and the resulting effects of the brain injury are also varied.

Until recently, a diagnosis of CP was generally made between 12 and 24 months based on a combination of clinical signs (e.g., lack of use of a limb), neurological symptoms (e.g., presence of spasticity*), and phys-

---

* A condition in which there is an abnormal increase in muscle tone or stiffness of muscle that can interfere with movement and speech, and be associated with discomfort or pain.

ical limitations (e.g., delayed independent sitting or walking). However, using certain standardized tests in combination with clinical examination and medical history, Novak and colleagues found that a diagnosis of CP can often accurately be made before six months corrected age.[*][21] They identified two distinct pathways in their International Clinical Practice Guideline for early diagnosis of CP:

- Before five months corrected age, for infants with newborn detectable risk factors (e.g., preterm):
  o MRI (magnetic resonance imaging)
  o GMs (Prechtl Qualitative Assessment of General Movements)[†]
  o HINE (Hammersmith Infant Neurological Examination)[‡]
- After five months corrected age for infants with infant detectable risk factors (e.g., delayed motor milestones)
  o MRI
  o HINE
  o DAYC (Developmental Assessment of Young Children)[§]

The presence of a brain injury is confirmed by MRI in many but not all children with CP. Imaging may also help determine when the brain injury occurred.[3] However, up to 17 percent of children diagnosed with CP have normal MRI brain scans.[3] For these children, best practice is to investigate further to rule out genetic and metabolic conditions.[3]

Successful implementation of early diagnosis programs has been demonstrated in different countries.[23-28] Early diagnosis is very important

---

* The term "corrected age" refers to how old an infant would be if they had been born on their due date rather than preterm. "Chronological age" refers to how old an infant is from their date of birth. Corrected age is often used when assessing growth and developmental skills usually up to a chronological age of two years. With preterm infants, it takes time to determine whether the delays are related to being preterm or are true delays.

† A standardized assessment of movement for infants, from birth to five months corrected age. It involves a video of an infant lying on their back while they are awake, calm, and alert. The recorded movements are then scored by a certified medical professional.

‡ A standardized neurological examination for infants age 2 to 24 months performed by a medical professional. There are three parts to the exam: carrying out a neurological examination (which is scored), noting developmental milestones, and observing behavior (both not scored).

§ A standardized assessment for infants and children from birth to five years, in which a medical professional scores a child's skills during observation of play or daily activity, asking a child to perform a skill, or by interviewing parents to measure ability in five domains: cognition, communication, social-emotional development, physical development, and adaptive behavior.

because it allows for early intervention, which helps to achieve better functional outcomes for the child.

Where a CP diagnosis is suspected but cannot be made with certainty, using the interim diagnosis of "high risk for CP" is recommended until a diagnosis is confirmed.[29] This allows the child to receive the benefits of CP-specific early intervention.[30]

These early interventions are designed to:[21]

- Optimize motor, cognition, and communication skills using interventions that promote learning and neuroplasticity
- Prevent secondary impairments and minimize complications that worsen function or interfere with learning (e.g., monitor hips, control epilepsy, take care of sleeping, feeding)
- Promote parent or caregiver coping and mental health

Neuroplasticity (also known as brain plasticity, neural plasticity, and neuronal plasticity) refers to the brain's ability to change. After a brain injury occurs, the brain will try to recover somewhat by creating new pathways around the injury, moving functions to a healthy area of the brain, or strengthening existing healthy connections. This potential for change and growth through practice and repetition allows the brain to develop new skills. [31,32]

Neuroplasticity is at its optimum during early brain development. The first thousand days are a critical time for brain development; this is a time when interventions are particularly effective.[33] This is also a time of extreme vulnerability: the same neuroplasticity that gives a child the potential to recover function also makes them very sensitive to any intervention, which can result in unwanted consequences unless the intervention has been proven safe.

Morgan and colleagues published an International Clinical Practice Guideline for early intervention for children from birth to two years of age with or at high risk of CP.[30] They followed this with another guideline in 2023 for children in the first year of life, which helps determine the most appropriate motor intervention to implement.[34]

These clinical practice guidelines for early diagnosis and early intervention should become standard of care[21,30,34] and be continually updated. The advancements in early diagnosis have resulted in multiple clinical trials in early interventions around the world, which will add to the research base in the coming years. (Further information on clinical trials is included in Chapter 6.)

Graham and colleagues noted that mothers of children with CP who have previously had a typically developing child often sense that something is wrong at a very early stage; they advised professionals to take the concerns of an experienced parent seriously.[3] Indeed, "parent-identified concern" is included in the International Clinical Practice Guideline for early diagnosis as a "valid reason to trigger formal diagnostic investigations and referral to early intervention."[21] Parent focus groups have also found that receiving early diagnosis or high risk for CP classification is a parent priority.[35]

Emily Perl Kingsley, who was a writer on the TV show *Sesame Street*, wrote a short essay titled "Welcome to Holland" in 1987 about parenting her son, born with Down syndrome. She described it as going on vacation and arriving at a different destination than what was expected. The essay resonates with many families on receiving a diagnosis of CP and is included in **Useful web resources**.

All mothers experience guilt, and I think the guilt of having a premature baby is magnified to infinity—What did I do wrong? Did I do too much? Did I work too hard? Was it because I missed that appointment? Was it because I went on that walk?

In many cases, *why* babies are born prematurely is not known. In my case, it was likely because I have a connective tissue disorder called Marfan syndrome. This sometimes leads to premature rupturing of the amniotic sac containing amniotic fluid around the baby in the uterus.

Function

That's one small step for man, one giant leap for mankind.

Neil Armstrong

"Function" means ability or capacity. "Motor function" refers to our ability to move, and "communication function" refers to our ability to transmit and receive information by whatever means. CP affects the development of movement, but it can also affect other areas, such as cognition. This section introduces the broad area of function and, again, lays groundwork for later sections.

Developmental milestones

The CDC published a series of developmental milestones that address typical development of the child from the age of two months to five years, in the following areas:[36]

- Social/emotional
- Language/communication
- Cognitive
- Movement/physical development

These milestones are an important reference when a child appears to be late in development compared with typically developing children. The CDC developmental milestones are included in **Useful web resources**.

Movement and physical development depend on the development and maturation of gross and fine motor function:

- **Gross motor function** (or gross motor skills): the movement of the arms, legs, and other large body parts. It involves the use of large muscles. Examples include sitting, crawling, standing, running, jumping, swimming, throwing, catching, and kicking. These movements involve maintaining balance and changing position.
- **Fine motor function** (or fine motor skills, hand skills, fine motor coordination, or dexterity): the smaller movements that occur in the wrists, hands, fingers, feet, and toes. It involves the control of small muscles. Examples include picking up objects between the thumb and forefinger, and writing. These movements typically involve hand-eye coordination and require a high degree of precision of hand and finger movement.

There is a usual sequence and timing to the achievement of gross motor developmental milestones in the typically developing child. A large study conducted by the World Health Organization (WHO) found that, with some variation, almost all typically developing children have achieved independent sitting by 9 months and independent walking by 18 months.[37] The average age and age range for achieving each of six gross motor developmental milestones are shown in Figure 1.5.1.

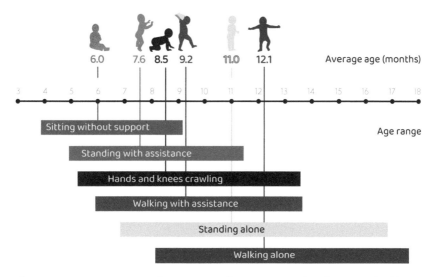

Figure 1.5.1 Average age and age range of gross motor developmental milestones.

The earlier motor development stages—sitting, standing, and sometimes, crawling—are important for the development of walking. Developmental stages build on each other. Early milestones in most cases are prerequisites to later ones, with crawling being the exception as not all children crawl.[37]

Milestones are an important reference when a child appears to be late in development compared with typically developing children. For example, one of the hallmarks of CP is that the child may be late in achieving gross motor developmental milestones. In fact, that may be what first alerts parents or professionals to a problem.

However, being late in achieving milestones does not mean that a child will never achieve them or that the child cannot progress.

The development of function is under the control of the nervous system and is affected to varying degrees in CP. Function may improve somewhat without treatment, but treatment is essential to maximize function as early as possible, which is why early intervention is so important.

Measuring function

A number of standardized measurement (assessment) tools may be used to measure function. Examples include:

- DAYC (Developmental Assessment of Young Children) for infants and children from birth to five years
- Peabody Developmental Motor Scales for infants and children from birth to five years
- Bayley Scales of Infant and Toddler Development for infants and children from 1 to 42 months
- Gross Motor Function Measure (GMFM) for children with CP aged five months to 16 years.

Information on these and other measurement tools is included in Appendix 1 (online).

Ally was a smaller version of any other typical baby, and we attended the physiotherapy appointments that are recommended for all premature babies. At that time, I was preoccupied with all the normal mum jobs and didn't have any concerns about Ally as she was alert and engaged and seemed to be following in her older sister Milly's footsteps, albeit at a slower pace. However, I did have a niggling concern that she was not using her right side as much as her left, and she was missing some milestones, but this, I was assured, would have been normal for a preemie like Ally.

At 10 months, Ally was admitted to hospital for a week due to a lung infection, called respiratory syncytial virus (RSV)/bronchiolitis. During that time, one of the pediatricians commented on an apparent right-side weakness Ally was displaying and recommended an MRI to rule out any brain anomalies. I didn't believe this was required but was grateful that an observant doctor was taking an interest in performing a thorough evaluation.

A couple of weeks later. I met with Ally's pediatrician to get her results, and that's when I learned the MRI showed damage in her brain and she had cerebral palsy. The doctor said that the diagnosis was "periventricular leukomalacia resulting in cerebral palsy with right-side hemiplegia."

All I could hear was the muffled sound of my own heartbeat in my ears as my blood pressure shot up as I desperately attempted to comprehend the diagnosis. This evolved into racing thoughts about Ally's future and whether she would ever talk, walk, or, most importantly, be happy.

Classification based on predominant motor type and topography

Order and simplification are the first steps toward the mastery of a subject—the actual enemy is the unknown.
Thomas Mann

Over the years, there has been much discussion of the classification of CP. Classification, or dividing into groups, is useful because it provides information about the nature of the condition and its severity (its level or magnitude). It also allows us to learn from people who have the condition at a similar level.

This section addresses classification of CP based on predominant motor type and topography. ("Predominant motor type" means predominant abnormal muscle tone* and movement impairment, and "topography" means area of the body affected). It also covers location of the brain injury and prevalence of CP by subtype. The next section looks at classification of CP based on functional ability.

---

* The resting tension in a person's muscles. A range of normal muscle tone exists. Tone is considered abnormal when it falls outside the range of normal or typical. It can be too low (hypotonia) or too high (hypertonia).

CP subtype based on predominant motor type

There are several subtypes of CP based on the predominant motor type. These include:

- Spasticity—spastic CP
- Dyskinesia—dyskinetic CP
- Ataxia—ataxic CP
- Hypotonia—hypotonic CP.[4]

See Table 1.6.1.

Table 1.6.1 CP subtypes based on predominant motor type

CP SUBTYPE	EXPLANATION
Spasticity—spastic CP	Spasticity is a condition in which there is an abnormal increase in muscle tone or stiffness of muscle that can interfere with movement and speech, and be associated with discomfort or pain.[22]
Dyskinesia—dyskinetic CP	Dyskinesia is a condition in which there are "abnormal patterns of posture and/or movement associated with involuntary, uncontrolled, recurring, occasionally stereotyped movement patterns."[8] ("Stereotyped movement patterns" means the movements are in a particular pattern, specific to that person, which is repeated.)
	Dyskinetic CP can be subdivided into either dystonic or choreo-athetotic CP.[38]
	• **Dystonic (dystonia):** Dystonia is characterized by involuntary (unintended) muscle contractions that cause slow repetitive movements or abnormal postures that can sometimes be painful.[39]
	• **Choreo-athetotic (choreo-athetosis):**
	○ Chorea is characterized by jerky, dance-like movements.[3]
	○ Athetosis is characterized by slow, writhing movements.[3]

Cont'd.

CP SUBTYPE	EXPLANATION
Ataxia—ataxic CP	Ataxia means "without coordination." People with ataxic CP "experience a failure of muscle control in their arms and legs, resulting in a lack of balance and coordination or a disturbance of gait."[40]
Hypotonia—hypotonic CP	Hypotonia is a condition in which there is an abnormal decrease in muscle tone.[22] The muscles are floppy.

It is worth noting that these abnormal muscle tone or movement impairments may be present in other conditions, not just CP.

CP subtype based on topography

There are two methods of classifying CP subtypes based on topography. One is older (historical), and one has been more recently adopted (SCPE).

With the first method, the names of all the subtypes have the suffix "plegia," which is derived from the Greek word for stroke, although there are causes of CP other than a stroke. The prefixes in the names of the subtypes—"mono," "hemi," "di," "tri," and "quad," also derived from Greek or Latin—indicate how many limbs are affected (see Table 1.6.2).*

---

* Occasionally, the terms "hemiparesis" for spastic hemiplegia, "diparesis" for spastic diplegia, and "quadriparesis" for spastic quadriplegia are used.[41]

Table 1.6.2 CP subtypes based on topography—historical

CP SUBTYPE	AREA OF BODY AFFECTED	
Monoplegia	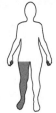	Mono = One. One limb, usually one of the lower limbs.
Hemiplegia	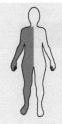	Hemi = Half. Upper and lower limbs on one side of the body. The upper limb is usually more affected than the lower limb.
Diplegia	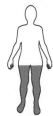	Di = Two. All limbs, but the lower limbs much more than the upper ones, which frequently show only fine motor impairment.
Triplegia	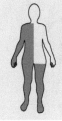	Tri = Three. Three limbs, usually the two lower limbs and one upper limb. The lower limb on the side of the upper limb involvement is usually more affected.
Quadriplegia	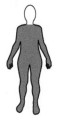	Quad = Four. All four limbs and the trunk; also known as tetraplegia.

One of the disadvantages of the historical classification system is a lack of precision.[8] However, this system has been and continues to be used extensively, particularly in the US.

The Surveillance of Cerebral Palsy in Europe network (SCPE) has developed a simpler classification method, also based on topography.[38] This method is now generally used in Europe and Australia. It identifies two main subtypes of CP: unilateral and bilateral (see Table 1.6.3).

Table 1.6.3 CP subtypes based on topography—SCPE

CP SUBTYPE	AREA OF BODY AFFECTED
Unilateral	One side of the body.
Bilateral	Both sides of the body.

Location of brain injury

Different subtypes of CP result from injury to different parts of the brain:

- Spasticity is associated with injury to the cerebrum.
- Dyskinesia is associated with injury to the basal ganglia and thalamus.
- Ataxia is associated with injury to the cerebellum.
- Hypotonia is associated with injury to the cerebrum and cerebellum.

Figure 1.6.1 summarizes CP subtypes, predominant motor types, topography, and location of brain injury.

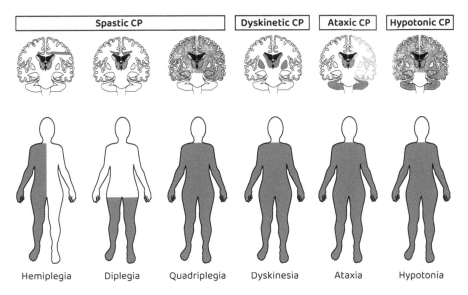

Figure 1.6.1 CP subtypes and location of brain injury (orange) and area of body affected (green).

Figure 1.6.1 shows:

- The extent of body involvement (green): regional involvement as in spastic hemiplegia and spastic diplegia; total body involvement as in spastic quadriplegia and the nonspastic forms of CP (i.e., dyskinesia, ataxia, and hypotonia).
- The location of the brain injury (orange) and CP subtype:
  - Injury primarily to the left cerebrum causing right-side spastic hemiplegia (and vice versa)
  - Injury to both left and right cerebrum causing spastic diplegia
  - More extensive injury to both left and right cerebrum causing spastic quadriplegia
  - Injury to the basal ganglia and thalamus causing dyskinesia
  - Injury to the cerebellum causing ataxia
  - Injury to both left and right cerebrum and cerebellum causing hypotonia

Note that this is a *very* simplified explanation. In reality, CP is much more nuanced. For example, there may be more than one area of brain injury. In addition, particularly with a preterm birth, brain injury may happen more than once. As well, the brain injury can vary from very mild to very severe.

Knowledge of the brain injury sometimes confirms the symptoms seen in a child. MRI scans are becoming more routine with CP. However, up to 17 percent of children with CP have normal MRI brain scans.[3]

Recall that the brain injury in CP is unchanging (i.e., the size and location do not change), but "unchanging" may be a bit misleading since with time, growth, and maturation of the brain and other structures, the effects of the brain injury become more apparent in the form of motor delays and problems with other body systems.

Prevalence of CP by subtype

Figure 1.6.2 shows the prevalence of CP by predominant motor type and topography for almost 11,000 Australian children with CP.[4,42] While precise percentages of prevalence are different in other countries, the data in Figure 1.6.2 is from a large dataset and is consistent with studies from other countries.[43,44,45,46] It shows that:

- The predominant motor type is spastic (78 percent).
- Hemiplegia, diplegia, and quadriplegia each represent approximately one-third of the total.

Note that only spastic CP is subdivided by topography because the other subtypes (i.e., dyskinetic, ataxic, and hypotonic CP) generally affect the whole body.

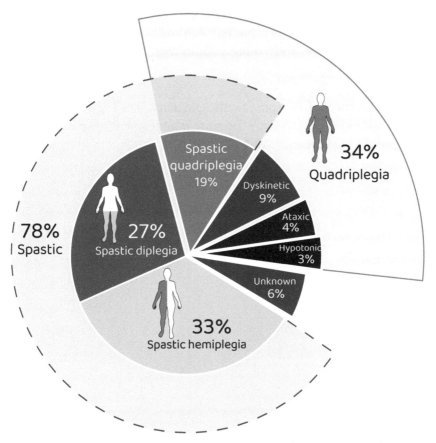

Figure 1.6.2 Predominant motor type and topography for Australian children with CP.[4,42]

It is important to note that different CP registers regard hypotonia differently. The Australian CP register includes hypotonia as a subtype of CP; the European CP register does not. Figure 1.6.2 shows that 3 percent of Australian children with CP were classified as having hypotonic CP.[4] One study found that only 46 percent of physicians who diagnose CP in the US and Canada would diagnose it in the case of hypotonia.[47] A diagnosis of CP is important because it may affect access to rehabilitation services in some countries.

Finally, it's important to understand that while CP is classified based on the predominant motor type, many individuals have secondary or co-occurring motor types. Data from the Australian CP register, for example, showed that 16 percent of individuals with spastic hemiplegia have co-occurring dyskinesia, and it is believed that the true prevalence of co-occurring motor types is higher.[4] A more recent report found that 50 percent of children and young people with CP had spasticity *and* dystonia.[48]

The co-occurrence of dystonia with spasticity has been underrecognized. This is important to know because management of spasticity and management of dystonia are different.

Classification based on functional ability

It is our choices, Harry,
that show what we truly are,
far more than our abilities.
J.K. Rowling

A series of functional ability classification systems has been developed, with each having the same structure and common language. These systems include classifying CP based on:

- Functional mobility (as in movement from place to place)
- Manual ability (ability to handle objects)
- Communication ability
- Eating and drinking ability
- Visual function

Functional mobility

The Gross Motor Function Classification System (GMFCS) is a five-level classification system that describes the functional mobility of children and adolescents with CP.[49] The GMFCS and the expanded, revised version—GMFCS E&R[50]—includes descriptions for five age groups:

- 0 to 2 years
- 2 to 4 years
- 4 to 6 years
- 6 to 12 years
- 12 to 18 years

The emphasis is on the child or adolescent's usual performance in their daily environment (i.e., their home and community).* By choosing which description best matches the child at their current age, they can be assigned a GMFCS level.

Table 1.7.1 describes the five levels. The severity of the movement limitations increases with each level, with level I having the fewest movement limitations and level V having the most. It is important to note, however, that the differences between the levels are not equal.

Table 1.7.1 Functional mobility across the five levels of the GMFCS[49,50]

GMFCS LEVEL	FUNCTIONAL MOBILITY
I	Walks without limitations
II	Walks with limitations
III	Walks using a handheld mobility device (assistive walking device)*
IV	Self-mobility with limitations; may use powered mobility†
V	Transported in a manual wheelchair

* Handheld mobility device (assistive walking device) includes canes, crutches, and walkers that do not support the weight of the trunk during walking.

† Powered mobility includes wheelchairs and scooters controlled by a joystick or electrical switch.

---

* In this context, "community" may be interpreted as "away from home." Moving about at home is generally easier since it is likely well suited or adapted to the person's needs. The community may be more challenging. It is important to keep in mind the impact of environmental and personal factors on what children and adolescents are able to do in their daily environment (home or community). See section 1.8, The International Classification of Functioning, Disability and Health.

The GMFCS levels are based on the method of functional mobility that best describes the child's performance after age six, but a child can be classified much earlier using these descriptions. They are relatively stable after age two.[49,51,52] In fact, stability into young adulthood has been demonstrated. McCormick and colleagues found that a GMFCS level observed around age 12 was highly predictive of motor function in early adulthood.[53]

Knowing a child's level offers insight into what the future may hold in terms of their mobility. It helps answer some of the many questions parents may have in the early days, such as, "Will my child walk?" or, "How serious is their CP?"

The full version of the GMFCS E&R is a short document and is included in **Useful web resources**. It contains further detail on functional mobility for each age and GMFCS level. It also includes a summary of the distinctions between each level to help determine which level most closely resembles a particular child's or adolescent's functional mobility. Useful illustrations have been developed based on the GMFCS for the two upper age bands (6 to 12 years and 12 to 18 years) by staff at the Royal Children's Hospital in Melbourne (see Figures 1.7.1 and 1.7.2).

GMFCS E & R between 6th and 12th birthday: Descriptors and illustrations

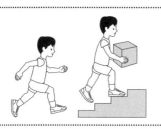

GMFCS Level I

Children walk at home, school, outdoors and in the community. They can climb stairs without the use of a railing. Children perform gross motor skills such as running and jumping, but speed, balance and coordination are limited.

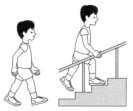

GMFCS Level II

Children walk in most settings and climb stairs holding onto a railing. They may experience difficulty walking long distances and balancing on uneven terrain, inclines, in crowded areas or confined spaces. Children may walk with physical assistance, a hand-held mobility device or used wheeled mobility over long distances. Children have only minimal ability to perform gross motor skills such as running and jumping.

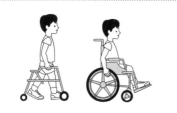

GMFCS Level III

Children walk using a hand-held mobility device in most indoor settings. They may climb stairs holding onto a railing with supervision or assistance. Children use wheeled mobility when traveling long distances and may self-propel for shorter distances.

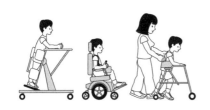

GMFCS Level IV

Children use methods of mobility that require physical assistance or powered mobility in most settings. They may walk for short distances at home with physical assistance or use powered mobility or a body support walker when positioned. At school, outdoors and in the community children are transported in a manual wheelchair or use powered mobility.

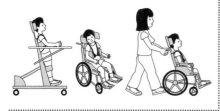

GMFCS Level V

Children are transported in a manual wheelchair in all settings. Children are limited in their ability to maintain antigravity head and trunk postures and control leg and arm movements.

GMFCS descriptors: Palisano et al. (1997) Dev Med Child Neurol 39:214-23
CanChild: www.canchild.ca

Illustrations Version 2 © Bill Reid, Kate Willoughby, Adrienne Harvey and Kerr Graham,
The Royal Children's Hospital Melbourne ERC151050

Figure 1.7.1 GMFCS E&R between 6th and 12th birthday: Descriptors and illustrations. Reproduced with kind permission from K. Graham and K. Willoughby, Royal Children's Hospital Melbourne, Australia.

GMFCS E & R between 12th and 18th birthday: Descriptors and illustrations

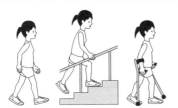

GMFCS Level I

Youth walk at home, school, outdoors and in the community. Youth are able to climb curbs and stairs without physical assistance or a railing. They perform gross motor skills such as running and jumping but speed, balance and coordination are limited.

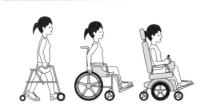

GMFCS Level II

Youth walk in most settings but environmental factors and personal choice influence mobility choices. At school or work they may require a hand held mobility device for safety and climb stairs holding onto a railing. Outdoors and in the community youth may use wheeled mobility when traveling long distances.

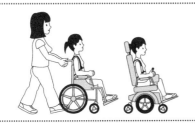

GMFCS Level III

Youth are capable of walking using a hand-held mobility device. Youth may climb stairs holding onto a railing with supervision or assistance. At school they may self-propel a manual wheelchair or use powered mobility. Outdoors and in the community youth are transported in a wheelchair or use powered mobility.

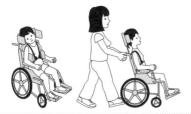

GMFCS Level IV

Youth use wheeled mobility in most settings. Physical assistance of 1-2 people is required for transfers. Indoors, youth may walk short distances with physical assistance, use wheeled mobility or a body support walker when positioned. They may operate a powered chair, otherwise are transported in a manual wheelchair.

GMFCS Level V

Youth are transported in a manual wheelchair in all settings. Youth are limited in their ability to maintain antigravity head and trunk postures and control leg and arm movements. Self-mobility is severely limited, even with the use of assistive technology.

GMFCS descriptors: Palisano et al. (1997) Dev Med Child Neurol 39:214-23
CanChild: www.canchild.ca

Illustrations Version 2 © Bill Reid, Kate Willoughby, Adrienne Harvey and Kerr Graham, The Royal Children's Hospital Melbourne ERC151050

Figure 1.7.2 GMFCS E&R between 12th and 18th birthday: Descriptors and illustrations. Reproduced with kind permission from K. Graham and K. Willoughby, Royal Children's Hospital Melbourne, Australia.

One use of the GMFCS has been classifying walking ability into three levels:[54]

- **Mild:** independent walker; GMFCS levels I–II
- **Moderate:** walker with aid; GMFCS level III
- **Severe:** wheelchair; GMFCS levels IV–V

In addition, the GMFCS led to the development of the gross motor development curves.[55,56] The curves show the change in gross motor function over time as measured by the Gross Motor Function Measure-66 (GMFM-66).[*] There are five curves, one for each GMFCS level (see Figure 1.7.3).

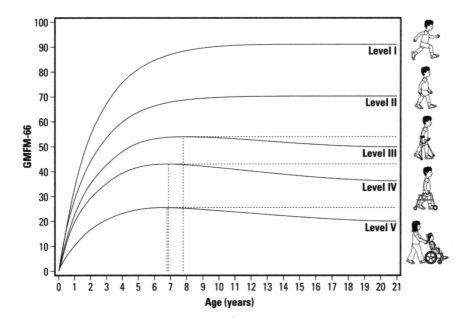

Figure 1.7.3 Gross motor curves in children with CP and the five levels of the GMFCS. Adapted with kind permission from *Cerebral Palsy: Science and Clinical Practice*, edited by B. Dan et al. (2014). Mac Keith Press.

The curves allow us to see how a child's gross motor function is likely to develop over time, as measured by the GMFM-66. The figure shows

---

[*] A standardized assessment tool used to evaluate the gross motor function of individuals with CP. It consists of 66 items that assess a wide range of gross motor skills. Also used is GMFM-88, which assesses 88 items. Each addresses five areas of increasing gross motor function: 1) lying and rolling, 2) sitting, 3) crawling and kneeling, 4) standing, and 5) walking, running, and jumping.

the average GMFM-66 score (vertical y-axis) at each GMFCS level by age (horizontal x-axis). Specifically, it shows:

- For each level there is an initial rapid rise in score to a peak, then it plateaus (levels I–II) or decreases (levels III–V).
- The score is highest for level I and lowest for level V.
- The dotted lines show the age at which the score peaks and the decrease from the peak to age 21 years for levels III–V (the oldest participants in the study were 21, so the shape of the curves after 21 are not known).
- Even a child at level I does not reach 100, the maximum, on the scale.

These curves are based on averages, and it is important to remember that some children were above and some below the line at each level.[55] Still, they are very useful. Why? Because they help answer some of the many questions parents have in the early days. Knowing a child's GMFCS level at age two, for example, allows parents to see how the child's gross motor function, as measured by the GMFM-66, is likely to develop over time. However, it is worth noting that the curves are not accurate before the age of two.

While remaining very realistic in expectations, the focus should be on helping the child reach their maximum possible gross motor function, not just hitting the average. The curves should guide, but not limit, a child's potential.

Manual ability

The Manual Ability Classification System (MACS) is a five-level classification system that describes how children and adolescents with CP age 4 to 18 years handle objects in daily activities.[57] The levels are based on the individual's ability to handle objects (relevant and age appropriate) and their need for assistance or adaptation. A separate Mini-MACS is available for children age one to four.[58]

Table 1.7.2 describes the five levels. Limitations of manual ability increase with increasing MACS level. As with the GMFCS, the differences between levels are not equal. The scale is used to classify overall ability to handle objects, *not* each hand separately. The emphasis is on the child's or adolescent's overall usual performance in their daily environment (their home, school, and community), rather than what is known to be their best performance.

Table 1.7.2 Ability to handle objects across the five levels of the MACS[57]

MACS LEVEL	ABILITY TO HANDLE OBJECTS
I	Handles objects easily and successfully
II	Handles most objects but with somewhat reduced quality and/or speed of achievement
III	Handles objects with difficulty; needs help to prepare and/or modify activities
IV	Handles a limited selection of easily managed objects in adapted situations
V	Does not handle objects and has severely limited ability to perform even simple actions

The full versions of the MACS and Mini-MACS are short documents and are included in **Useful web resources.** They provide further detail on each level and a summary of the distinctions between adjacent levels to help determine the most appropriate level for the individual.

An alternative to the MACS is the Bimanual Fine Motor Function (BFMF) [59,60,61] (see Figure 1.7.4). Unlike the MACS (and Mini-MACS), the BFMF assesses the child's ability to grasp, hold, and manipulate objects in *each* hand separately.[60] More information on the BFMF is included in **Useful web resources.**

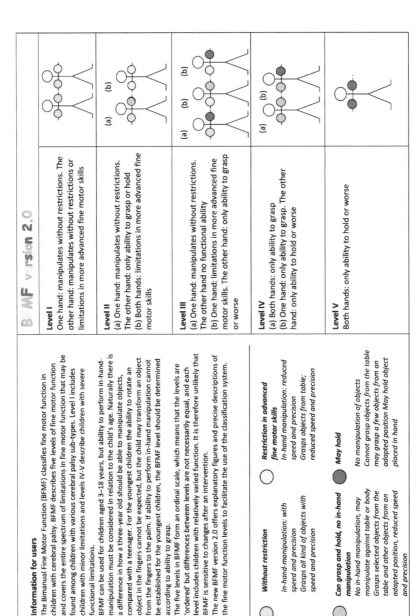

Information for users

The Bimanual Fine Motor Function (BFMF) classifies fine motor function in children with cerebral palsy. BFMF describes five levels of fine motor function and covers the entire spectrum of limitations in fine motor function that may be found among children with various cerebral palsy sub-types. Level I includes children with minor limitations and levels IV–V describe children with severe functional limitations.

BFMF can be used for children aged 3–18 years, but ability to perform in-hand-manipulation must be considered in relation to the child's age. Naturally there is a difference in how a three-year old should be able to manipulate objects, compared with a teenager. For the youngest children the ability to rotate an object in the fingers cannot be expected, but the child may transform an object from the fingers to the palm. If ability to perform in-hand manipulation cannot be established for the youngest children, the BFMF level should be determined according to ability to grasp.

The five levels in BFMF form an ordinal scale, which means that the levels are 'ordered' but differences between levels are not necessarily equal, and each level includes children with relatively varied function. It is therefore unlikely that BFMF is sensitive to changes after an intervention.

The new BFMF version 2.0 offers explanatory figures and precise descriptions of the fine motor function levels to facilitate the use of the classification system.

○ *Without restriction*

In-hand-manipulation: with speed and precision
Grasps all kind of objects with speed and precision

○ *Restriction in advanced fine motor skills*

In-hand manipulation: reduced speed and precision
Grasps objects from table; reduced speed and precision

◔ *Can grasp and hold, no in-hand manipulation*

No in-hand manipulation, may manipulate against table or body
Grasps selected objects from the table and other objects from an adapted position, reduced speed and precision

● *May hold*

No manipulation of objects
Cannot grasp objects from the table may grasp a few objects from an adapted position May hold object placed in hand

B FMF v rsion 2.0

Level I
One hand: manipulates without restrictions. The other hand: manipulates without restrictions or limitations in more advanced fine motor skills

Level II
(a) One hand: manipulates without restrictions. The other hand: only ability to grasp or hold
(b) Both hands: limitations in more advanced fine motor skills

Level III
(a) One hand: manipulates without restrictions. The other hand no functional ability
(b) One hand: limitations in more advanced fine motor skills. The other hand: only ability to grasp or worse

Level IV
(a) Both hands: only ability to grasp
(b) One hand: only ability to grasp. The other hand: only ability to hold or worse

Level V
Both hands: only ability to hold or worse

Figure 1.7.4 BFMF level identification chart. Reproduced with kind permission from Dr. Kate Himmelmann and Dr. Ann-Kristin Elvrum.

Communication ability

The Communication Function Classification System (CFCS) is a five-level classification system that describes everyday communication performance for children with CP.[62] Table 1.7.3 describes the five levels. Hidecker and colleagues have defined some key concepts used in this classification system:

> Communication occurs when a **sender** transmits a message, **and a receiver** understands the message ... **Unfamiliar conversational partners** are strangers or acquaintances who only occasionally communicate with the person. **Familiar conversational partners** such as relatives, caregivers, and friends may be able to communicate more effectively with the person because of previous knowledge and personal experiences ... All methods of communication performance are considered ... These include speech, gestures, behaviors, eye gaze, facial expressions, and augmentative and alternative communication (AAC).[62]

Table 1.7.3 Communication ability across the five levels of the CFCS[62]

CFCS LEVEL	COMMUNICATION ABILITY
I	Effective sender and receiver with unfamiliar and familiar partners
II	Effective but slower-paced sender and/or receiver with unfamiliar and/or familiar partners
III	Effective sender and receiver with familiar partners
IV	Inconsistent sender and/or receiver with familiar partners
V	Seldom-effective sender and receiver even with familiar partners

An alternative to the CFCS is the Viking Speech Scale (VSS),[63,64,65] but it addresses just speech. It is a four-point scale, with level I having the fewest limitations and level IV the most (see Table 1.7.4).

Table 1.7.4 Viking Speech Scale

VSS LEVEL	SPEECH UNDERSTANDABILITY
I	Speech is not affected by motor disorder.
II	Speech is imprecise but usually understandable to unfamiliar listeners.
III	Speech is unclear and not usually understandable to unfamiliar listeners out of context.
IV	No understandable speech.

More information on both the CFCS and VSS is included in **Useful web resources.**

Eating and drinking ability

The Eating and Drinking Ability Classification System (EDACS) is used for individuals with CP who are age three and older.[66] The EDACS assesses eating and drinking from two perspectives across the five levels:[66]

- **Safety:** For example, aspiration (food or liquid entering the airway or lungs instead of the esophagus) and choking (blockage of the airway by food)
- **Efficiency:** Amount of food and liquid lost from the mouth and time taken to eat.

Table 1.7.5 describes the five levels.

Table 1.7.5 Eating and drinking ability across the five levels of the EDACS[66]

EDACS LEVEL	EATING AND DRINKING ABILITY
I	Eats and drinks safely and efficiently
II	Eats and drinks safely but with some limitations to efficiency
III	Eats and drinks with some limitations to safety; there may be limitations to efficiency
IV	Eats and drinks with significant limitations to safety
V	Unable to eat and drink safely—tube-feeding may be considered to provide nutrition

Useful illustrations for the EDACS from age three years have been developed focusing on the safety and efficiency aspects of feeding (see Figure 1.7.5).

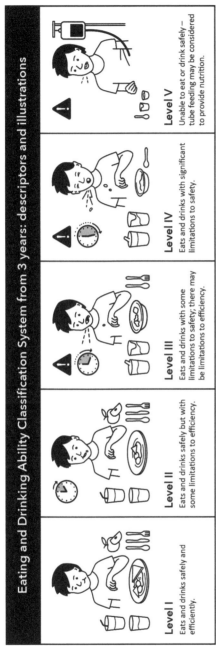

Eating and Drinking Ability Classification System from 3 years: descriptors and illustrations

Level I
Eats and drinks safely and efficiently.

Level II
Eats and drinks safely but with some limitations to efficiency.

Level III
Eats and drinks with some limitations to safety; there may be limitations to efficiency.

Level IV
Eats and drinks with significant limitations to safety.

Level V
Unable to eat or drink safely – tube feeding may be considered to provide nutrition.

Sellers, D., Mandy, A., Pennington, L., Hankins, M. and Morris, C. (2014). Development and reliability of a system to classify the eating and drinking ability of people with cerebral palsy. Dev Med Child Neurol, 56: 245-251. https://doi.org/10.1111/dmcn.12352

Illustrations © Jane Coffey

Figure 1.7.5 EDACS from three years of age. Reproduced with kind permission from Dr. Diane Sellers; © Jane Coffey.

A Mini-EDACS has been developed for children with CP from age 18 to 36 months.[67] More information on the EDACS and Mini-EDACS is included in **Useful web resources.**

Visual function

The Visual Function Classification System (VFCS) is for individuals with CP from the age of one. Table 1.7.6 describes the five levels.

Table 1.7.6 Visual function across the five levels of the VFCS[68]

VFCS LEVEL	VISUAL FUNCTION
I	Uses visual function easily and successfully in vision-related activities
II	Uses visual function successfully but needs self-initiated compensatory strategies
III	Uses visual function but needs some adaptations
IV	Uses visual function in very adapted environments but performs just part of vision-related activities
V	Does not use visual function even in very adapted environments

More information on the VFCS is included in **Useful web resources.**

Using classification systems

Together, the various classification systems provide a lot of information, and each is valid and reliable.[*68,69] Because families can understand (and assign) classification system levels,[69,70] the systems can help with communication between medical professionals and families. They also help with good planning of care both in the present and into the future since they are stable over time.[69] However, it is because they are stable over time that they should not and cannot be used to detect change after an intervention.[70] Robust research is one of the backbones for improving clinical care for individuals with CP. The classification systems are very useful for research since participants can be better identified for research studies.

Finally, although CP is a single diagnosis, it is far from a uniform condition. Similar to autism, a name change, from "cerebral palsy" to "cerebral palsy spectrum disorder," has been suggested.[71]

> If the guilt I felt when Ally was born was all encompassing, the guilt I experienced when she was diagnosed was incomprehensible and insurmountable. I know that balanced people will insist on the uselessness in dwelling on such issues, and there is no doubt they are right. This is, of course, much more challenging when you are immersed in the situation and feeling so out of control and alone. My advice is to acknowledge the feeling of crushing guilt, admit it is present, and let it pass through you. The challenge is in moving forward and not staying in inertia.

---

* A good classification system must be:
  - **Valid:** It measures what it claims to measure.
  - **Reliable:** It provides the same answer when used by different people or by the same person at different times.
  - **Accurate:** It measures how close a value is to its true value (e.g., how close an arrow gets to the target).
  - **Precise:** It measures how repeatable a measurement is (e.g., how close the second arrow is to the first one, regardless of whether either is near the target).

These same principles also apply to measurement (assessment) tools. A kitchen scale (weighing scale) can be used to illustrate the different concepts:
  - If the scale claims to measure weight and does so, then the scale is valid.
  - If it provides the same reading regardless of who uses it or when they use it, then the scale is reliable.
  - If the reading is correct when a known standard weight is weighed, then the scale is accurate.
  - If repeated weighings of the same item give the same reading (whether accurate or not), then the scale is precise.

That's the place I launched my own challenge from, determined to do everything in my power to "fix" Ally.

I began to feverishly study up on CP, read every piece of googled literature available, and questioned and challenged everything I heard. Other mums with CP kids were always very generous with their advice and helped me enormously. It's a challenge to find specific advice on the type of cerebral palsy that you're dealing with as it is such a broad area, but I encourage every parent to read, follow up, get the physiotherapy with your child, and most important, be their advocate.

The International Classification of Functioning, Disability and Health

*The individual is rarely going to be altered very much,
whereas the environment slowly but surely can.*

Tom Shakespeare

The International Classification of Functioning, Disability and Health (ICF), a framework briefly addressed in the Introduction, is considered here in more detail and in the context of CP. The ICF was developed by WHO[*] in 2001 to help show the impact of a health condition at different levels and how those levels are interconnected. It tells us to look at the full picture—to look at the person with a disability in their life situation. The "F" in the short-form name of the framework (the ICF) stands for "functioning," which shows where its emphasis lies.

The framework provides a way of looking at the concepts of health and disability. It shows that every human being can experience a decrease in health and thereby experience some disability. That is, disability is not

---

[*] When WHO (the World Health Organization) was established in 1948, it defined health as "… a state of complete physical, mental, and social well-being and not merely the absence of disease or infirmity." This interesting and broad definition has stood the test of time: it has never been amended.

something that happens only to a minority of people. The ICF thus "mainstreams" disability and recognizes it as a widespread human experience. See Figure 1.8.1.

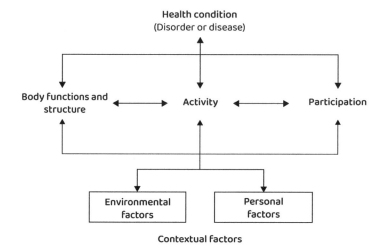

Figure 1.8.1 International Classification of Functioning, Disability and Health (ICF). Reproduced with kind permission from WHO.

The framework describes three levels of human functioning and disability as difficulty functioning at one or more of these three levels:[1]

- **Body functions and structure** refers to functioning at the level of the body or a body part.[*] For example, spasticity, muscle weakness, pain, and cognition are at this level. Impairments are defined as problems in body functions and structure.
- **Activity** is performing a task or action by an individual; for example, walking or getting dressed. Activity limitations are difficulties an individual may have in performing activities.
- **Participation** is involvement in life situations. Playing sports with friends or attending school are examples. Participation restrictions are difficulties an individual may experience being involved in life situations.

---

* WHO formally defines "body functions" as physiological functions of body systems (including psychological functions). "Body structures" are defined as anatomical parts of the body such as organs, limbs, and their components.

The framework also includes factors that influence any of the three levels of functioning (termed "contextual factors"):

- **Environmental factors** make up the physical, social, and attitudinal environment in which people live. Examples include structural barriers at home and in the community, such as steps or stairs without handrails in the house, or a school with stairs but no elevator.
- **Personal factors** include gender, age, social background, education, past and present experiences, and other factors that influence how the person experiences disability. Examples include a person's attitude, determination, motivation, and resilience.

The three levels of human functioning, plus environmental and personal factors, are all interconnected with the health condition. The ICF shifts the focus from the *cause* to the *impact* of a health condition at the different levels.

Regarding activity, the ICF distinguishes between motor capacity and motor performance:

- **Motor capacity** is what a person can do in a standardized, controlled environment (e.g., a child at an appointment and walking on a smooth surface with the medical professional and parent watching and encouraging them).
- **Motor performance** is what a person actually does in their daily environment (e.g., a child walking in a crowded playground on uneven surfaces).

There is a third concept to keep in mind when considering activity: motor capability, which is what a person can do in their daily environment.[72] For example, a child may be able to ride a bike to school—they have the capability—but they may choose not to. Their performance is influenced by their choice. Physical and social environment and personal factors such as motivation influence the relationship between capacity, capability, and performance.[72]

A series of "F-words" has been developed and inserted into the different areas of the ICF, providing a useful adaptation of the framework (see Figure 1.8.2).[73] "Fitness," "functioning," "friends," "family," "fun," and "future" are highlighted as areas of focus for the child with a health condition. Indeed, these also apply to adults. A number of useful videos on the F-words are included in **Useful web resources.**

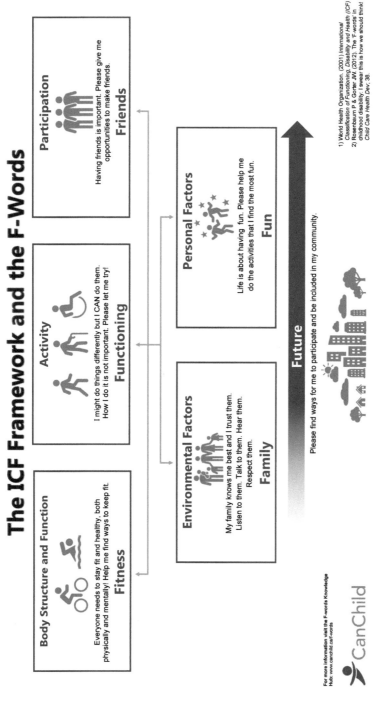

Figure 1.8.2 The ICF framework[1] and the F-words.[73] Reproduced with kind permission from CanChild.

Key points Chapter 1

- CP is a group of conditions caused by an injury to the developing brain that can result in a variety of motor and other problems that affect how the child functions. Because the injury occurs in a developing brain and growing child, problems often change over time, even though the brain injury itself is unchanging.
- CP is a lifelong condition. There is currently no cure, nor is one imminent, but good management and treatment can help alleviate some or many of the effects of the brain injury.
- Seventy to 80 percent of CP cases are associated with prenatal factors, and birth asphyxia (insufficient oxygen during birth) plays a relatively minor role.
- Infants who are born preterm (earlier than 37 weeks) or who have low birth weight have a higher risk of CP.
- The current CP birth prevalence for high-income countries is declining and is now 1.6 per 1,000 live births. It is higher for low- and middle-income countries.
- The most recent report from the Australian Cerebral Palsy Register shows a decrease in both prevalence and severity of CP.
- Using certain standardized tests in combination with clinical examination and medical history, a diagnosis of CP can often accurately be made before six months corrected age.
- Confirmation of the presence of a brain injury by magnetic resonance imaging (MRI) occurs in many but not all individuals with CP. Up to 17 percent of children given the diagnosis of CP have normal MRI brain scans.
- Early diagnosis is very important because it allows for early intervention. Early intervention helps to achieve better functional outcomes for the child.
- CP can be classified based on the predominant motor type (the predominant abnormal muscle tone and movement impairment) and topography (area of the body affected).
- A number of classification systems describe the functional mobility (as in movement from place to place), manual ability (ability to handle objects), communication ability, eating and drinking ability, and visual function of individuals with CP.

Chapter 2

Spastic hemiplegia

Section 2.1 Introduction 63

Section 2.2 The brain injury 73

Section 2.3 Growth 77

Section 2.4 Bones, joints, muscles, and movements 80

Section 2.5 Typical hand function and typical walking 90

Section 2.6 Primary problems 95

Section 2.7 Secondary problems 104

Section 2.8 Tertiary problems 123

Section 2.9 Motor function in individuals with spastic hemiplegia 125

Section 2.10 Associated problems 132

Key points Chapter 2 139

Introduction

Nothing in life is to be feared,
it is only to be understood.
Now is the time to understand more,
so that we may fear less.
Marie Curie

The title of this book is *Spastic Hemiplegia—Unilateral Cerebral Palsy*. "Spastic hemiplegia" is the term historically used to describe this condition, and it remains in use today in the US. The term derives from "spastic" (the type of high tone), "hemi" (half, referring to one side of the body affected), and "plegia" (the Greek word for stroke). Over the past 20 years, the term "unilateral spastic CP," or simply "unilateral CP," has been adopted in Europe and Australia because it is thought to provide a more accurate description of the condition. "Unilateral" refers to one side of the body being affected. The three terms "spastic hemiplegia," "unilateral spastic CP," and "unilateral CP" are all used in the scientific literature. In this book, written in the US, we use the term "spastic hemiplegia," and since spastic hemiplegia is often referred to simply as hemiplegia, we use both terms interchangeably.

Spastic hemiplegia affects the upper and lower limbs of one side of the body. The upper limb is usually more affected than the lower limb. Spasticity is the most common type of atypical tone present in individuals with hemiplegia, although dystonia can be present as well.

As noted in Chapter 1, the Gross Motor Function Classification System (GMFCS) offers an indication of the severity of the condition. This book is relevant to those at GMFCS levels I and II: those who are capable of walking independently or with an assistive walking device. GMFCS levels I and II account for the majority of individuals with spastic hemiplegia.

Spastic hemiplegia is a complex and lifelong condition. There is currently no cure. However, good management and treatment can help reduce its effects. This chapter explains spastic hemiplegia from birth through adolescence. It should contribute to your understanding of how the condition arises and develops over time. It provides information intended to help parents understand the diagnosis and what to anticipate as their child grows to adulthood. It provides adolescents and adults with an understanding of their condition. Chapter 3 addresses the management of the condition during childhood and adolescence. Chapter 4 is devoted to spastic hemiplegia in adulthood.

Spastic hemiplegia is caused by injury mostly, but not exclusively, to the cerebrum on one side of the brain—the parts of the brain that control voluntary movement, and receive and process sensory information for the opposite side of the body.

Physical features

Gage, an orthopedic surgeon, described the main features of hemiplegia as follows:[74]

> In hemiplegia ... there is a relatively intact unilateral sensory and motor system; there is not such a problem with overall body balance. The upper extremity is more severely involved than the lower. Typically, the individual walks with a postured upper extremity which is internally rotated at the shoulder, flexed at the elbow, and flexed ... at the wrist. The hand is frequently clenched

with the thumb in the palm ... Sensory deprivation is the major problem in the upper extremity ... The individual depends totally on the other limb and seems to be almost unaware of the hemiplegic side ... The flexed and motionless arm is one of the most distinctive features of hemiplegia ...Internal rotation of the lower limb and equinus of the foot and ankle [are typical features].

He added that the affected arm generally remains motionless, unlike the unaffected arm, which swings freely during walking.[74]

Table 2.1.1 explains and illustrates the typical physical features of hemiplegia. Together, these features paint a picture of an individual holding the weaker arm in a flexed position and who walks leading with their stronger leg. Individuals with hemiplegia can have some, but not necessarily all, of these features.

Table 2.1.1 Typical physical features of spastic hemiplegia GMFCS levels I and II

TERM USED IN DESCRIPTIONS	EXPLANATION	ILLUSTRATION
Adducted shoulder	The arm is moved inward toward the middle of the body (midline).	
Inwardly rotated shoulder	The upper arm is turned internally toward the body.	

Cont'd.

TERM USED IN DESCRIPTIONS	EXPLANATION	ILLUSTRATION
Flexed elbow	The arm is bent at the elbow. It is difficult to extend and straighten the elbow.	
Pronated forearm	The hand is in the palm-down position	
Flexed wrist	The wrist is bent downward. It is difficult to extend and straighten the wrist.	
Adducted and flexed thumb	The thumb is bent and positioned toward the middle finger. This is also termed "thumb in palm."	
Flexed fingers	The fingers are folded in toward the palm.	
Lumbar lordosis	An exaggerated inward curve in the lumbar region of the spine, often called a swayback.	
Anterior pelvic tilt	A tipping forward of the pelvis to the front. (The triangle indicates the pelvis.)	
Adduction and internal rotation at the hips	Adduction is movement toward the middle of the body. Internal rotation is a twisting movement around the long axis of a bone toward the middle of the body. With adduction and internal rotation at the hips, the thigh turns inward and toward the middle of the body. The right side shows these features.	

Cont'd.

TERM USED IN DESCRIPTIONS	EXPLANATION	ILLUSTRATION
Flexed hips	The hips are bent.	
Hyperextended knee	"Hyperextended" means beyond straight or over-straightened ("back-kneeing"). This is also termed "genu recurvatum." The knee on the left is hyperextended; the knee on the right is typical.	
Flexed knee	The knee is bent. Note that the knee may be *either* hyperextended or flexed.	
Abducted forefoot	The front part (forefoot) of the right foot moves away (outward) from the back part of the foot. The right forefoot is abducted; the left forefoot is typical.	
Valgus hindfoot	The right heel (hindfoot) is turned *away* from the middle of the body to an atypical degree (valgus). The right hindfoot is in a valgus position; the left hindfoot is typical. This is also termed "everted foot" or "eversion."	

Cont'd.

TERM USED IN DESCRIPTIONS	EXPLANATION	ILLUSTRATION
Varus hindfoot	The right heel (hindfoot) is turned *toward* the middle of the body to an atypical degree (varus). The right hindfoot is in a varus position; the left hindfoot is typical. This is also termed "inverted foot" or "inversion."	
Plantar flexed foot	The right toes are pointed downward; the left foot is typical. In walking, this is referred to as toe walking or equinus gait.	

Distribution across classification systems

The effects of the brain injury can extend beyond movement and posture. Several classification systems for individuals with CP were introduced in section 1.7, including classification on the basis of:

- Functional mobility: Gross Motor Function Classification System (GMFCS)
- Ability to handle objects: Manual Ability Classification System (MACS)
- Communication ability: Communication Function Classification System (CFCS)
- Eating and drinking ability: Eating and Drinking Ability Classification System (EDACS)
- Visual function: Visual Function Classification System (VFCS)

Figure 2.1.1 summarizes the percentage distribution of children with hemiplegia across the five levels of the GMFCS, MACS, CFCS, and the EDACS.[43–46,75–78] No data was found for the VFCS.

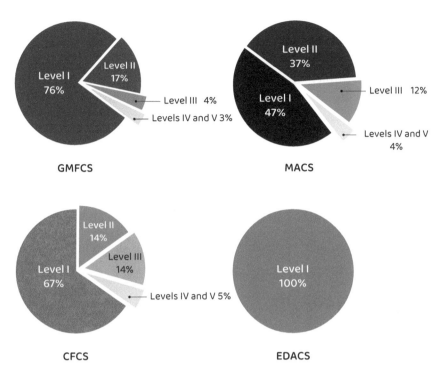

Figure 2.1.1 Distribution of children with hemiplegia across the GMFCS,[43-46,75-78] MACS,[46,76,78] CFCS,[46,78] and EDACS.[78]

Figure 2.1.1 shows that in the studies cited:

- Children with hemiplegia have a high level of gross motor function; almost all (93 percent) were functioning at GMFCS levels I and II.
- Children with hemiplegia have some problems with fine motor ability; however, 84 percent were functioning at MACS levels I and II.
- Children with hemiplegia have some problems with communication; however, 81 percent were functioning at CFCS levels I and II.
- Although the sample size was small (34 children), all children with hemiplegia were eating and drinking safely and efficiently; all were functioning at EDACS level I.

Furthermore, the level at which an individual functions on one of these classification systems can sometimes, though not always, be related to how they function on another. More specifically, one study reported a moderate correlation between GMFCS and MACS but a strong correlation between GMFCS and CFCS in children with hemiplegia.[46]

Co-occurring motor type

With spastic hemiplegia, the predominant motor type is spasticity. However, individuals with spastic hemiplegia sometimes also have co-occurring, or secondary, motor types. Data from the Australian CP register shows that 16 percent of individuals with spastic hemiplegia[*] have co-occurring dyskinesia, while 1 percent have co-occurring hypotonia.[4] It is believed that the true prevalence of co-occurring motor types is higher[4] and the presence of dystonia with spasticity has been underrecognized.[48] A recent study found that 50 percent of children and young people with CP (all subtypes) had spasticity *and* dystonia.[48] This finding is important because the management of spasticity and dystonia is different.

Associated problems

A large Australian study reported on the prevalence of associated problems (i.e., problems with other body systems) among children aged five with hemiplegia (all GMFCS levels).[79] See Figure 2.1.2.

---

[*] For those who acquired CP in the prenatal or perinatal period only; also includes monoplegia.

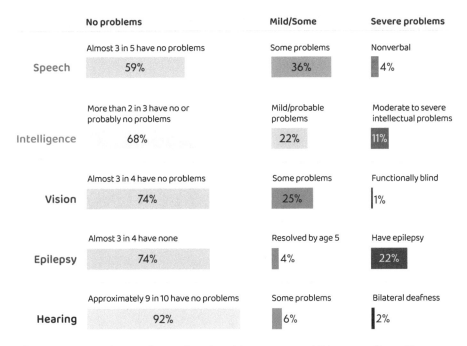

Figure 2.1.2 Prevalence of associated problems among children age five with hemiplegia (all GMFCS levels; data also includes monoplegia).

Figure 2.1.2 shows that a proportion of children with hemiplegia (all GMFCS levels) have problems in the areas of speech, intelligence (cognition), epilepsy, vision, and hearing of varying severity. Not shown in the figure is that more than 90 percent of children had none or only one severe associated problem.[79] As well, the prevalence and severity of associated problems were found to be greater in children at higher GMFCS levels compared with those at lower GMFCS levels.[79] Section 2.10 addresses associated problems in more detail.

Finally, where possible, we cite research studies relevant to those with hemiplegia GMFCS levels I and II. Where studies include multiple subtypes, we aim to give an indication of the proportion of individuals with hemiplegia and/or GMFCS level. Sometimes, we include information about CP in general, where this is deemed useful.

USEFUL WEB RESOURCES

The brain injury

The greater danger for most of us lies not in
setting our aim too high and falling short;
but in setting our aim too low,
and achieving our mark.

Michelangelo

In terms of brain injuries, *when* and *where* (i.e., the timing in development and the location in the brain) an injury occurs determines the effects and severity of that injury, which translates to the subtype of CP.

There are two types of brain injury commonly associated with hemiplegia: periventricular leukomalacia (PVL) and lesions following middle cerebral artery stroke:[80]

- **Periventricular leukomalacia (PVL):** "Peri" means around, "ventricular" means relating to the ventricles* in the brain, "leuko" means "white," and "malacia" means abnormal softening of tissue.

---

* Interconnected fluid-filled cavities that produce, circulate, and contain cerebrospinal fluid, which protects the brain and spinal cord.

The full term, "periventricular leukomalacia," describes the injury and means softening of the white tissue (white matter) around the ventricles. The ventricles are the black areas shown in Figure 2.2.1. The injury (orange area) occurs near these ventricles.

- **Middle cerebral artery stroke**. The injury or damage is to the gray matter and/or white matter, following middle cerebral artery stroke.[*] There are two types of strokes: ischemic and hemorrhagic:
    - An ischemic stroke occurs when a blood vessel supplying the brain is blocked, leading to a lack of oxygen and nutrients to the affected area. "Ischemia" means an inadequate supply of blood to an organ or part of the body.
    - A hemorrhagic stroke occurs when a blood vessel in the brain ruptures and causes bleeding. "Hemorrhage" means the escape of blood from a ruptured blood vessel.

Figure 2.2.1 shows the areas of the body that may be associated with the brain injury of hemiplegia. The white matter in the area of injury includes the motor tracts (that control movement and posture; pink lines in Figure 2.2.1) and sensory tracts (that deliver sensory information; green lines) between the spinal cord and brain. In hemiplegia the brain injury occurs *mostly, but not exclusively*, on one side of the cerebrum.

Because most (though not all) motor tracts cross over at the brain stem and sensory tracts at the spinal cord, an injury to the left cerebrum generally causes right-sided hemiplegia and vice versa. The tracts in the area associated with the brain injury affect both the upper and lower limb on the opposite side.

---

[*] The main artery is also commonly associated with adult hemiplegic stroke.

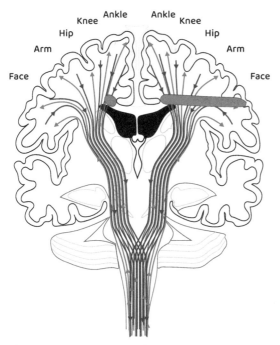

Face   Arm   Hip   Knee   Ankle   Ankle   Knee   Hip   Arm   Face

Figure 2.2.1 An example of brain injury resulting in hemiplegia. The motor tracts (pink) descend from the cerebrum to the spinal cord, and the sensory tracts (green) ascend from the spinal cord to the cerebrum. The ventricles are the black areas. The orange area indicates the injury.

It is important to remember that this is a simplified explanation and, in reality, it is much more nuanced, unique to the individual, and complex. For example, there may be more than one area of brain injury. In addition, particularly with preterm birth, brain injury may happen more than once. The timing in development when the injury occurs is important because the areas of the brain that are developing at the time of the injury are the most vulnerable.

Ally's diagnosis of cerebral palsy due to periventricular leukomalacia as given by the pediatrician was very matter of fact and technical. While understanding the technicalities of CP is very important, it is essential to remember that every child is different, and assessments must be part of a holistic overview of a child's development. Over the years, Ally has had a variety of such assessments, including measurements, gait analysis,* etc. These are very important, especially during growth spurts, which in Ally's case, really have had an impact on her physical development. I can certainly see that as she is coming into her teenage years and growing weekly that there is a significant impact on her gait and tone. This makes these measurements extremely important as they give a continual overview of changes and allow for modifications to orthoses.

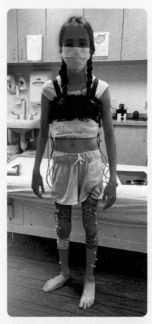

Ally having her gait analysis before surgery, age 11.

---

* A measurement tool used to evaluate gait. Within gait analysis, multiple variables are evaluated using different measurement tools.

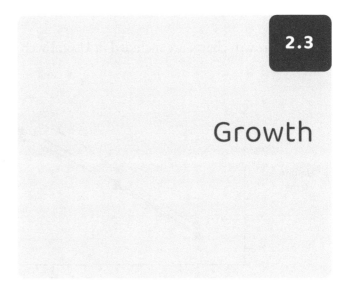

Growth

You have to do your own growing no matter
how tall your grandfather was.
Abraham Lincoln

The musculoskeletal problems in spastic hemiplegia develop in proportion to growth; therefore, an understanding of growth is helpful.

Growth occurs in three major phases during a child's life: birth to age
three, three years to puberty, and puberty to maturity. Of the three
phases, two are of *rapid* growth: from birth to three years and during
puberty.[81] The rate of growth that occurs in these two phases is particularly important for the child with spastic hemiplegia because musculoskeletal problems emerge with growth.

It is worth noting that there are slight differences in growth between
boys and girls with CP and typically developing peers. A large US study
of growth in children and adolescents with CP led to the development
of growth charts for boys and girls with CP age 2 to 20. These were
developed for each GMFCS level.[82,83] The study found that children and
adolescents with CP (all subtypes) are shorter than typically developing

peers (see Figures 2.3.1 and 2.3.2). Similar trends in height difference among children and adolescents with CP have been observed in other parts of the world.[84]

These growth charts are included in **Useful web resources.**

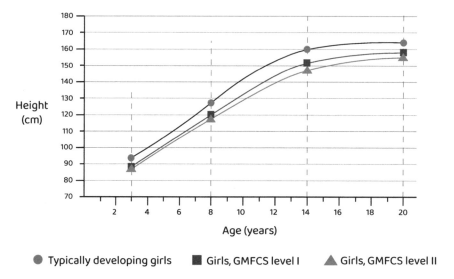

Figure 2.3.1 Height of girls with CP compared with typically developing peers. Data shows the 50th percentile height at various ages. Data collated and compiled from references.[82,83,85,86]

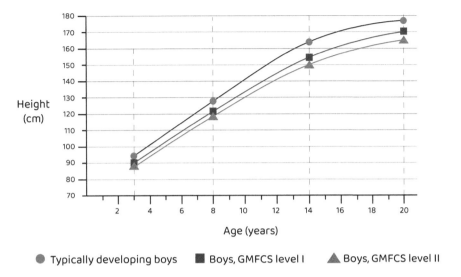

Figure 2.3.2 Height of boys with CP compared with typically developing peers. Data shows the 50th percentile height at various ages. Data collated and compiled from references.[82,83,87,88]

Bones, joints, muscles, and movements

It is not by muscle, speed, or physical dexterity that great things are achieved, but by reflection, force of character, and judgment.

Marcus Tullius Cicero

This section may seem like a physics and biology lesson, but because spastic hemiplegia affects the bones, joints, muscles, and movements, a basic understanding of them all helps enormously in understanding both the condition and its treatment.

Bones form the framework of the body, with the bones, joints, and muscles working together as levers to perform movement. In physics, a lever is a simple machine with four key components:

- A lever (a rigid bar)
- A fulcrum (a point about which the lever pivots)
- A resisting force (or load, such as a weight to be moved)
- An applied force (or effort; something that is doing the moving) (see Figure 2.4.1)

An example of a lever in humans is the arm lifting a weight:

- The forearm bones are the lever.
- The elbow joint is the fulcrum.
- The object being lifted is the resisting force.
- The contraction of the elbow flexor muscles creates the applied force.

Muscles provide the action; the bones just follow.

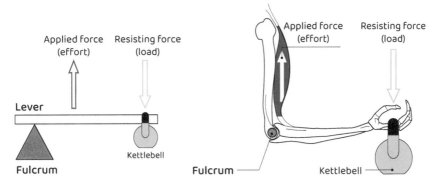

Figure 2.4.1 A lever (left) and the corresponding parts in the human arm (right).

Both the resisting force and applied force act on the lever at a distance from the fulcrum, which creates a torque or rotation (also called a "moment") about the fulcrum. This distance is called the force's "lever arm" (or "moment arm"). Even if the force stays constant, when the lever arm increases in length, the torque increases, and vice versa. Using the example in Figure 2.4.1, if the kettlebell were moved closer to the fulcrum (elbow), effectively shortening the lever arm, a smaller applied force (i.e., muscle contraction) would be required to lift it.

As explained, muscles contract to produce force. The force produced can be very small (e.g., to pick up a feather) or very large (e.g., to pick up a kettlebell).

There are three types of muscles in the body:

- **Cardiac:** Muscle that forms the bulk of the wall of the heart
- **Smooth:** Muscle located in the walls of hollow internal structures such as the blood vessels, stomach, and intestines
- **Skeletal:** Muscle attached (mostly) to bones

Spastic hemiplegia primarily affects skeletal muscle.* Skeletal muscles contract to produce movement or maintain posture. The bones cannot stand up on their own; gravity would pull them down. When muscles contract, in addition to causing movement, they exert force, which keeps the body erect. Without these forces opposing gravity, the bones would collapse in a heap on the ground.

In a sense, the bones are like the limbs of a marionette (or puppet, see Figure 2.4.2). The marionette cannot stand up on its own.

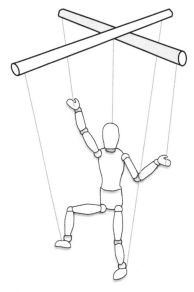

Figure 2.4.2 A marionette (puppet).

There are three types of muscle contractions:

- **Concentric (shortening):** For example, when going up a flight of stairs, the quadriceps (the muscles in front of the knee joint) contract concentrically—they shorten so that the knee extends.
- **Eccentric (lengthening):** For example, when going down a flight of stairs, the quadriceps (the same muscle that is involved in going up the stairs) contract eccentrically—they lengthen so that the knee bends. The lengthening contraction controls the bending of the knee against gravity.

---

* There are some reports of smooth muscle being affected in CP.[89,90,91]

- **Isometric (no change in length):** For example, when maintaining a posture (i.e., opposing the force of gravity), the muscles contract isometrically, without getting longer or shorter.

Every muscle has its own length when it is at rest. Muscles produce optimal force in the middle of that resting length.

While the details of the different types of contractions are not important in understanding hemiplegia as such, it is helpful to keep in mind that during most movements (e.g., walking), muscles move in fractions of a second between these different types of contractions.

Muscles also contain noncontractile elements—that is, elements that are incapable of contracting. These form the tendon and various sheaths (enveloping or covering tissue). The tendon is the cord-like structure that attaches the muscle to the bone. The Achilles tendon, for example, attaches the gastrocnemius and soleus muscles—both calf muscles—to the heel. The combination of the muscle, tendon, and various sheaths is collectively known as the muscle-tendon unit (MTU).

Note also that there is a difference between muscle strength and muscle power: both are important for everyday activities like walking and running. Muscle strength is the amount of force that a muscle can generate during a specific movement—for example, the weight you can lift at the gym in a single repetition. Muscle power is the rate of force production (i.e., how fast the force is being produced). There is a strength aspect to power, but it is also about the speed of the movement. Jumping is an example of a power-based activity.

Something else to consider is range of motion (ROM), also called "range of movement," which is a measure of joint flexibility. The actual ROM through which a joint can be passively moved is measured in degrees. An instrument called a goniometer* is used to measure the ROM of a joint. (See Figure 2.4.3). A video about measuring ROM is included in **Useful web resources.**

---

* A goniometer is like a movable protractor, used for measuring angles, as shown in Figure 2.4.3.

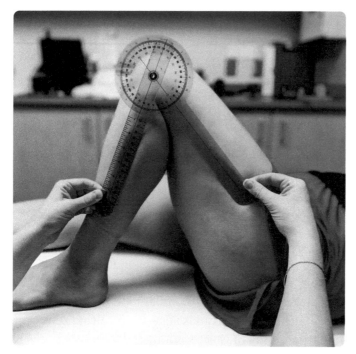

Figure 2.4.3 Measuring the ROM of the knee joint using a goniometer.

Tables 2.4.1 and 2.4.2 explain the movements, joint ROMs, and key muscles for both the upper and lower limbs. These tables are included as a reference and may be helpful at different times; for example, it may be useful to take them to some appointments. Below are some relevant points:

- Muscles are generally arranged in pairs around a joint. The muscles on one side of the joint move the joint in one direction, while the muscles on the other side of the joint move the joint in the opposite direction. Key muscles are identified at each joint, but minor muscles have not been included.
- Movements typically affected by spasticity are shown on the left side of the tables and are indicated **with a green background**. *Some, but not necessarily all, of the muscles responsible for those movements may be affected by spasticity.* The tables show the movements typically affected by spasticity, but there may be some variation between individuals.
- Two-joint muscles play a role in movement at two joints. (Some muscles in the hand and foot cross more than two joints.) The most

significant movements affected by two-joint muscles *and* spasticity **are indicated in orange** on the left side of the tables.

- Typical ROMs for each joint are shown. The closer a joint's ROM is to typical, the better. A muscle contracture is a limitation of a joint's ROM.[92] The terms "muscle contracture" and "tight muscle" are used interchangeably in the CP field and in this book.

To stretch a muscle, we do the opposite of that muscle's action. To stretch a flexor muscle, for example, we must extend the joint. To stretch an extensor muscle, we must flex the joint. To fully stretch a muscle, we must move the joint through its full ROM. Because some muscles cross two joints rather than one, both joints are involved in the stretching of two-jointed muscles. To stretch the two-jointed hamstrings, for example, we have to extend the knee while flexing the hip. Long sitting (sitting with the legs extended) is a good method of stretching the hamstrings because the knees are extended while the hips are flexed.

Table 2.4.1 Upper limb movements, joint ROMs,[93] and key muscles

MOVEMENT (Green background indicates movements affected by spasticity *on the involved side* in hemiplegia)		KEY MUSCLES RESPONSIBLE FOR THE MOVEMENT (Two-jointed muscles are indicated in orange)
Shoulder adduction Movement of the arm toward the middle of the body (midline) **ROM 0 to 140 degrees**		**Shoulder adductors** • Latissimus dorsi • Teres major • Pectoralis major
Shoulder flexion Movement of the arm upward toward the face **ROM 0 to 180 degrees**		**Shoulder flexors** • Pectoralis major • Deltoid
Shoulder internal rotation Movement of the upper arm internally toward the middle of the body (midline) **ROM 0 to 70 degrees**		**Shoulder internal rotators** • Latissimus dorsi • Teres major • Pectoralis major
Elbow flexion Movement of the forearm toward the upper arm **ROM 0 to 150 degrees**		**Elbow flexors** • Biceps • Brachialis • Brachioradialis
Forearm pronation Internal rotation of the forearm that results in the hand moving from the palm-up to the palm-down position **ROM 0 to 80 degrees**		**Pronators** • Pronator teres • Pronator quadratus
Wrist flexion Movement of the palm of the hand toward the inside of the forearm **ROM 0 to 80 degrees**		**Wrist flexors** • Flexor carpi radialis • Flexor carpi ulnaris • Palmaris longus
Thumb adduction Movement of the thumb toward the fingers **ROM 0 to 80 degrees**		**Thumb adductors** • Adductor pollicis
Thumb flexion Movement of the thumb into palm **ROM 0 to 50 degrees**		**Thumb flexors** • Flexor pollicis longus • Flexor pollicis brevis
Finger flexion Movement of the fingers toward the palm **ROM 0 to 90 degrees**		**Finger flexors** • Flexor digitorum superficialis • Flexor digitorum profundus

OPPOSITE MOVEMENT		KEY MUSCLES RESPONSIBLE FOR THE OPPOSITE MOVEMENT
Shoulder abduction Movement of the arm away from the middle of the body (midline) **ROM 0 to 45 degrees**		**Shoulder abductors** • Supraspinatus • Deltoid
Shoulder extension Movement of the arm to the back of the body **ROM 0 to 60 degrees**		**Shoulder extensors** • Deltoid • Latissimus dorsi • Teres major
Shoulder external rotation Movement of the upper arm externally away from the middle of the body (midline) **ROM 0 to 90 degrees**		**Shoulder external rotators** • Infraspinatus • Teres minor
Elbow extension Movement of the forearm away from the upper arm **ROM 0 to 150 degrees**		**Elbow extensors** • Triceps
Forearm supination External rotation of the forearm that results in the hand moving from the palm-down to the palm-up position **ROM 0 to 80 degrees**		**Supinators** • Supinator
Wrist extension Movement of the palm of the hand away from the inside of the forearm **ROM 0 to 70 degrees**		**Wrist extensors** • Extensor carpi radialis • Extensor carpi ulnaris • Extensor carpi radialis brevis
Thumb (radial) abduction Movement of the thumb away from the fingers **ROM 0 to 80 degrees**		**Thumb abductors** • Abductor pollicis longus • Abductor pollicis brevis
Thumb extension Movement of the thumb away from the palm **ROM 0 to 50 degrees**		**Thumb extensors** • Extensor pollicis longus • Extensor pollicis brevis
Finger extension Movement of the fingers away from the palm **ROM 0 to 90 degrees**		**Finger extensors** *Individual muscles not listed*

Table 2.4.2 Lower limb movements, joint ROMs,[94,95] and key muscles

MOVEMENT (Green background indicates movements affected by spasticity)		KEY MUSCLES RESPONSIBLE FOR THE MOVEMENT (Two-jointed muscles are indicated in orange)
Hip flexion Movement of the thigh up toward the pelvis **ROM 0 to 125 degrees**		**Hip flexors** • Iliopsoas • Rectus femoris
Hip adduction Movement of the thigh toward the midline **ROM 0 to 20 degrees**		**Hip adductors** • Adductor longus • Adductor magnus • Adductor brevis • Gracilis
Hip internal rotation Rotary movement of the thigh toward the midline; also known as inward or medial rotation **ROM 0 to 45 degrees**	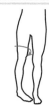	*Individual muscles not listed*
Knee flexion Increasing the angle between the thigh and lower leg **ROM 0 to 140 degrees** Note: Reference point is the straight leg. The angle increases the nearer the lower leg moves to the thigh.	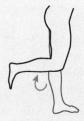	**Knee flexors** • Hamstrings • Gastrocnemius
Ankle plantar flexion Movement of the foot away from the lower leg **ROM 0 to 45 degrees** Note: Reference point is the 90-degree angle between the lower leg and the foot.	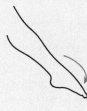	**Ankle plantar flexors** • Gastrocnemius • Soleus

OPPOSITE MOVEMENT	KEY MUSCLES RESPONSIBLE FOR THE OPPOSITE MOVEMENT
Hip extension Movement of the thigh away from the pelvis **ROM 0 to 10 degrees** 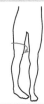	**Hip extensors** • Gluteus maximus • Hamstrings
Hip abduction Movement of the thigh away from the midline **ROM 0 to 45 degrees**	**Hip abductors** • Gluteus medius
Hip external rotation Rotary movement of the thigh away from the midline; also known as outward or lateral rotation **ROM 0 to 45 degrees** 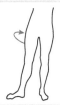	*Individual muscles not listed*
Knee extension Decreasing the angle between the thigh and lower leg **ROM 140 to 0 degrees** Note: Reference point is the flexed leg. The angle decreases the further the lower leg moves away from the thigh.	**Knee extensors** The quadriceps (quads) consist of four muscles: • Rectus femoris • Vastus intermedius • Vastus lateralis • Vastus medialis
Ankle dorsiflexion Movement of the foot toward the lower leg **ROM 0 to 20 degrees** Note: Reference point is the 90-degree angle between the lower leg and the foot.	**Ankle dorsiflexors** • Tibialis anterior • Toe extensors

Typical hand function and typical walking

The hand is the cutting edge of the mind.

Jacob Bronowski

Typical hand function

Our hands are the tools we use to play and do work and to perform many activities of daily living (ADLs), which are the essential self-care tasks typically performed daily, such as bathing, dressing, grooming, eating, and toileting. Our hands are important because they provide sensation and movement. Effective development of hand skills depends on adequate postural mechanisms, cognition, visual perception, and tactile ability.* Hand use is complex and involves intricate coordination of the senses and muscles to perform tasks, such as:

---

* **Postural mechanisms** are the system of muscles, joints, and sensory feedback that the body uses to maintain balance and upright posture while sitting, standing, or moving about. **Visual perception** is interpreting and making sense of visual information from the environment by the brain. **Tactile ability** refers to the sense of touch and the ability to perceive and interpret physical sensations through the skin, providing information such as light touch, deep touch, temperature, vibration, and pain.

- **Grasping:** Using the fingers and thumb to hold onto an object. There are several types of grasps, such as palmar, pincer, and lateral, which depend on the shape and size of the object being grasped:
  - ○ Palmar grasp: Holding an object using the palm and fingers
  - ○ Pincer grasp: Holding an object between the tips of the index finger and thumb
  - ○ Lateral grasp: Holding an object between the side of the index finger and the thumb (such as someone might hold a key)
- **Carrying:** Transporting a handheld object from one place to another
- **Releasing:** Letting go of an object. There are two types of releases: power and precision release:
  - ○ Power release: quick and forceful
  - ○ Precision release: more controlled and gradual
- **Manipulating:** Moving and positioning an object within the hand (e.g., turning a key, opening a door, using a pen).

Bilateral hand use involves both hands in a task. The term "bimanual activities" is also used to describe activities that involve both hands.

In addition, the task of maintaining balance, while sitting, for example, is very important for reaching and grasping. In the sitting position the body functions as an anchor for all the levers that are used in arm movements.

Typical walking

In general, we take walking for granted. It is only when we encounter a problem that we stop to think about what walking entails. The term "gait" refers to a person's manner of walking. "Typical" gait refers to the typically developing person's manner of walking, which has been studied extensively. Because having problems with walking is one of the hallmarks of spastic hemiplegia, this section briefly looks at the features of typical walking.

Walking is a phenomenal achievement. It involves generating forces, managing gravity, speed, balance, and more. In evolutionary terms, walking on two limbs was advantageous because it freed our upper limbs for other tasks. It is no surprise that crawling comes before walking in human gross motor development: a crawling child has four limbs on the floor and is therefore more stable. Walking, which involves balancing on two limbs, is a more advanced and more demanding form of movement.

a) The requirements of walking

Walking has four requirements:[96]

- **A control system:** The nervous system provides the control system for walking.
- **An energy source:** The energy required is supplied by oxygen[*] and the breakdown of food.
- **Levers providing movement:** The levers are the bones.
- **Forces to move the levers:** Muscle contraction provides the forces for walking. As we saw in the previous section, movement is generated by muscle forces acting on the levers (the bones).

b) The gait cycle

One complete gait (or walking) cycle refers to the time between two successive occurrences of the same event in walking—for example, the time between when one foot strikes the ground and when that same foot strikes the ground again. Figure 2.5.1 shows what is happening with each limb during a complete gait cycle. The gait cycle is divided into two major phases:

- **Stance phase:** The period of time the foot of interest (green in Figure 2.5.1) is on the ground
- **Swing phase:** The period of time the foot of interest is in the air

Stance phase occupies approximately 60 percent of the gait cycle, and swing phase occupies approximately 40 percent.[96] There are two periods in the gait cycle when both limbs are on the ground; this is termed "double stance" (or "double support"). Single stance (or single support) is when just one limb is on the ground. Walking involves alternately balancing on each single limb as we move forward.

---

[*] Energy can be produced without oxygen in some cases; for example, for short bursts of quick walking. This is termed "anaerobic metabolism."

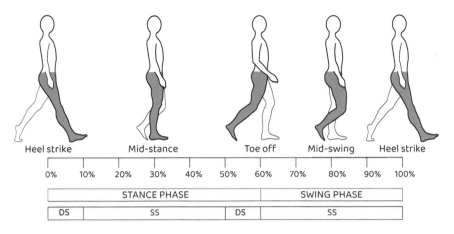

| Heel strike | Mid-stance | Toe off | Mid-swing | Heel strike |

0%   10%   20%   30%   40%   50%   60%   70%   80%   90%   100%

| STANCE PHASE | SWING PHASE |
| DS | SS | DS | SS |

Figure 2.5.1 A complete gait cycle. "DS" is double stance; "SS" is single stance.

c) Attributes of typical walking

The following are attributes of typical walking that are frequently lost in individuals with spastic hemiplegia:[96]

- **Stability in the stance phase:** A reflection of controlled movement and good balance
- **Foot clearance in the swing phase:** Movement of the foot forward without dragging the toe
- **Pre-positioning of the foot for initial contact (heel strike):** Preparation of the foot to strike the ground with the heel (see Figure 2.5.1)
- **Adequate step length:** A sufficiently long step taken
- **Energy conservation:** Energy-efficient walking

Problems with the first four of these attributes contribute to problems with the fifth, the energy cost of walking.

When a typically developing child begins to walk, they do so without these attributes. The knees are relatively stiff and they walk with a wide base of support (i.e., the legs are far apart). But as the child develops balance and their motor system matures, their gait evolves toward the adult pattern, generally by about three and a half years of age.[97] It appears that walking is innate rather than learned, and it depends on the progressive maturing of the central nervous system.

I would say to parents that you do need great patience with children with CP as they have to put so much energy into physical movement and development. This can sometimes slow down their development in other areas such as speaking or with their schoolwork. I've gone to parent-teacher meetings over the years and been given feedback about concerns regarding Ally's reading, maths, or executive functioning, and then been amazed the following year when, quite often, Ally has caught up.

People may assume that kids with CP have the same capabilities as everyone else when they are in mainstream school. In many ways they do, and certainly for Ally, her tenacity and determination support this perception. But we also need to be conscious, understanding, and supportive of their limitations. Our physiotherapist joined me for a school appointment with Ally's teacher on one occasion, and as we walked out to the car together after the meeting, she remarked that she wasn't sure that people understand how much harder Ally has to work just to sit up straight or to try to keep up with the other kids. This level of effort can be formally measured through oxygen consumption levels when children with CP carry out normal activities. When Ally was assessed, her oxygen consumption (a measure of energy expenditure) was approximately one and a half times higher than for kids with typical development. This measurement is an excellent way to show how much harder children with CP have to work to accomplish everyday tasks.

Primary problems

Divide each difficulty into as many parts as is
feasible and necessary to resolve it.

René Descartes

The motor system or neuromusculoskeletal system involves the nervous system, muscles, bones, joints, and their related structures. Based on clinical expertise, Gage proposed a useful framework for classifying the neuromusculoskeletal problems that occur in children with spastic CP.[74,98] Problems are categorized into primary, secondary, and tertiary problems:

- Primary problems are caused by the brain injury and are therefore present from when the brain injury occurred. Many are neurological problems but may also include alterations in the structure of the muscles themselves.
- Secondary problems develop over time in the growing child. They are problems of atypical muscle growth and bone development and are referred to as "growth problems."
- Tertiary problems are the "coping responses" that arise to compensate for or counteract the primary and secondary problems.

Classifying the problems of hemiplegia in this way is helpful because:

- For families, it may aid in their understanding of the many problems encountered. The classification helps explain how and when the problems likely develop and change over time.
- For medical professionals, it is important to separate out the different problems to decide what can, cannot, and should not be treated, providing a road map for treatment.

A very useful tool for classifying the problems, which can sometimes be difficult to separate, is motion analysis. Motion analysis is addressed in Chapter 3. This section covers primary problems, and the next two cover secondary and tertiary problems.

The primary neuromusculoskeletal problems are problems present from when the brain injury occurred. In general, the primary problems are difficult to change or improve. However, with diligent management, the impact of these primary problems can be minimized, and function can be maximized.

Understanding the primary (this section), secondary (next section, 2.7), and tertiary (section 2.8) problems and how they combine to affect motor function (section 2.9) is key to understanding hemiplegia. These sections are long, but they are worth reading in order to gain a full understanding of the condition. Your physical therapist or physician may be able to answer any questions you may have. It may also help to use Tables 2.4.1 and 2.4.2 as references.

The primary problems include the following, which are examined each in turn, adapted from Gage:[74,98,99]

- **Lack of selective motor control**
- **Poor balance**
- **Abnormal tone**
- **Muscle weakness**
- **Sensory problems**

Even though primary problems are discussed separately, the problems exist together and they trend in similar directions (the level of effect of one is mirrored in others, plus they can exacerbate one another).

Primary problems should be evaluated and considered separately while recognizing that they may trend together. In other words, if impairment is greater in one area (e.g., selective motor control), it tends to be greater in other areas (e.g., weakness). In general, the severity of primary problems is a significant predictor of GMFCS level.

Lack of selective motor control

In simple terms, selective motor control refers to the ability to isolate a muscle or combination of muscles to produce a particular movement. This includes being able to contract a muscle without the opposite muscle contracting (which is termed "co-contraction"). For example, some people cannot wink one of their eyes, no matter how hard they try because they do not have good selective motor control over the muscles responsible for winking. Another example is ankle dorsiflexion/plantar flexion (moving the foot up and down) without moving knees or hips. A child with hemiplegia has problems with selective motor control and therefore has difficulty performing some movements.

Selective motor control can be checked by asking the child to perform certain movements, such as moving the foot up and down. Each limb and joint is tested separately. This evaluates whether the child:

- Can do the full movement in both directions
- Can do the movement without involving other body movements
- Can do the movement without doing a mirror movement, or other movement, in the same or the other limb.

The severity and number of muscles affected by lack of selective motor control in hemiplegia depends on the extent of the brain injury.

The muscles further away from the brain (hand and ankle) are generally more affected than muscles that are closer (shoulder and hip). In addition, from the standpoint of selective motor control, muscles that cross more than one joint are more severely involved than muscles that cross only one joint.[99]

Poor balance

Balance is generally understood as the ability to not fall. More specifically, it's about controlling our body within our base of support.[100] Good balance is needed to be able to function in our environment.

About half of our body mass is in our trunk,[101] so good balance largely relies on controlling our trunk position within the support base whether we are lying, sitting, standing, or walking. When we are lying down, our whole body is in contact with the surface, so balance is easy. When we are standing or walking, only our feet are in contact with the surface (ground), so balance is more challenging.

To control our body position, we also must sense where our body is and then move as appropriate. This means our motor and sensory systems are involved in balance. The motor system is the neuromusculoskeletal system already described, including the nervous system, muscles, bones, joints, and their related structures. Sensory systems involved include vision, vestibular input, proprioception, and tactile feedback:[102]

- Vision involves sensory receptors in the eyes.
- Vestibular input involves sensory receptors in our ears.
- Proprioception involves sensory receptors in our muscles and joints.
- Tactile feedback involves sensory receptors in our skin.

Our brain combines the information from all these sensory receptors to interpret our body position and motion relative to itself and our surroundings.[102] Individuals with CP, including those with hemiplegia, may have deficits in one or more of the sensory or motor systems, any of which can impact balance.[3,103]

A gentle push (forward, backward, and/or side to side) of a child tests balance reactions. A child with typical balance will easily maintain their balance and, if necessary, take a compensatory step to regain it. A child with balance problems may fall over or take longer to regain their balance (more than one step).

Conflicting views exist in the literature on whether poor balance reactions can be improved by training and/or therapy.[103]

Ally fell a lot when she was younger because she has balance issues. She broke her collarbone twice, her foot once (in seven places), and experienced a couple of concussions. We learned that bone health is extremely important for kids with CP, and we do try and encourage a healthy diet and vitamin supplements notwithstanding that Ally remains very slim. Ally now sees an endocrinologist who reviews Ally as she grows.

Ally never wants to move slowly, and we always had our hearts in our mouth when she would run rather than walk! This was explained to us by her physiotherapist and it seems that running was easier than walking. Her balance has improved as she has gotten older, and she is increasingly more stable on her feet, but her friends joke that she is the one that is most likely to fall over or definitely spill her milkshake! Ally is a very determined girl, and when there is something she wants to do, it is very difficult, if not impossible, to stop her. I'm never sure if this is as a result of her prematurity, her CP, or just her natural personality, but it certainly helps her to achieve the results she wants.

Abnormal tone

Muscle tone is the resting tension in a muscle. A range of "normal" muscle tone exists. Tone is considered "abnormal" when it falls outside the range of normal or typical. It can be too low (hypotonia) or too high (hypertonia). Abnormal muscle tone occurs in all types of CP. In children with hemiplegia, tone is typically too high in the involved arm and leg due to spasticity.

a) Spasticity

Spasticity is one type of high tone. There are several definitions of spasticity. One is that it is a condition in which there is an abnormal increase in muscle tone or stiffness of muscle that can interfere with movement and speech, and be associated with discomfort or pain.[22] Another definition highlights the velocity-dependent nature of spasticity.[104]

A muscle reacts to rapid stretching by contracting in opposition (i.e., the muscle tightens rather than continuing to stretch or lengthen). This protects the muscle from overstretching when quickly stretched. See Figure 2.6.1.

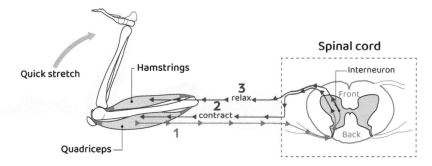

Figure 2.6.1 Example of a "normal" stretch reflex. **1.** Quadriceps are stretched quickly, and information is sent via sensory neurons to the spinal cord. **2.** Motor neurons cause the quadriceps to contract to resist the quick stretch. **3.** Motor neurons cause the hamstrings to relax to allow the quadriceps to contract.

- A **"normal" stretch reflex** is a rapid, involuntary muscle contraction (in the quadriceps in Figure 2.6.1) in response to a sudden stretch of the muscle.*
- A **"hyperactive" stretch reflex** is an exaggerated reflex response that leads to excessive muscle contraction and increased muscle tone. Spasticity is a hyperactive stretch reflex (the excessive muscle contraction can be felt as resistance by a person doing a quick passive stretch of the muscle).†

The speed of the rapid stretch is important because the spastic reaction happens only with a *quick* stretch. If the stretch is slow, it does not elicit a spastic reaction. (The effect of speed can be noted by comparing a muscle's response to slow versus quick passive stretching.) The muscle stretching that occurs, during walking for example, is quick (an entire gait cycle occurs in about one second); thus, the spastic response can happen in people with hemiplegia while walking.

---

* Doctors routinely perform a knee-jerk reflex test using a small rubber hammer to check for healthy reflex responses.

† Passive stretching is when another person stretches an individual's muscle.

Spasticity results from a loss of inhibition—the dampening input from specific nerve cells in the brain to nerve cells in the spinal cord, and hence to certain muscles.

Clonus is the most extreme form of spasticity, defined as a series of involuntary, rhythmic muscular contractions and relaxations. It can be seen in the gastrocnemius (one of the calf muscles); for example, when an examiner quickly dorsiflexes the foot (moves the foot up), the foot may then plantar flex (move down) and continue to move up and down uncontrollably for a number of beats (contraction and relaxation cycles). A video depicting clonus is included in **Useful web resources**.

b) Dystonia

As noted in section 2.1, individuals with hemiplegia sometimes have secondary or co-occurring motor types in addition to spasticity. The Australian CP register found that 16 percent of individuals with hemiplegia (all GMFCS levels) have co-occurring dyskinesia.[*4] It is believed that the true prevalence of co-occurring motor types is higher.[4] A more recent study found that 50 percent of children and young people with CP had spasticity *and* dystonia.[48] The presence of dystonia with spasticity has been underrecognized, which is important to note because the management of spasticity and dystonia is different.

Dystonia is a disorder characterized by involuntary (unintended) muscle contractions that cause slow repetitive movements or abnormal postures that can sometimes be painful.[39] Some define dystonia as muscles that "contract that you do not want to contract when you try to move." In contrast to spasticity, dystonia does not occur as a result of rapid stretch. Examples of dystonia include the leg muscles tightening or uncontrolled, posturing movements of the fingers or toes when surprised, talking, or playing a video game (where there is excitement or tension).

Abnormal muscle tone can be measured using different measurement tools. See Table 2.6.1.

---

* For those who acquired CP in the prenatal or perinatal period only, and also includes monoplegia.

Table 2.6.1 Measurement tools for abnormal muscle tone

MEASUREMENT TOOL	TYPE OF ABNORMAL MUSCLE TONE
Modified Ashworth Scale (MAS)[105,106]	Spasticity
Modified Tardieu Scale (MTS)[106,107]	Spasticity
Barry-Albright Dystonia Scale (BADS)[108]	Dystonia
Hypertonia Assessment Tool (HAT)[109,110]	Dystonia and spasticity (and rigidity*)

* Rigidity is another type of high tone in which the muscles have the same amount of stiffness irrespective of the degree of movement. It is uncommon and practically does not exist in CP.

Muscle weakness

In general terms, muscle weakness is the inability to generate muscle force. (Refer to Tables 2.4.1 and 2.4.2, which show the main upper and lower limb muscles arranged in pairs around each joint.) Studies have found that the strength of the major muscle groups of both the involved and uninvolved upper and lower limbs in children with hemiplegia was less than that of those of age-matched, typically developing peers.[111,112] The causes of the muscle weakness resulting from the brain injury are varied and include:

- Smaller muscles[113]
- Atypical muscle composition (i.e., more fat and collagen)[114]
- Poor selective motor control or co-contraction of muscles on the opposite side of the joint[3]
- Incomplete voluntary activation of the muscle[115]
- Decreased muscle lever arms, often due to bony malalignments or related problems[116,117,118]

Muscle strength can be measured by manual muscle testing, by a hand-held machine called a dynamometer, or with more sophisticated tests as might be done in a sports clinic. Measuring muscle strength for people with CP is challenging because of the lack of selective motor control and contractures.

Sensory problems

A full discussion of sensory problems is included in section 2.10.

Secondary problems

The human foot is a masterpiece of
engineering and a work of art.
Leonardo da Vinci

The secondary problems in hemiplegia develop slowly over time and in direct proportion to the rate of bone growth. They also depend on the amount and type of usage of the muscles. We saw earlier that the periods of most rapid growth are from birth to age three and during puberty. These are, therefore, periods of great challenge and change in the child with hemiplegia.

Secondary problems arise as a result of the atypical forces imposed on the growing skeleton by the effects of the primary brain injury and movement. In other words, the primary problems drive the secondary problems. The good news is that the secondary problems have more treatment options.

This section covers:

- Atypical muscle growth
- Atypical bone development

Atypical muscle growth

What follows is a simplified explanation of atypical muscle growth in hemiplegia. This is a very complex subject, and more is still being learned about the differences between muscles in typically developing individuals and in people with spastic CP. Also, as noted in the last section, the primary problems may also include alterations in the structure of the muscles themselves. A muscle grows in length in response to stretch. It has been shown that for normal muscle lengthening to occur, two to four hours of stretching per day is required.[98] Bones grow during sleep,[119] and in a typically developing child, this required amount of stretching occurs when the child gets up in the morning and starts to move about, to run, and to play. This typical movement moves the joints and results in normal stretching of the muscles, which provides the stimulus for laying down new muscle cells and is how a muscle grows in length. Thus, bone growth leads to stretching of the muscle, which leads to the muscle growing in length.

Because the primary problems predominantly affect the neuromusculoskeletal systems in children with hemiplegia, they usually have decreased physical activity levels compared to typically developing children.[120] The reduced amount of physical activity can then affect their capacity to actively stretch their muscles. Even with movement, the child with hemiplegia may not fully stretch out their muscles through the typical ROM of the joints. Thus, the reduced stretching range for many muscles may become the norm.

As a result, the muscles fail to grow adequately in length and width[*] and contractures develop, [†] which result in joints having reduced ROM. Indeed, in the past, CP was called "short muscle disease," although it's

---

[*] Muscles also grow in width. Growth in width has been shown to be decreased as well.[121]

[†] More precisely, the contracture occurs in the muscle-tendon unit (MTU) and/or capsule of the joint, not just the muscle.

worth noting that despite this title, the problem arises from muscles failing to grow in length and width rather than from becoming shortened. With lack of movement, the muscles also become stiff.

For young children with hemiplegia, their muscles may still achieve full ROM when they are relaxed; for example, during sleep. Over time, however, they may develop contracture, meaning that the full joint ROM cannot be achieved at any time. One study found decreasing ROM in the lower limb muscles in children with CP (34 percent unilateral) from age 2 to 14 years.[122]

Contractures particularly affect the two-joint* muscles.[3] They interfere with positioning and movement. For example, an elbow flexion contracture may result in limited ability to extend the elbow in reaching. Contractures may also interfere with the typical movements that lead to achieving gross motor milestones. Decreased mobility at any age may lead to activity limitation and reduced participation. Nordmark and colleagues described the nature of the problem: a decrease in ROM with age may result in decreased mobility, which in turn results in a further decrease in ROM—a vicious circle.[122]

In addition to the factors outlined above that may cause contractures to develop over time, there may be differences at a tissue level between the muscles of individuals with CP and those of the typical population. These differences include:[3,121,123,124,125]

- **Smaller muscles** in both diameter and length, which may partially explain muscle weakness
- **Lengthened and fewer sarcomeres** (the functional unit of contraction of a muscle), though the muscle itself is shortened, this could also contribute to muscle weakness
- **Muscles being stiffer,** which is believed to be caused by atypical extracellular matrix (the network surrounding the muscle cells, consisting of collagen, proteins, and more)
- **Decrease in the number of satellite cells,** which are responsible for the majority of muscle growth
- **Increased fat and collagen,** which could contribute to muscle weakness even if the muscle is the same size

---

* Including multi-joint muscles.

In summary, muscle quality and size may be different. Muscles may become smaller (less muscle bulk) and stiffer (less elastic) compared with those of typically developing children. Smaller muscle size has been reported in children with spastic CP compared to typically developing children and in children as young as 15 months.[126,127] It is to be expected that the muscles of a 14-year-old with spastic CP would be very different from those of a 1-year-old with spastic CP. There is still more to learn about altered muscle composition in spastic CP.

To compensate for atypical muscle growth in a child with CP, parents have to ensure that their child gets adequate opportunity to stretch and move their spastic muscles. Traditionally, this included the parent doing daily slow stretches of the child's spastic muscles through their full ROM. (This is called passive stretching; the slow stretching does not elicit the spastic response.) However, passive stretching is no longer recommended in isolation. The current evidence places a greater emphasis on other methods of stretching, including positioning, orthoses, casting,* and especially active movement. Because of its importance, a detailed section on stretching is included in the next chapter. The aim is to keep full ROM for as long as possible to prevent contractures from developing to the greatest possible extent. Working on ROM is not something that can begin when the child is older. It has to start right at the time of diagnosis. However, despite best efforts, it is often inevitable that some contractures may develop.

The rate of development of contractures often mirrors the rate of growth of the child; that is, contractures tend to develop during periods of rapid growth (which is why keeping a growth chart is useful). While great attention needs to be paid to stretching and activity during periods of active growth, stretching is needed throughout childhood and adolescence. Even in the "quieter" growth years, the child will still gain height.

Note that the situation can be even more complicated. It is possible for some muscles to become too long in response to abnormal postures and movement. One example is crouch gait (persistent flexed-knee gait).

---

* Casting consists of stretching a muscle by applying a plaster of paris or a fiberglass cast; for example, a below-knee cast to stretch the tight gastrocnemius and/or soleus muscles (calf muscles) to hold the muscle in a position of maximum stretch. After a few days to one week, the cast can be removed. A series of casts is typically needed to gain the desired effect.

The one-joint muscles responsible for upright posture and alignment (gluteus maximus, vasti, and soleus) are stretched repetitively and for prolonged periods of time during growth. As a result, they gradually become too stretched, too long, and less effective in maintaining upright posture. This sequence can result in progressively worsening crouch gait.

Atypical bone development

This section addresses:

a) Lever-arm dysfunction
b) Scoliosis
c) Leg length discrepancy
d) Bone health

a) Lever-arm dysfunction

Atypical bone development is interlinked with atypical muscle growth in hemiplegia. The long bones of the body (the bones of the upper and lower limbs) grow in a particular area called the "growth plates" (see Figure 2.7.1), but it is the forces acting on the bones that play a part in their ultimate shape—termed "bone modeling."[99]

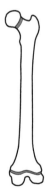

Figure 2.7.1 Growth plates (orange) in a long bone.

Growing bone is "plastic," or "malleable," which is what allows the forces to model the bone. The expressions "If you put a twist on a growing bone, it will take the twist" and "Just as the twig is bent the tree's inclined" illustrate this concept.

If the muscle forces and bone forces are typical and occur at the correct time in development, then the final shape of the bone will be typical as well (e.g., the femoral head and the hip socket helping to shape each other). If forces are atypical or mistimed in relation to a child's development, the bones may be misshaped.

The movements that help the child achieve the six main gross motor milestones* described in Chapter 1 and the time in development at which they occur are part of the typical forces acting on the bones. It is important to understand that the bones of younger children are more malleable than the bones of older children. One of the hallmarks of hemiplegia is that the child can be late in achieving gross motor milestones when the bones are less malleable with less ability to remodel or reshape. This is in addition to the influences of altered muscle forces and tone. We can compare this to providing opportunities for our children: we have to provide them at the right time. Peekaboo will delight your six-month-old infant, but your six-year-old child will likely roll their eyes if you try to play Peekaboo with them. In the presence of hemiplegia, typical bone modeling (shaping) may not occur as the bone grows.

In addition to bone modeling, a certain amount of bone *remodeling* (reshaping) occurs in development.

Ally is always slower than other kids of her age group in meeting her milestones, and we have been vigilant in monitoring her progress. I will never forget the day that Ally first crawled when she was 16 months old. She had completed months of physiotherapy to develop her supporting abdominal muscles; we had also consistently worked with her at home on positional strengthening exercises and motivational games to follow and mimic with her toys. She had a toy snail that she was particularly attached to and was very determined to move like him.

We were at an appointment with her physio and occupational therapist on the day she finally crawled. They were taking a video to map her progress,

---

* The milestones are significant, but so are the movements leading up to the milestones. For example, when a child is able to stand holding on to furniture, they may also be able to hold on with one hand and turn their body to bend down and pick up an object. All these movements, not just the main movements, contribute to the normal forces that act on the bones.

and in true Ally style, she seemed determined to impress everyone and crawled across the room out of nowhere! It was one of the best days of our lives as it was a beacon of hope for Ally's future as she showed she had the ability to strengthen herself and develop all those muscles in her limbs. She walked at two years of age, again ensuring an audience was present. This time, she was in the pharmacy with her dad and was wearing a snowsuit when she decided to walk across the room to get something off a shelf. This was again a momentous occasion.

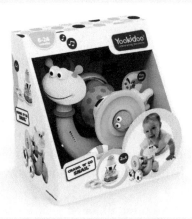

The toy that encouraged Ally to crawl, a Yokidoo Crawl 'N' Go Snail.

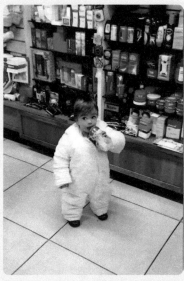

Ally's first time walking.

The effectiveness of a muscle action to produce movement depends not only on the muscle but also on the shape and length of the bones and the position of the joints. If the position or shape of the bone and joint is not typical, the bone is less effective as a lever. For example, if the femur (thigh bone) is misshapen, the hip abductors cannot work as effectively because the pulling force of the muscle will be in an incorrect direction. Gage coined the term "lever-arm dysfunction" to describe the influence of bone problems on movement.[74] These problems include lever arms (bones) that are short, flexible, twisted, and/or in the wrong position.

The following are common problems in hemiplegia; each is explained below:

i)   **Hip displacement (subluxation and dislocation)**
ii) **Excessive femoral anteversion**
iii) **Tibial torsion**
iv) **Pes valgus or pes varus**
v)   **Upper limb problems**

i) Hip displacement (subluxation and dislocation)

The hip joint is a ball-and-socket joint that is formed by the head (ball) of the femur and the acetabulum (socket) of the pelvis. Under the influence of bone growth and spastic muscles, a child's hip may become displaced: the ball moves partially out of the socket. This can be progressive and can lead to complete displacement. There are two stages of hip displacement:

- **Subluxated hip (hip subluxation)** is when the ball is partially out of the socket but is still in contact with it—the ball is still partially covered by the socket.
- **Dislocated hip (hip dislocation)** is when the ball has moved completely out of the socket.

The development of hip displacement is a slow process. Even though it starts out silently (it is painless), it can lead to pain and reduced function in the longer term. See Figure 2.7.2.

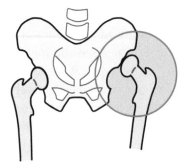

Figure 2.7.2 A dislocated hip. The right hip is normal. The left hip is dislocated: the head of the femur (ball) has moved completely out of the acetabulum (socket) of the pelvis.

Research has shown that the risk of hip displacement increases with GMFCS level.[128,129] The risk for children with CP has been found to be:

- The same as typically developing children, for GMFCS level I with one important exception (addressed in section 3.3)
- 15 percent for GMFCS level II

The measure used in X-rays for hip surveillance (monitoring) is called the "migration percentage" (MP), also known as the Reimer's migration index (RMI). Both terms refer to the percentage of the ball that has moved out of the socket, which can range from 0 to 100. "Normal" is less than 10 percent,[3] and hip displacement (subluxation) is anything greater than that. Mild abnormalities may not be problematic, but once the MP is greater than 30 percent, the likelihood of further displacement is almost certain (if there is growth remaining). Hip dislocation is defined as MP over 90 and up to 100 percent.[130]

See section 3.3 for more information on hip surveillance.

You may also come across the term "dysplasia," which means abnormal growth. Though closely related to hip displacement, it is not the same thing. Acetabular dysplasia is when the hip socket doesn't develop correctly and becomes shallow. It both results from and contributes to hip displacement.

ii) Excessive femoral anteversion

The important parts of the femur for the purposes of this discussion are the head (ball), neck, and shaft. The neck connects the head with the shaft. See Figure 2.7.3.

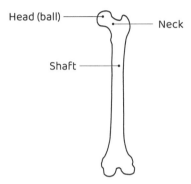

Figure 2.7.3 A femur.

The term "femoral anteversion" comes from "femoral" referring to the femur (thigh bone) and "version" referring to the angle of the neck of the femur relative to the shaft. "Ante" means "forward." "Femoral anteversion," therefore, is a condition where the neck of the femur is rotated relatively forward.

Figure 2.7.4 is a view of a hip and leg from the top down. The range of "normal" values for femoral anteversion varies depending on the reference used, but typically it's around 0 to 30 degrees in adults.[131,132] The mean value for adult females is 15 degrees and for men it's 10 degrees.

At birth, a typically developing infant has approximately 40 degrees of femoral anteversion.[133] With typical movement, the anteversion they have at birth rapidly decreases in the first three to four years and further reduces until puberty to typical adult values.

In children with hemiplegia, in the involved leg, femoral anteversion may not be corrected with growth. In fact, the femoral anteversion present at birth not only fails to reduce with growth but may increase. This is termed "excessive femoral anteversion."

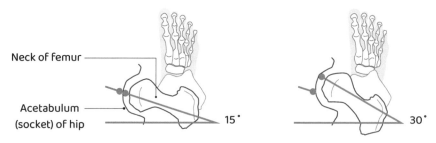

Neck of femur

Acetabulum
(socket) of hip

15°

30°

Figure 2.7.4 Femoral anteversion, top-down view: normal (left), with the neck of the femur correctly aligned with the acetabulum (socket) of the hip, and excessive (right), with the neck of the femur not correctly aligned.

The mean femoral anteversion for children with CP increases with GMFCS level, and is:[129]

- 30 degrees for GMFCS level I
- 36 degrees for GMFCS level II

Excessive femoral anteversion often leads to walking with inward knee rotation and the foot turned in (intoeing). This helps the hip abductors be in a better position to act more effectively because it increases the muscle's lever arm. However, this turning in of the knee and foot leads to functional difficulties such as tripping and falling.

"Femoral torsion" means a twisted femur. While technically it is not the same as "femoral anteversion," the effect on function and treatment is similar, which is why the two terms are often used interchangeably.

iii) Tibial torsion
The tibia is the main bone in the lower leg, often called the shinbone. Tibial torsion is a twist in the tibia. At birth, the typically developing child has about five degrees of internal tibial torsion (i.e., an inward twist of the tibia).[134] As with the femur, with the right forces acting at the right time and in the right sequence, the internal tibial torsion present in the infant turns into 10 to 15 degrees of external tibial torsion in the adult.[135] However, in the child with hemiplegia, the internal tibial torsion may not correct (persistent internal tibial torsion causing intoeing) or may overcorrect over time and become "excessive external" tibial torsion, with the foot turning out too much. See Figure 2.7.5.

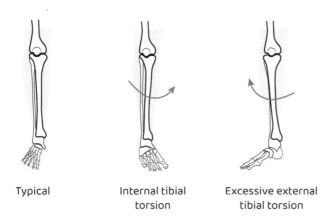

Typical   Internal tibial   Excessive external
                     torsion   tibial torsion

Figure 2.7.5 Tibial torsion of the right leg. Left: typical—foot exhibiting 10 to 15 degrees of external tibial torsion. Middle: internal tibial torsion—foot slightly turned in. Right: excessive external tibial torsion—foot excessively turned out.

The internal tibial torsion present at birth sometimes persists in children with hemiplegia, but as noted above, it often develops into an excessive external twist. Persistent internal tibial torsion may be seen in the younger child with hemiplegia, while excessive external tibial torsion may be seen in the older child with hemiplegia.

It is worth noting that in a child with femoral torsion *and* external tibial torsion, the femur (upper leg) is turned inward, but the tibia (lower leg) is turned outward. In addition, excessive external tibial torsion can occur in either leg for an individual with hemiplegia.

iv) Pes valgus or pes varus

The terms "pes valgus" and "pes varus" originate from "pes," meaning foot, and "valgus" or "varus," turning away from midline (valgus) and toward the midline (varus). Pes valgus and pes varus are a series of complex hindfoot, midfoot, and forefoot malalignments. (The hindfoot is the heel. The midfoot is the middle of the foot around the arch. The forefoot comprises the toes and the long bones leading up to the toes). Tables 2.7.1 and 2.7.2 explain the components of pes valgus and pes varus.

With pes valgus *or* pes varus, the three segments of the foot develop malalignments over time in response to the atypical forces exerted on the bones, and in each case (i.e., with either pes valgus *or* pes varus) they are commonly seen together. These malalignments reduce the effectiveness of the bones as lever arms and thus interfere with movement. Think of a person whose foot is turned outward as they attempt to walk forward. The foot needs to be stiff and extended in the last part of the stance phase of the gait cycle to propel the body forward. If the foot is too flexible, it becomes ineffective at doing its job. This is an example of a lever arm that is too flexible.

Table 2.7.1 Pes valgus

COMPONENT	ILLUSTRATION
Valgus hindfoot: The heel is turned outward from the midline of the body to an abnormal degree.	The left foot has a valgus hindfoot; the right foot is normal.
Pronation of the midfoot: This is a rotation of the bones on the inside of the arch at the midfoot so that in walking, the arch rolls inward to the floor.	The left foot has a pronated midfoot; the right foot is normal.
Abduction of the forefoot: The front of the foot is turned outward from the midline of the body to an abnormal degree.	The forefoot on the left is abducted; the forefoot on the right is typical.

Table 2.7.2 Pes varus

COMPONENT	ILLUSTRATION
Varus hindfoot: The heel is turned inward, toward the midline of the body, to an abnormal degree.	The left foot has a varus hindfoot; the right foot is normal.
Supination of the midfoot: There is a rotation of the bones, creating a higher arch that results in distributing weight primarily on the outer side of the foot in walking.	The left foot is supinated; the right foot is normal.
Adduction of the forefoot: The front of the foot is turned toward the midline of the body to an abnormal degree.	The forefoot on the left is adducted; the forefoot on the right is typical.

You may also come across the terms "equinovalgus" and "equino-varus." Equinovalgus or equinovarus includes the features of pes valgus or pes varus, but a tightness in the calf muscle may cause a pull on the heel to raise it off the ground. The midfoot and forefoot remain on the ground when standing or walking. However, at their most extreme, these conditions cause the individual to walk on their forefoot.

v) Upper limb problems

Muscles also affect the growth of bones in the upper limb. Examples of upper limb problems include:

- Forearm pronation: Spasticity in forearm pronator muscles may lead to the radius and ulna (long bones of the forearm) developing a twist along the length of the bones, resulting in forearm pronation (internal rotation of the forearm that results in the hand moving from the palm-up to the palm-down position).
- Wrist flexion: Spasticity in wrist flexor muscles may lead to wrist flexion (movement of the palm of the hand toward the inside of the forearm).

See Figure 2.7.6.

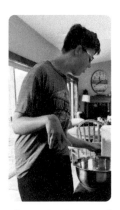 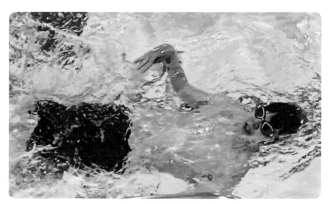

Figure 2.7.6 Upper limb posture in individual with right-side hemiplegia.

b) Scoliosis

Scoliosis is a three-dimensional rotation and curvature of the spine. When viewed from the back, the spine of a person with scoliosis is a C- or S-shaped curve instead of a straight line. See Figure 2.7.7.

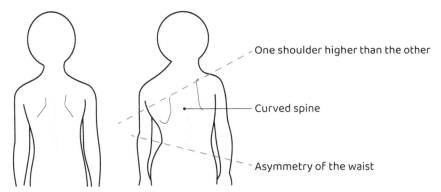

Figure 2.7.7 A typical spine (left) and a spine with scoliosis (right, showing a C-shaped curve). Note that one shoulder is higher than the other and there is asymmetry at the waist.

The angle of the scoliosis curve, the Cobb angle (also referred to as the curve magnitude) is measured on an X-ray image. The Cobb angle is the angle between the two most tilted vertebrae[*] at the upper and lower ends of a spinal curve (see Figure 2.7.8). A diagnosis of scoliosis is made when the Cobb angle is 10 degrees or greater. The Cobb angle is also used to monitor scoliosis progression and to guide treatment recommendations.

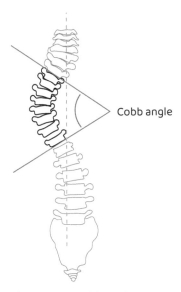

Figure 2.7.8 Cobb angle measurement.

---

[*] The spine consists of vertebrae (the plural of vertebra) and intervertebral discs. Vertebrae are bony structures with a hole in the middle for the spinal cord to pass through.

The prevalence and severity of scoliosis in individuals with CP increases with GMFCS level.[136,137] The prevalence of scoliosis was found to be:[137]

- 14 percent for GMFCS level I
- 15 percent for GMFCS level II

However, for those with CP GMFCS levels I and II, most scoliosis curves are small, mostly nonprogressive, and with minimal or no symptoms.[137]

c) Leg length discrepancy

Leg length discrepancy is where one leg (the involved leg) is shorter than the other. This is usually treated when the difference in length is greater than 2.5 cm (1 inch).[138]

d) Bone health

Bone is a living tissue that is constantly being created, removed, and replaced. The term "osteoporosis" means "porous bones" (i.e., bones with low bone density*). Low bone density arises when either insufficient new bone is created or the rate of absorption of bone is greater than the rate of formation.

As people age, more bone is naturally lost than replaced. People with osteoporosis, however, have greater bone loss than is normal for their age. Figure 2.7.9 shows a normal bone and one with osteoporosis; the latter has much less bone material (i.e., less bone density).

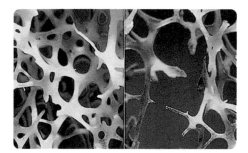

Figure 2.7.9 Cross-section of normal (left) and osteoporotic bone (right). Reproduced from Wikipedia user Gtirouflet, used under a Creative Commons license.

---

* The terms "bone density" and "bone mineral density" are used interchangeably.

Bones can become so weak that a break (fracture) may occur with stress (such as a fall). A break may even occur spontaneously. Osteoporosis is a "silent" disease in that it is often diagnosed only when a bone fracture occurs. It is the most common cause of bone fractures among elderly people.

"Osteopenia" is the term used to define bone density that is not normal but not as low as in osteoporosis.[139] It can be regarded as the midpoint between healthy bone and osteoporosis. Having osteopenia places a person at risk of developing osteoporosis.

Bone health is determined by measuring bone mineral density (BMD) with a Z-score, which represents the number of standard deviations* an individual's bone density differs from the average for their age and sex. The cutoff for low bone density is a Z-score of -2.0. A study of BMD levels in children with CP (all subtypes) found evidence of low BMD for those at GMFCS level II but not GMFCS level I.[140] When data for 22 children with hemiplegia was analyzed, the mean BMD Z-scores for the femur was significantly lower for the affected limb compared to the unaffected one. The study also found that approximately two-thirds of the children (all CP subtypes and all GMFCS levels) had insufficient vitamin D, which is important for calcium metabolism in the body and for bone development.[140]

As kids with CP get older, they are more affected by the issues that arise, and the most frustrating part is we will never know the effect CP ultimately has on them. I remember Ally as a tiny baby with no tone issues, and while we're very lucky her CP is mild and she is not badly affected, she does still experience spasticity in her leg. Her physiotherapist recently commented that it's also becoming more apparent in her right arm. Stretching is really important, and I can see the benefits of encouraging your child to be active and do as much exercise as they can comfortably tolerate. As Ally gets older, it has become easier for more fun and natural stretches to happen. She has done a significant variety of stretch-inducing activities over the years through gymnastics, reformer

---

* The extent to which a point differs from the mean or average.

Pilates, and swimming, and at home we encourage any type of stretching including hanging from the door!

CP also impacts long-bone growth due to spasticity caused by tight muscles, which needs to be managed to avoid impaired growth and bone/muscle problems (again, a significant incentive to do the physio). For Ally, this has manifested in one leg being shorter than the other, and she has to have various lifts in her shoes or AFOs depending on what she is wearing. Leg length discrepancy, if untreated, can be very damaging and can affect the hips and pelvis, in particular. Ally, now at age 12, is due to have surgery in the coming months, which will hopefully equalize her limb lengths and avoid lifelong complications.

Epiphysiodesis is a surgical procedure on the physeal growth plate that slows the growth of the lower limb long bone on the unaffected side. It is important for people to know that this surgery is time sensitive. In Ally's case, she has had a series of X-rays of both legs and of the left elbow and hand, which informed the surgeon of the bone age and allowed them to predict the leg length discrepancy that will be present at end of growth.

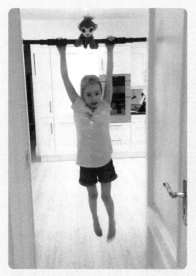
Ally stretching at home.

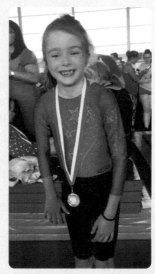
Ally at gymnastics.

Tertiary problems

> Our greatest glory is not in never falling,
> but in rising every time we fall.
> **Confucius**

The tertiary problems in hemiplegia are the coping responses or compensations that arise due to the individual's need to deal with or get around the primary and secondary problems.[99] Following are some examples of tertiary problems that may arise on the affected side in hemiplegia:

- **Nonuse of the affected arm:** Using the mouth, legs, or any other body part or environmental support to complete a bilateral (two-handed) task, or avoiding bilateral tasks altogether. This may also be termed "developmental disregard."
- **Pelvic obliquity:** One hip being higher than the other when viewed from the front. This may be the result of the individual being up on the toes of the affected limb (asymmetric equinus). The asymmetry at the feet causes the hips to be at different levels. A difference in leg lengths is another cause.

- **Truncal sway (also referred to as trunk sway):** A side-to-side swaying of the trunk in walking, generally a compensation for hip abductor weakness on the affected side.
- **Retracted pelvis:** Walking with the pelvis on the affected side rotated back (retracted) and rotated forward on the unaffected side (protracted).
- **Vaulting:** Rising up on the toes during stance on the unaffected side in order to help clear the affected leg during swing. The term "vault" means "jump" or "leap over." Vaulting is a common compensation and can be mistaken as a primary or secondary problem.

To correct the tertiary problems, the root cause (i.e., the primary and secondary problems), not the compensation, needs to be addressed. In the case of truncal sway, for example, addressing hip abductor weakness on the affected side may reduce the sway.

While compensations are often the most visually apparent features of CP, they do not require treatment; these compensations—the tertiary problems—may be reduced or eliminated when the underlying cause is treated and they are no longer required.[*99]

---

* It is worth noting that these compensations are general gait compensations that may be found in other disabilities, not just CP.

Motor function in individuals with spastic hemiplegia

> I get up. I walk. I fall down.
> Meanwhile I keep dancing.
> **Daniel Hillel**

The combination of the primary, secondary, and tertiary problems affects overall function in hemiplegia. That is, how a person with hemiplegia uses their involved upper limb and how they walk results from a combination of the neurological problems present from birth (the primary problems), the muscle and bone problems that develop with growth (the secondary problems), and any coping responses that they develop as a result (the tertiary problems).

Upper limb use

We saw in section 2.1 that children with hemiplegia have a high level of gross motor function—almost all (93 percent) are functioning at GMFCS levels I and II,[43–46,75–78] which is why the focus of this book is on those two levels. Children with hemiplegia have more problems with fine motor function; as noted in section 2.1, 84 percent were functioning at MACS levels I and II while 12 percent were functioning at level III.[46,76,78]

In a study of 45 children with hemiplegia across all GMFCS levels, Hidecker and colleagues found only a moderate correlation between GMFCS and MACS.[46] Therefore, although a child may be GMFCS levels I or II, they may be functioning at a lower level on the MACS.

Problems with fine motor control in individuals with hemiplegia means that functional everyday tasks are more difficult to perform, such as dressing (e.g., buttoning a shirt, zipping up a jacket), toileting, feeding (e.g., holding silverware, cutting food), carrying a tray, getting soap from a dispenser, turning the pages of a book, and typing (a very important skill as technology advances). Many of these tasks involve grasp, pinch, and release.[141]

House and colleagues developed a nine-level classification system to describe the functional use of the upper limb.[142] See Table 2.9.1.

Table 2.9.1 House upper limb functional use scale[142]

LEVEL	CATEGORY	DESCRIPTION
0	Does not use	Does not use
1	Poor passive assist	Uses as stabilizing weight only
2	Fair passive assist	Can hold object placed in hand
3	Good passive assist	Can hold object and stabilize it for use by other hand
4	Poor active assist	Can actively grasp object and hold it weakly
5	Fair active assist	Can actively grasp object and stabilize it well
6	Good active assist	Can actively grasp object and manipulate it
7	Spontaneous use, partial	Can perform bimanual activities and occasionally uses the hand spontaneously
8	Spontaneous use, complete	Uses hand completely independently without reference to the other hand

This scale is a useful communication tool for families and medical professionals. Going about our ordinary life, we may not be tuned into different levels of functioning of the upper limb. There is no treatment available that will fully restore the involved upper limb in hemiplegia to full and normal function. However, if treatment improves function by even a few levels, it can greatly assist in the activities of daily living that involve the two hands (e.g., unscrewing the lid on a jar, carrying multiple objects) and improve the appearance of the limb, which is important to many individuals.

Another tool to measure upper limb function is the Functional Independence Measure of Children (WeeFIM), commonly used to assess functional daily living activities in children[143] in the areas of eating, grooming, bathing, dressing, and toileting.

Table 2.9.2 shows the scores from a study that measured self-care among children (mean age 11) with hemiplegia and diplegia GMFCS levels I and II.[144] Higher scores indicate greater independence. The table shows that children with hemiplegia had more problems with self-care than did children with diplegia. Children with hemiplegia with greater mobility problems (GMFCS level II) had more problems with self-care than those with better mobility (GMFCS level I).[144]

Table 2.9.2 WeeFIM self-care scores for children with hemiplegia and diplegia

HEMIPLEGIA GMFCS LEVEL I	HEMIPLEGIA GMFCS LEVEL II	DIPLEGIA GMFCS LEVEL I	DIPLEGIA GMFCS LEVEL II
91	79	94	89

When Ally was 11, her teacher suggested to us that Ally should transition to using a computer at school. She noticed that Ally tires as the requirement for writing increases, and this fatigue had been increasing over the past few years.

We had previously resisted this suggestion to use a computer because we didn't want Ally to be seen or treated differently. However, when I discussed her teacher's recommendation with her, she was delighted. She saw the opportunity to get a computer for school as a big help.

This is a reminder to me that we do need to listen and be guided by our kids, especially as they get older, and not always make assumptions about what they are thinking.

Walking

The manner in which a person with hemiplegia walks results from a combination of the neurological problems present from birth (the primary problems), the muscle and bone problems that develop with growth (the secondary problems), and any coping responses that develop as a result (the tertiary problems).

In a typically developing child, once mature walking has developed by around three and a half years of age,[97] their manner of walking changes little. The development of mature walking takes longer in children with CP and is dependent on GMFCS level. The gait of a person with spastic hemiplegia may also change over time as growth occurs and more atypical muscle and bone problems accumulate.

Winters and colleagues developed a four-group classification system for the sagittal gait patterns in individuals with spastic hemiplegia, which is still in use today.[145] They are termed "sagittal gait patterns" because they are best observed when looking at a person from the side. These patterns build on each other, impacting more muscle groups.

It is important to identify each individual's walking patterns as the management, interventions, and treatments used are very different. Group I is the least affected and group IV is the most affected. (Note that groups I to IV should not be confused with GMFCS levels.) Table 2.9.3 explains each of these gait patterns.

Table 2.9.3 Gait patterns in spastic hemiplegia.[145]

GAIT PATTERN	IMAGE*	EXPLANATION
Group I **Drop foot**		Those in group I have problems at ankle level during both stance and swing. Drop foot is characterized by weakness or inability to lift the foot during the swing phase of gait. This is the mildest gait pattern and affects only the ankle of the involved leg and only during swing.
Group II **True equinus** **This gait pattern is the most common in spastic hemiplegia**		Those in group II have problems at ankle level. True equinus is when the individual stands and walks on their toes (equinus) of the involved leg due to the limited ROM at the ankle joint. Within this gait type, there are two subcategories: • IIA—equinus (toe walking) with a typical knee and extended hip. • IIB—equinus (toe walking) with hyperextension of knee and hip. Beginning with group II, the involved leg may not grow as long as the uninvolved leg, which may lead to limb-length discrepancy. Foot malalignments may be present— equinovarus or equinovalgus (see section 2.7).

Cont'd.

GAIT PATTERN	IMAGE*	EXPLANATION
Group III **Equinus/jump knee**		Those in group III have problems at ankle and knee levels. Crouch gait is defined as persistent flexed-knee gait. The exact degree of knee flexion that constitutes crouch gait varies in the literature but is typically greater than or equal to 20 degrees. The term "jump knee" comes from the fact that the person appears to be jumping with each step, as if they are trying to clear an obstacle on the ground.
Group IV **Equinus/ jump knee/ hip flexed, adducted and internally rotated**		Those in group IV have problems at ankle, knee, and hip levels. In addition to problems of group III above, there is also a lack of extension at the hip. Importantly, hip problems are also associated with excessive adduction and internal rotation of the hip.

* In the images the three small circles represent the hip, knee, and ankle joints. The triangle represents the hip.
Images reproduced with kind permission from the Cerebral Palsy Foundation.

A video explaining different gait patterns is included in **Useful web resources**.

We saw in section 2.5 that energy conservation is one of the five attributes of typical walking. Walking with spastic hemiplegia is less energy efficient than typical walking. Think of energy expenditure during walking like the fuel efficiency of a car. A more efficient car will consume less fuel while traveling a set distance. People can generate energy at a finite rate. A person with spastic hemiplegia, with their energy-inefficient gait, travels a shorter distance for a given amount of energy or gets tired more easily when they have to walk a set distance. This has important consequences for activity and participation.

Can the child or adolescent keep up with their peers in terms of speed or the distance they cover? Do they frequently feel fatigued and need to rest? All the factors that cause the increased energy expenditure of walking for all children with CP are not yet fully understood.

Three-dimensional (3D) computerized motion analysis is a very important tool for understanding the gait deviations that arise in spastic hemiplegia and for planning treatment, and is addressed in Chapter 3. Two children with spastic hemiplegia may walk similarly, but the mechanisms behind their walking may differ, and 3D computerized motion analysis helps understand each child's gait and the problems contributing to it.

It's important to keep in mind that kids with CP work two to three times harder than other kids to accomplish the same tasks and therefore use significantly more energy than their peers. I recommend employing little tricks to help when you are traveling or doing errands; for example, bringing a trunkie (ride-on suitcase) or folding scooter to the airport, or parking closer to a venue so your child won't get tired walking. These small accommodations can make the experience easier for them.

It's also important that you accept the disability to ensure they enjoy the event; sometimes treating them like another child may mean they are exhausted before the event even starts.

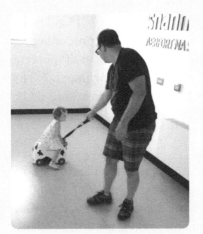

Ally being pulled through the airport on a trunkie.

Associated problems

Create the highest, grandest vision possible for your life, because you become what you believe.

Oprah Winfrey

We have addressed the neuromusculoskeletal issues that arise in spastic hemiplegia and their effects on motor function. In section 2.1, we saw that a minority of children with spastic hemiplegia (all GMFCS levels) have problems in the areas of speech, intelligence (cognition), epilepsy, vision, and hearing of varying severity. However, more than 90 percent of children have none or only one severe associated problem.[79] The prevalence and severity of associated problems have been found to be greater in children at higher GMFCS levels compared with those at lower GMFCS levels.[79]

This section looks at associated problems that children and adolescents with spastic hemiplegia may have. These problems are important to consider because for some individuals with spastic hemiplegia, they may reduce their well-being far more than any of their motor problems.

- **Speech, language, communication, and feeding:** Approximately two in five children with spastic hemiplegia have some level of speech challenge.[79] Due to the motor, sensory, and cognitive problems caused by the brain injury, children may have difficulties with:

  o Oral motor movements* that affect speech production, including imprecise articulation† and slowed speech production
  o Respiratory strength or control affecting voice or speech loudness
  o Manipulation of food and swallowing

  These problems, if present, are typically mild. Associated conditions such as hearing problems and seizures can further impact speech and swallowing skills.

- **Sensory problems:** "Sensory" refers to the senses that include vision, hearing, taste, smell, and touch. "Sensation" can be defined as the physical feeling or perception arising from something that happens to or that comes in contact with the body. "Decreased sensation" means a reduction in the ability to perceive sensory stimuli. "Tactile problems" are ones related to the sense of touch. Sensory input gives us much information about the outside world, which we then incorporate into learning and actions. For instance, if we feel the heat from sitting too close to a fire, we learn to move to a comfortable distance away. Similarly, if we feel that we have sticky fingers from having had ice cream drip on them, the sensation reminds us to wash our hands. These are examples of how a sensation allows us to take information from the world, incorporate it into our learning, and finally to choose an action in response to that sensation. When sensation is diminished, the information from the environment is therefore diminished, and the opportunity for using that information for learning and for subsequent action is diminished.

  Feedback from the hand's sensation is integral to hand action and use. The injury to the brain in hemiplegia affects the sensory input from the affected hand and this greatly affects the development of the affected hand's use. Individuals with hemiplegia may be able to

---

* These relate to the muscles and structures involved in speech and other oral (mouth related) tasks; for example, chewing and swallowing.

† Production of clear and distinct sounds.

identify sensory deficits since only one side of the body is primarily involved; they may notice a difference between the two sides of their body. The use of the affected hand may be limited, at least in part because of weakness and decreased sensation. Then, because of the limited use, it may cause further weakness and decreased sensation. This creates a chain of circumstances that can reduce hand function.

Sensory problems can also include the inability to sense where a limb is in space (**proprioception**), and the inability to identify an object by feeling it (**stereognosis**).

Proprioception testing can be carried out with a finger proprioception test. The individual, without looking, is asked to indicate whether a specific finger (e.g., the index finger) is pointed upwards or downwards. This test evaluates the individual's ability to sense where their finger is in space.

Stereognosis testing can be carried out by asking an individual to perform a tactile object recognition (TOR) test.[146] Common objects (e.g., key, pencil, coin, spoon) are placed in the hand of the individual or they are asked to pick them up. The person's eyes are closed or the objects are hidden from them. They are asked to identify each object by feel. See Figure 2.10.1.

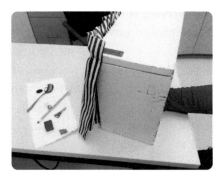

Figure 2.10.1 Stereognosis testing.

Van Heest and colleagues found that in children with spastic hemiplegia, 97 percent had problems with stereognosis and 46 percent with proprioception in the involved hand.[146] They also noted that children with severe stereognosis problems had significantly smaller limbs than those with mild or moderate.[146]

Sensory challenges can also include **cold extremities**. This can affect hands and feet, and for many it can be independent of ambient temperature. Fifty-six percent of ambulatory (able to walk) children with CP (all subtypes) reported cold extremities.[147] In some individuals, temperature changes can be associated with color changes of the hand and arm.

Approximately one in four children with spastic hemiplegia has some level of **vision** challenge.[79] Strabismus, where the eyes do not look in the same direction at the same time, is more common among individuals with CP than in the typical population.[148] (Strabismus is often referred to as having crossed eyes or a squint.)

Approximately 1 in 10 children with spastic hemiplegia has some level of **hearing** challenge.[79]

- **Epilepsy:** Approximately one in four children with spastic hemiplegia has epilepsy.[79] Epilepsy can be diagnosed if an individual experiences at least two unprovoked seizures (not stemming from any identifiable cause such as illness or fever) occurring more than 24 hours apart. A seizure is "uncontrolled, abnormal electrical activity of the brain that may cause changes in the level of consciousness, behavior, memory, or feelings."[149]

- **Pain:** Pain has been extensively reported in individuals with CP. Forty-eight percent of ambulatory children with CP (all subtypes) reported pain.[147] Common causes in children with CP include hip displacement, muscle spasms, procedures, headaches, neuropathic pain,[*] and visceral pain.[†][150] Pain in childhood *or* adolescence has been strongly associated with low quality of life.[151,152]

- **Urinary dysfunction:** Urinary dysfunction includes problems such as late-achieving continence (being toilet trained) and involuntary nighttime urination (bed-wetting).[153] However, urinary dysfunction is uncommon in children with spastic hemiplegia.[90]

---

[*] A type of chronic pain caused by damage to the nervous system. It can be experienced as a burning, or stabbing sensation unrelated to any external stimulus.

[†] A type of pain in the internal organs. It can be experienced as a dull, aching, or cramp-like pain and is difficult to precisely locate.

- **Constipation:** Twenty-two percent of ambulatory children with CP (all subtypes) reported constipation.[147]

- **Sleep:** Sleep problems have been reported in 36 percent of ambulatory children with CP (all subtypes).[147] They include delayed insomnia, disrupted sleep, early awakening, or a combination. Suggested causes include difficulty to relax and calm down or presence of spasticity, anxiety, epilepsy, and pain.[147]

- **Cognition:** Approximately one in three children with spastic hemiplegia has some level of cognitive challenge.[79] Children may have difficulties related to processing, comprehension, learning, attention, expressive language, memory, organization, and problem-solving. To help identify and better understand specific cognitive or behavioral challenges, individuals with CP may be referred for neuropsychological evaluation.* This testing is valuable in identifying individual strengths and needs associated with coordinated brain functioning, assisting with securing additional resources and interventions as needed, and following progress over time or changes after interventions.

- **Sexual relationships:** Young adults with CP (49 percent unilateral, 87 percent GMFCS levels I to II, 18 to 22 years, average intelligence) had less experience in romantic and sexual relationships than their age-matched peers.[154] In addition, young adults with CP (49 percent unilateral, 84 percent GMFCS levels I to II, 20 to 24 years, average intelligence) experienced various problems or challenges with sexual relationships, including inability to achieve orgasm (20 percent), physical problems with sex† related to CP (80 percent), and emotional inhibition to initiate sexual contact (45 percent). Many have reported wanting information, including the impact of CP on sexual function and fertility.[155]

---

* Neuropsychology is a specialty that focuses on understanding brain functioning as it relates to cognition and behavior. Neuropsychological testing helps evaluate broad areas of cognitive function; for example, intelligence, language, visuospatial function, executive function, attention, memory, and processing speed. These areas frequently work in collaboration for efficient cognitive functioning.

† Includes spasticity, difficulty positioning, stiffness of joints and muscles, and fatigue.

- **Quality of life:** Quality of life (QOL) is defined as "the individual's perception of their position in life in the context of the culture and value system in which they live, and in relation to their goals, expectations, standards, and concerns."[156] A large European QOL study of 500 children with CP (44 percent unilateral spastic, 68 percent GMFCS levels I to II) age 8 to 12, who could self-report, found they have similar QOL to their peers.[151] A follow-up study of 431 adolescents with CP (all subtypes) age 13 to 17 found that they had significantly lower QOL than the general population in only 1 of the 10 domains measured—social support and peers,[152] and that adolescents with CP need help to maintain and develop peer relationships.[152]

  Looking at the severity of impairments for children with CP:[151]

  o Children with poorer walking ability had poorer *physical well-being.*
  o Those with intellectual impairment had lower *moods and emotions* and less *autonomy.*
  o Those with speech difficulty had poorer *relationships with their parents.*

  Among adolescents with CP, severity of impairment was significantly associated with reduced QOL for moods and emotions, autonomy, and social support and peers.[152] Pain in childhood or adolescence was also strongly associated with low QOL.[151,152]

- **Mental and behavioral health:** Mental health has been defined as "a state of mental well-being that enables people to cope with the stresses of life, realize their abilities, learn well and work well, and contribute to their community."[157] While mental and behavioral health are closely related, they are different. Mental health has more to do with thoughts and emotions. Behavioral health has more to do with how people react in a situation—two people in the same situation may react in very different ways. Both mental and behavioral health strongly contribute to QOL.

  The QOL study noted above observed no differences between children and adolescents with CP and peers in psychological well-being and moods and emotions (aspects of mental health). However, a number of studies have reported a higher level of mental and behavioral health symptoms and disorders among children and adolescents with CP.[158,159,160,161,162]

- ○ A 1996 UK study of a large sample of children with spastic hemiplegia age 2 to 16 found a high level of psychiatric problems* reported by parents and teachers (54 percent and 42 percent respectively).[158] When a large subset of the children was individually assessed, over half (61 percent) were found to have psychiatric problems, which was higher than the typical population (15 percent). The most common were conduct, emotional (anxiety and fears), and hyperactivity problems. These problems went untreated in the majority of individuals.[158]
- ○ A 2018 review of studies concluded that mental health symptoms are common in children and adolescents with CP. Those with an intellectual disability had a higher risk of mental health symptoms.[159]
- ○ A 2020 Danish study reported that the prevalence of mental health disorders was significantly higher in children and adolescents with CP (all subtypes) (22 percent) compared with peers (6 percent).[160]
- ○ Children and adolescents with CP (subtype not reported) experienced bullying and social exclusion at school and that this affects mental health.[161]
- ○ Adolescents and young adults with spastic hemiplegia had lower self-esteem than peers and upper extremity differences correlated more strongly with lower self-esteem than lower extremity differences.[162]

Noritz and colleagues suggested that the higher prevalence of mental and behavioral health problems in children and adolescents with CP may be due to the underlying brain injury, pain and physical difficulties, and limitations with participation.[163] It is important that problems with mental and behavioral health be addressed.

---

* Psychiatry is the branch of medicine that diagnoses and treats mental health problems. Mental health is a more inclusive term that encompasses a range of problems, including those that may not necessarily be diagnosed or treated within a psychiatric setting. Sometimes, however, the two terms ("mental health" and "psychiatric problems") are used interchangeably.

Key points Chapter 2

- Spastic hemiplegia affects the upper and lower limbs of one side of the body. The upper limb is usually more affected than the lower limb.
- Studies show that children with hemiplegia have a high level of gross motor function—93 percent were functioning at GMFCS levels I and II. They have more problems with fine motor ability; however, 84 percent were functioning at MACS levels I and II.
- Spasticity is the most common type of atypical tone present in individuals with hemiplegia, although dystonia can be present as well.
- Spastic hemiplegia is caused by injury mostly, but not exclusively, to the cerebrum on one side of the brain—the parts of the brain that control voluntary movement and receive and process sensory information for the opposite side of the body.
- There are two types of brain injury commonly associated with hemiplegia: periventricular leukomalacia (PVL) and lesions following middle cerebral artery stroke.
- A minority of children with hemiplegia (all GMFCS levels) have problems of varying severity in the areas of speech, intelligence (cognition), epilepsy, vision, and hearing. However, more than 90 percent of children have none or only one severe associated problem. These and other associated problems may reduce well-being far more than motor problems.
- A useful framework for classifying the musculoskeletal problems that occur in children with spastic CP categorizes them into primary, secondary, and tertiary problems. Primary problems are caused by the brain injury and are therefore present from when the brain injury occurred. Secondary problems develop over time in the growing child. They are problems of atypical muscle growth and bone development and are referred to as "growth problems." Tertiary problems are the "coping responses" that arise to compensate for or counteract the primary and secondary problems.
- A nine-level classification system describes the functional use of the involved upper limb, and a four-group classification system describes the gait patterns in individuals with spastic hemiplegia.

Chapter 3

Management and treatment of spastic hemiplegia to age 20

Section 3.1 Introduction 143

Section 3.2 What does best practice look like? 145

Section 3.3 Overall management philosophy 153

Section 3.4 Therapies 158

Section 3.5 The home program 181

Section 3.6 Assistive technology 196

Section 3.7 Tone reduction 218

Section 3.8 Orthopedic surgery 229

Section 3.9 Managing associated problems 243

Section 3.10 Alternative and complementary treatments 248

Section 3.11 Community integration, education, independence, and transition 251

Key points Chapter 3 266

Introduction

Knowing is not enough; we must apply.
Willing is not enough; we must do.
Johann Wolfgang von Goethe

The difference between management and treatment is subtle. "Management" is the broader term, taking into account all aspects of an individual's life, whereas "treatment" refers to the use of a specific intervention; for example, physical therapy, orthoses, or orthopedic surgery. The terms "treatment" and "intervention" are largely interchangeable.

Rosenbaum and colleagues summed up the distinction as follows:[164]

Management implies looking at the child's day from a 24-hour perspective and ensuring that all aspects of their life are being given appropriate attention and intervention, hence the need to integrate therapy into the total management package and to appreciate the contribution of the many team members. We provide treatment to achieve management in order to enhance function and life quality.

The overall goal of management is to help the individual with hemiplegia reach their true potential—to promote their self-confidence and independence to the greatest possible extent. This is no different from the goal parents have for any of their children. However, when it comes to the young person with hemiplegia, the family and professionals must work hard to ensure the condition does not hold them back from achieving their potential. Reflecting the International Classification of Functioning, Disability and Health (ICF) model addressed in section 1.8, the aim of management is to promote optimal participation in daily life by enhancing activities and minimizing problems with body functions and structure. At the same time, environmental and personal factors are also considered.

This chapter examines what good management and treatment look like. It addresses management and treatment to age 20, and Chapter 4 then addresses hemiplegia in adulthood. This age cutoff is appropriate for a couple of reasons:

- Growth is an important factor in hemiplegia. As we saw in the growth charts in Chapter 2, growth is generally complete by age 20.
- Around age 18 to 20, health services in most countries transition from pediatric to adult. Sadly, health services for adults with CP are generally much less developed than those for children.

USEFUL WEB RESOURCES

What does best practice look like?

Medicine is a science of uncertainty
and an art of probability
Sir William Osler

It is important to understand what best practice in the medical care of individuals with hemiplegia looks like. This section provides an overview of the generally accepted principles underpinning best practice in the management and treatment of hemiplegia at the time of writing. Best practice is likely to continue to evolve over time. It currently includes:

- Family-centered care and person-centered care
- A multidisciplinary team approach
- Evidence-based medicine and shared decision-making
- Data-driven decision-making
- The importance of specialist centers
- Early intervention
- Setting goals
- Using measurement tools and measuring outcome

Family-centered care and person-centered care

When a child is diagnosed with hemiplegia, the whole family is affected: parents, siblings, and extended family members. Family-centered care is a way of ensuring that care is planned around the whole family, not just the child with the condition.* It can be thought of as a meeting of experts who pool their knowledge to jointly develop the most appropriate plan of care for the child. The parent is the expert on their child, while the professional is the expert on the condition and its treatment. Professionals who practice family-centered care see themselves not as the sole authority but as a partner with the parent in the provision of care for the child.

Family-centered care and person-centered care are closely related. The latter evolves from the former as the child grows. In person-centered care, the individual is an active participant and decision-maker in their own medical care. A few points on person-centered care:

- Person-centered care involves the professional engaging the child from an early stage in conversations. A study of factors that predict whether a child will answer questions during primary care pediatric visits found that if a doctor simply looks at a very young child when they ask a question, that child is more likely to engage in the medical process.[166]
- Person-centered care promotes the opposite of "learned helplessness," the belief that nothing one chooses to do can affect what is happening.[167] Learned helplessness can be regarded as a secondary disability.
- One study found that having learned how to take personal responsibility for personal health during childhood was significantly associated with regular physical activity in adults with CP.[168]

---

* Family-centered care is also termed "family-centered service." CanChild defines family-centered care as being "made up of a set of values, attitudes, and approaches to services for children with special needs and their families. Family-centred service recognizes that **each family is unique**; that the family is the **constant in the child's life**; and that they are the **experts on the child's abilities and needs**. The family works with service providers to make informed decisions about the services and supports the child and family receive. In family-centred service, the strengths and needs of all family members are considered."[165]

The change from family-centered care to person-centered care is gradual, and parents and medical professionals can help facilitate the shift over time.

A multidisciplinary team approach

A multidisciplinary team approach means the individual is being treated by medical professionals from several disciplines working together as a team, although each stays within their own professional boundaries. Optimal treatment for individuals with CP may include physical therapy (PT); occupational therapy (OT); speech and language pathology (SLP), also termed "speech and language therapy" (SLT); nursing; orthotics; pediatrics; neurology; neurosurgery; orthopedic surgery; physical medicine and rehabilitation (PM&R), also termed "physiatry"; and more.*

A more detailed explanation of the role of the team members is included in *Cerebral Palsy Road Map: What to Expect as Your Child Grows*[169] (included in **Useful web resources**).

Evidence-based medicine and shared decision-making

Evidence-based medicine (or evidence-based practice) is "the conscientious, explicit, and judicious use of current best evidence in making decisions about the care of individual patients."[170] It combines the best available external clinical evidence from research with the clinical expertise of the professional.[170] Family priorities and preferences are also considered.[171] Since clinical expertise can vary, it is important to know that recommendations made in this book may be different at other hospitals and treatment centers.

---

* The role of PT, OT, and SLP is explained in section 3.4. **Orthotics** is concerned with the design, manufacture, and management of orthoses), devices designed to hold specific body parts in position to modify their structure and/or function. **Pediatrics** deals with children and their medical conditions. **Neurology** deals with disorders of the nervous system. **Neurosurgery** involves surgical management of disorders of the nervous system. **Orthopedic surgery** involves surgical management of disorders affecting the musculoskeletal system: the muscles, bones, joints, and their related structures. **PM&R** aims to enhance and restore functional ability and quality of life among those with physical disabilities.

Best practice management of CP is by a multidisciplinary team that is skilled in this condition and that engages with the family in a shared decision-making model. Shared decision-making is a process in which the family is actively involved in making the medical decisions. It incorporates the principles of evidence-based medicine.[172]

Unfortunately, though evidence-based practice is the goal, several authors in the field of CP have noted that there is a long way to go to achieve it.[173,174] The translation of research into clinical practice can be slow: this applies to all medical fields, not just CP. It has been found that it takes an average of 17 years for research evidence to reach clinical practice.[175] For example, the GMFCS was first published in 1997, but a 2015 published survey of 283 pediatric physical therapists found that fewer than half used the GMFCS consistently,[176] and a 2018 study found that fewer than half of 303 caregivers knew their child's GMFCS level.[177]

Implementation science is an emerging field of health care science that focuses on bridging the gap between research and its effective implementation in clinical practice. Factors that influence successful implementation include organizational behavior, clinician behavior, and patient preferences. An example is the successful implementation of the guideline for early detection of CP across a network of five US high-risk infant follow-up programs.[24] Another is the development and rollout of COVID-19 vaccines.

Funding for CP research is low, which makes the choice of research conducted very important. A 2018 US initiative to set a person-centered research agenda for CP involved a collaboration among all stakeholders—including caregivers and people with CP—based on the belief that a research agenda developed collaboratively would be more useful to the entire community than one developed by professionals alone. It was built around the concept of "nothing about us without us."[*178]

---

* Sixteen top research priorities were identified. Leading themes included the comparative effectiveness of interventions, physical activity, and understanding aging. It also highlighted the need to focus on longitudinal research that includes outcomes related to participation and quality of life.

Data-driven decision-making

Best practice demands decision-making be data-driven. (This can also be called "data-informed decision-making.") For example, in orthopedic surgical decision-making in CP (e.g., for lower limb single-event multi-level surgery, or SEMLS, addressed in section 3.8), data is drawn from multiple sources, including:

- The individual's history
- Functional outcome measures and self-reported outcome measures
- Physical examination
- Imaging
- Gait analysis*
- Examination under anesthesia

The skilled evaluation of multiple sources of data is essential for good decision-making.

The importance of specialist centers

Specialist centers, also known as centers of excellence, are on the rise in many areas of medicine across the developed world. Consider, for example, specialist centers for breast cancer. Research has shown that outcomes in breast cancer treatment improve with the number of breast cancer cases a particular center has treated (this is known as centralization).[179] The annual number of operations per center and per surgeon (specialization) is also important, and the multidisciplinary team is of paramount importance.[179]

A specialist center for the treatment of individuals with CP:

- Has a multidisciplinary team that includes the specialties described earlier
- Treats a high volume of patients with CP on a routine or daily basis
- Provides the full range of evidence-based treatment options, allowing the most suitable ones to be chosen for each child

---

* A measurement tool used to evaluate gait. Within gait analysis, multiple variables are evaluated using different measurement tools (see section 3.8).

- Conducts research and publishes in peer-reviewed journals
- Ideally, offers a lifetime of care; CP is not just a "children's condition"

Early intervention

Early intervention is essential in the management of CP. Early intervention is usually from birth to age three in the US[180] and may continue beyond that age elsewhere. We have already seen that:

- Early diagnosis is necessary for early intervention.
- Early intervention offers the best opportunity to tap into neuroplasticity.
- Early intervention is important for minimizing the secondary problems as the child grows. Remember, growth is most vigorous in the first three years of life.

Though the emphasis with intervention is on early implementation, intervention continues to be required during childhood, adolescence, and adulthood.

Setting goals

Treatment goals should be collaboratively agreed upon by the child, parent, and professional as part of family-centered care and shared decision-making. The achievement of goals should be evaluated after treatment. One widely used goal-directed system used in rehabilitation is known as SMART, a system applied in many industries in areas like project management and employee performance. It is also used in personal development.

The SMART system goals are designed to be Specific, Measurable, Achievable, Relevant, and Time-bound:[181]

- **Specific** and **Measurable:** Goals that are specific and measurable should contain five elements:
  - Who
  - Will do what
  - Under what conditions

- ○ How well
- ○ By when
- **Achievable:** Goals should match the child's prognosis and be attainable.
- **Relevant:** Goals should hold meaning for the child and family. Goals should be functional; that is, not solely based on impairment (problems with body functions and structure).
- **Time-bound:** Goals must have a specific date for achievement.[*]

The following are some examples of SMART goals:

- Adeline will reciprocally creep 30 feet independently in order to move between rooms of her home within three months.
- Maris will use her helper hand to hold the paper while coloring with her dominant hand within three weeks.
- Sarah will use a step-through pattern on stairs (rather than a compensatory step pattern)[†] within her home within six weeks.
- William will zip up his coat independently within one month.
- Sydney will place a coin in the toy piggy bank with her affected hand within three weeks.
- Henrik will produce the "s" phoneme (sound) at the beginning of the word at a sentence level with 85 percent accuracy within one month.

Research has shown that:

- Therapies that focus on achieving functional goals in everyday life result in measurable improvements in gross motor skills compared to therapies that are not goal-directed.[182]
- The development of fewer and more meaningful goals is imperative for adherence, improved outcomes, and greater individual and family satisfaction.[183]
- Children can be trusted to identify their own goals, thereby influencing their involvement in their own treatment programs. If the child creates their own goal, they will likely be more motivated to achieve it. Children's self-identified goals were found to be as

---

[*] Typically, a goal would include a specific date for achievement, rather than the less specific "within three months."

[†] A step-through pattern on stairs involves alternating placing one foot on the next step; a compensatory step pattern involves placing both feet on the same step before one foot proceeds to the next step.

achievable as parent-identified goals and remained stable over time (i.e., achievements were maintained).[184]

- A family-centered approach to intervention has been shown to improve motivation and outcome.[185]

A number of tools are available to incorporate family goals. Some of the more common ones are the Canadian Occupational Performance Measure (COPM),[186] the Goal Attainment Scale,[187] and the Gait Outcomes Assessment List (GOAL).[188,189,190,191]

Using measurement tools and measuring outcome

Many variables can be measured, including height, grip strength, walking speed, and upper limb functional use. Some variables can be measured using equipment, others by parent or self-report (e.g., by completing a questionnaire). A tape measure, dynamometer, timed walk test, and the House upper limb functional use scale (see Table 2.9.1) are all examples of measurement tools used to measure these variables. A measurement can be taken at any point in time to establish a person's status at that point in time.

An outcome is defined as a result or an effect; thus, "measuring outcome" means measuring a result or an effect. If a person's walking speed is measured before a treatment, such as orthopedic surgery, and then again afterward, the effect or result—the outcome—of the surgery on the person's walking speed can be evaluated.

Variables used to measure outcome can be classified as technical, functional, or by patient/parent satisfaction. For example, lower limb orthopedic surgery is commonly evaluated using many technical variables (joint ROM, gait deviations, energy consumed in walking) as well as functional variables (gross motor function, walking ability). Each variable provides different but complementary information. Variables can be measured in each domain of the ICF (body functions and structure, activity, and participation). A range of variables covering different domains of the ICF provides the most comprehensive evaluation of outcome. Appendix 1 (online) includes more information on measurement tools.

Overall management philosophy

When there is no turning back,
then we should concern ourselves only
with the best way of going forward.
Paulo Coelho

In the journey to adulthood, reflecting the ICF model, the overall goal is to promote optimal participation in daily life by enhancing activities and minimizing problems with body functions and structure. The definition of CP describes it first as a disorder of the development of movement and posture, causing activity limitation that is often accompanied by disturbances of sensation, perception, cognition, communication, and behavior, by epilepsy, and by secondary musculoskeletal problems.[2] While a lot of attention is given to development of movement and posture and secondary musculoskeletal problems, for some individuals with hemiplegia, difficulties with communication or learning may pose bigger barriers to participation. In section 2.1, we saw that children with hemiplegia:

- Have a high level of gross motor function—almost all (93 percent) functioning at GMFCS levels I and II
- Have some problems with fine motor ability; however, 84 percent still function at MACS levels I and II

We saw that across all GMFCS levels, many children age five with hemiplegia had some level of problem with speech (40 percent), hearing (8 percent), vision (26 percent), intellectual status (33 percent), and epilepsy (22 percent).[79] Problems with, for example, speech, language, and cognition, if present, may be more challenging for the individual with hemiplegia than their upper or lower limb functional limitations.

The following are some pointers in the overall management of hemiplegia in childhood and adolescence:

- CP-specific early interventions are designed to:[21]
  - Optimize motor, cognition, and communication skills using interventions that promote learning and neuroplasticity
  - Prevent secondary impairments and minimize complications that worsen function or interfere with learning (e.g., monitor hips, control epilepsy, take care of sleeping, feeding)
  - Promote parent or caregiver coping and mental health
- Morgan and colleagues published an International Clinical Practice Guideline for early intervention for children age 0 to 2 with or at high risk of CP.[30] They followed this with another guideline in 2023 for children in the first year of life, which helps decide what kind of motor intervention to choose from based on the motor problem.[34] Earlier, Novak and colleagues summarized the state of the evidence as of 2019 for interventions for children with CP. They used a traffic light system:[14]
  - Green means go because high-quality evidence indicates the effectiveness of that intervention.
  - Red means stop because high-quality evidence indicates the ineffectiveness or harm from that intervention.
  - Yellow means measure clinical outcome (i.e., measure the effect of the intervention on the individual) because the evidence either does not exist or is yet unclear on the benefit of the intervention.

The above guidelines help therapists support families, and links to them are included in **Useful web resources.**

- Early treatment of speech and language delays has many benefits. Improving the child's ability to communicate is not only important for the child's language development, but also for their social-emotional development and ongoing learning ability.
- Naturally, a child with hemiplegia tends to favor using their unaffected hand because it functions so well. Both constraint-induced movement therapy (CIMT) and bimanual therapy are recommended to encourage and promote the use of the affected upper limb. CIMT involves restraint of the unaffected hand combined with intensive structured therapy. The restraint may be soft, such as a mitten. The child then participates in games and activities that require use of their affected hand. Bimanual therapy consists of games and activities designed to improve the child's ability to use both arms and hands together.
- As children reach school age, hand function is increasingly necessary for schoolwork and is supported with therapy services to facilitate school participation.
- Primary, secondary, and tertiary problems are addressed in sections 2.6. to 2.8. Other than high tone and to a limited extent weakness, the primary problems (the neurological problems) are difficult to treat. The secondary problems (the growth problems) can often be treated, and treatment for the tertiary problems (coping responses or compensations) is generally not necessary.
- Monitoring musculoskeletal development is a constant throughout childhood and adolescence. It includes, for example, physical examination, X-rays, and gait analysis.
- Treatment of musculoskeletal concerns in hemiplegia generally begins at diagnosis with physical and occupational therapies. Over time, orthoses and casting may be added, and tone reduction* may be considered as well. Different treatments, when used together, can amplify the effect of individual treatments; for example, attending therapies to achieve a new functional goal following botulinum neurotoxin A (BoNT-A) injections.† The saying, "The whole is greater than the sum of its parts" applies.

---

* An **orthosis** (also termed "brace" or "splint") is a device designed to hold specific body parts in position in order to modify their structure and/or function. **Casting** consists of applying a plaster of paris or a fiberglass cast; for example, a below-knee cast to stretch the tight gastrocnemius and/or soleus muscles (calf muscles) to hold the muscle in a position of maximum stretch. **Tone reduction** is addressed in detail in section 3.7.

† BoNT-A is a tone-reducing medication that is injected directly into the muscle.

- Hip surveillance and spine surveillance are structured approaches to monitoring the development of the hips and spine respectively in individuals with CP and should start early in life:
  - The risk of hip displacement for children with hemiplegia at GMFCS level I is the same as typically developing children with one important exception—children who have hip involvement (Winters group IV, see section 2.9) have a substantial risk.
  - The risk of hip displacement for children with hemiplegia at GMFCS level II is 15 percent.[128,129]
  - The AACPDM (American Academy for Cerebral Palsy and Developmental Medicine) has developed a care pathway to monitor hip development in children and adolescents with CP (included in **Useful web resources**). It includes recommendations for the timing of clinical examination and X-rays. This also includes special considerations for Winters group IV because of their higher risk.
  - Formal hip surveillance programs for children and adolescents with CP have been implemented in a number of countries, including Australia and Sweden.[3,192]
  - Unlike hip surveillance, no formal guidelines exist for spine surveillance at this time. However, we saw in Chapter 2 that for individuals at GMFCS levels I and II, scoliosis curves (Cobb angle greater than 10 degrees) are uncommon, generally small, mostly nonprogressive, and with minimal or no symptoms.[137] However, Willoughby and colleagues recommend that small curves be monitored.[137] Management of scoliosis for individuals with hemiplegia is included in Appendix 2 (online).
- Despite best efforts, and for the reasons described in Chapter 2, the development of some muscle and bone problems is largely inevitable in individuals with hemiplegia. Depending on the degree to which they impact function and participation, orthopedic surgery may be recommended. Single-event multilevel surgery (SEMLS)—a single operation to address all muscle and bone problems at once—is often used. An intensive period of rehabilitation can help achieve a higher level of function following surgery. Orthopedic surgery is addressed in section 3.8.
  - SEMLS is more frequently required for the lower rather than the upper limb. Unpublished data from Gillette Children's indicate that approximately 45 percent of children with hemiplegia require lower limb SEMLS while 20 percent require upper limb

SEMLS. If SEMLS is required for both, they may be carried out at the same time or separately. SEMLS for the lower limb is best carried out between the ages of 6 and 12.[193] For the upper limb, soft tissue surgeries are best carried out between the ages of 7 and 10.[194]

- o SEMLS does not alter the primary problems of CP, and a gradual recurrence of some muscle and bone problems may occur in a small proportion of individuals post-SEMLS.

- Overall, minimizing the amount of orthopedic surgery needed remains an important goal. Because growth is a major factor in musculoskeletal care, once growth ceases at around age 20, a certain stabilization of the condition occurs. No treatment should ever be viewed as an end point. All treatments are aids in the pursuit of the overall goal of getting to skeletal maturity (i.e., adulthood) with the fewest possible problems.

- It is also worth noting that no treatment (with today's treatments) will give full function to the affected limbs. However, with the upper limb for example, if treatment improves function by even a few levels on the House upper limb functional use scale, the affected upper limb can greatly assist in the activities of daily living that involve the two hands.

Finally, the home program (addressed in section 3.5) is a constant in the life of the child and adolescent with hemiplegia.

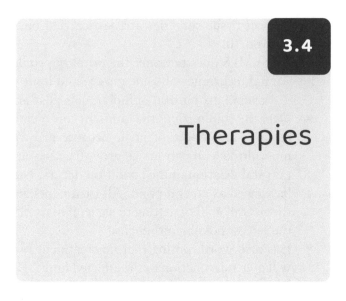

Therapies

The nice thing about teamwork is that
you always have others on your side.
Margaret Carty

Many children with hemiplegia attend physical therapy, occupational therapy, and/or speech and language pathology at various points during their development. Therapy is defined by Rosenbaum and colleagues as:

> *A process of helping a family (and a child) to learn ways for a child to function optimally in their many environments. It ... involves using the therapist's expertise to explore ways that will enable the child and the family to live as fully and functionally as possible.*[164]

Obviously, this definition extends to the adolescent and adult with CP as well. Improvement in function should be the primary goal of therapy.

This section covers:

- **Physical therapy**
- **Occupational therapy**
- **Speech and language pathology***
- **Delivery of therapy services**
- **Getting the most out of appointments**

From the day Ally was diagnosed, the importance of physiotherapy and early intervention was stressed to me over and over. I strongly encourage all parents to engage with the services offered and do all the exercises and stretches at home. Ally began intensive physiotherapy with public services when she was released from hospital and with private services at 10 months following her diagnosis. She was assigned an amazing physiotherapist at our local CP support center when she left the hospital. On the day of Ally's diagnosis with her pediatrician, this physio drove to our house to explain cerebral palsy and the implications, which was an act of caring that I will not forget. It is the unselfishness of people like this that stay with you forever and make this challenging journey so much easier. Ally has been very fortunate to meet many "superstars" along the way, from the NICU nurse who came in on the weekend to ensure I was producing breast milk to her current fabulous physiotherapist who gets into the pool with her most Friday mornings to make the therapy fun!

Physical therapy

Physical therapists provide services that develop, maintain, and restore a person's maximum movement and functional ability.[195] Physical therapists have different titles in different countries: in many countries they

---

* There are other types of therapy offered by specialists: for example, play therapists, music therapists, and recreational therapists. A recreational therapist is qualified to provide recreational therapy services in the US and Canada. There may be an equivalent professional in other countries.

are called physiotherapists. In this book, we use the terms "physical therapist" and "physical therapy."*

Services that pediatric physical therapists provide for children and adolescents with CP may include:[171]

- Developmental activities
- Movement and mobility
- Strengthening
- Motor learning
- Balance and coordination
- Recreation, play, and leisure
- Daily care activities and routines
- Equipment design, making, and fitting
- Tone management
- Assistive technology (including orthoses)
- Posture, positioning, and lifting

Physical therapists work as part of the multidisciplinary team taking care of the child or adolescent.

Though physical therapists may select treatments designed to improve functional activities, the treatments themselves are often not strictly functional activities. For example, a child's goal may be to be able to get up from the floor without holding on to anything for support. During the evaluation, the physical therapist may identify limited ankle range of motion (ROM) and weak hip and knee extensors on the affected side as the underlying problems preventing the child from meeting their goal. As a result, the physical therapist might include casting (to address the limited ROM) and isolated strengthening exercises (to address the weak extensors) on the affected side in the plan of care for that child with hemiplegia. These treatments address the underlying problems, but they themselves are not functional activities. However, as the underlying problems are reduced, the treatment will shift to *task-specific functional activities*. In this example, the child begins to practice moving from the floor to standing.

---

* In Ireland, the terms "physical therapist" and "physiotherapist" are not interchangeable. There, a "physical therapist" is someone trained specifically in the manual treatment of soft tissues, mostly massage.

Another example is if the child's PT goal is to walk more independently, then the therapy might primarily involve walking and the many activities that form the building blocks for walking.

Thus, treatments are often task-specific functional activities. Research supports task-specific training (green light) for improved gross motor function.[14]

We now address some elements of physical therapy (PT) in more detail.

a) Strengthening

Lack of muscle strength is one of the primary problems, but muscle strength is further affected by the development of the secondary problems (abnormal muscle growth and bone development). We saw in Chapter 2 that muscle strength was reduced in children with hemiplegia.[111,112] Historically, strengthening was frowned upon because it was thought to increase spasticity. However, it now is known to increase the force-producing capability, not the spasticity, of the muscle,[196] and therefore strengthening is recommended.

The physical therapist can determine which strengthening exercises are appropriate for the child at their developmental stage. Muscles can be strengthened in different positions. Strengthening may be functional, like moving into sitting from standing, or from standing to sitting, or stair climbing.

In addition to doing focused muscle strengthening exercises, strengthening has to be built into normal life. For the small child, a variety of positions can provide an opportunity to strengthen the muscles during play. Often, those same positions can be used to achieve both stretch and strength. Strength training targets the more involved side, which can be challenging due to compensatory movements (e.g., the child succeeds in completing the activity without symmetrical use of the limbs). The need for strengthening also applies to the older child and adolescent.

Research supports strength training for improved lower limb strength (green light) and upper limb strength (yellow light).[14]

b) Functional mobility and gait training

Physical therapists specialize in movement, and a significant amount of PT is focused on practicing functional mobility. The physical therapist selects specific mobility activities or tasks based on the individual's age, function, as well as the family's goals.

For very young children, physical therapists emphasize practicing developmental activities such as rolling, creeping, and crawling. Later, they may emphasize moving from one position to another such as moving in and out of standing positions or moving with support (e.g., cruising—when the child walks alongside a sofa while holding on for support). Depending on the child's function and environmental demands, physical therapists may teach children to use different movements[*] or recommend the use of orthoses or mobility aids[†] to maximize the child's independence.

For older children, adolescents, and adults, functional mobility includes how a person moves in and out of bed, transfers (stands up and sits down or moves from chair to chair) and moves around in their environment (walking or using a wheelchair).

Another area of focus is gait training, an intervention to work on developing or improving walking skills. As with other aspects of functional mobility, physical therapists may recommend the use of orthoses or mobility aids to maximize the child's independence. Physical therapists (in collaboration with the multidisciplinary team) are a great source of guidance on mobility aids and orthoses to use in daily life.

Gait training is often a progression. It may initially require more assistance and more-supportive mobility aids, but progress to less assistance and less-supportive mobility aids. Physical therapists (in collaboration with other members of the multidisciplinary team) are a great source

---

[*] For example, nonreciprocal rather than reciprocal crawling. Reciprocal crawling involves coordinated movements of opposite hands and knees to move forward; nonreciprocal crawling refers to any form of movement (e.g., using a single hand to drag themselves forward without coordinating both sides of the body).

[†] Mobility aids (also termed "assistive mobility devices," "assistive devices," "walking aids," and "gait aids") vary in the level of support they provide. Some are used in therapy to help the child who is newly learning to walk. For the most part, however, people with hemiplegia, GMFCS levels I and II, walk without mobility aids. A scooter and wheelchair are examples of mobility aids used in hemiplegia for longer distances.

of guidance on mobility aids and orthoses to use in daily life. Gait may progress to increasing distance walked (endurance for walking) and walking in more challenging environments. In addition, following surgery or based on environmental demands (e.g., moving between classes in a busy high school hallway), may necessitate temporary or periodic use of a posterior walker for balance and safety. Or on a large college campus, a wheelchair or scooter may be necessary so as not to fatigue the student moving between classes—if the individual is spending a great deal of their energy on walking a long distance to get from class to class, they may be fatigued compared with their peers when they arrive to learn. More-supportive mobility aids or orthoses might be recommended to reduce fatigue, pain, and/or falls, which speaks to the competing goals: there is a balance to be struck between independent walking and intermittently using mobility aids and orthoses to allow the person to participate more fully in everyday life.

Specific gait training interventions used during therapy may include treadmill training, body weight support treadmill training, and various forms of assisted and even robotic training. Using a treadmill can be helpful to focus on increased speed or symmetry. Harnesses can be used to provide body weight support or for safety when walking on the floor or treadmill. Lower limb robotics is a growing aspect of CP therapy.[197] For example, robotic-assisted training may involve using an exoskeleton* to provide some assistance to move the legs while walking. The emphasis during these interventions is on practicing a high number of repetitions or steps, providing the opportunity to learn from errors, decreasing support, and getting practice in a variety of environments.

With hemiplegia, particular attention needs to be paid to more weight-bearing on the weaker lower limb and to symmetrical walking. This can help prevent overuse syndrome and osteoarthritis† in the long term.

Research supports treadmill training for improved walking speed, endurance, and gross motor function (green light) and improved weight-bearing (yellow light).[14]

---

* A wearable robotic device designed to help with walking by providing external support to the wearer's lower limbs.

† The breakdown of cartilage in the joints.

c) Electrical stimulation

Neuromuscular electrical stimulation (NMES), also simply termed "electrical stimulation" (ES), is a treatment (and not a task-specific functional activity) that involves the electrical stimulation of nerves to produce a muscle contraction. Functional electrical stimulation (FES), a subtype of NMES, involves electrical stimulation that produces a contraction to obtain a functionally useful movement. Electrodes are placed on the muscle and a device transmits the electrical current through a wired or wireless connection.

Electrical stimulation is usually used in combination with functional activities and for muscle strengthening. It may also be used during gait training (e.g., to stimulate the ankle dorsiflexor during swing phase).

An FES orthotic to correct for footdrop in the swing phase of gait may be useful (see Figure 3.6.1). Here, the physical therapist will work with an orthotist. The utility of an FES orthotic, however, may be limited by the individual's tolerance of the stimulation. In addition, the device does not work very well for footdrop where there is very high tone in the plantar flexors. The person's ankle ROM must also be sufficient to use an FES orthotic.

Research supports electrical stimulation for improved walking and strength (yellow light).[14]

d) Stretching

Stretching is not a task-specific functional activity, but it is still important in hemiplegia; it helps to improve or maintain joint ROM and alignment.

The physical therapist can provide guidance, but stretching must be built into the activities of normal life. We saw in Chapter 2 that two to four hours of stretching per day is required for normal muscle growth, and the typically developing child gets this amount of stretch during the day when they get up and start to move about, run, and play using a normal movement pattern. We also saw that lack of muscle growth leads to contractures in people with hemiplegia.

Stretching is required throughout growth for the young child, the older child, and the adolescent with hemiplegia. How this stretching is achieved may vary over the years, but the need for it remains constant. There are also critical periods when stretching is especially important during the periods of most rapid growth: the first three years and the adolescent growth spurt.

Though we refer to stretching muscles, what is actually being stretched is the muscle, the tendon, and all the tissues that surround them called the muscle-tendon unit (MTU) and the associated joint. Muscles responsible for the movements (left columns of Tables 2.4.1 and 2.4.2) are in particular need of stretching because they are affected by spasticity. It is worth becoming familiar with these.

The methods used for stretching depend on a number of factors, including level of spasticity, muscle tightness, age, and developmental stage.

Traditionally, stretching was done by performing slow *passive* stretching* of spastic muscles. However, due to weak evidence supporting the efficacy of passive stretching, greater emphasis is now placed on other, active methods of achieving muscle stretch.[198] Novak and colleagues concur that passive stretching in isolation appears to be ineffective and do not recommend it since effective substitutes exist.[14] While passive stretching is sometimes still needed, it should not be the only method used.

The following describes different methods of stretching (any number of which may be used simultaneously).

i) Positioning

A variety of positions can be used throughout the day to achieve sustained muscle stretching to promote muscle growth. It is important that the child or adolescent get a variety of positions throughout the day and not spend too much time in one. They may have favorite positions, but it is important to vary them. For the small child, moving between positions may require parental support.

---

* When another person stretches an individual's muscle.

"W-sitting" is the term used to describe the sitting position in which the child's bottom is on the floor while their legs are out to each side. Looking from the top, the legs form a "W" shape. (See Figure 3.4.1.) Children with hemiplegia like W-sitting because it is a stable position, requires less balance, and leaves the hands free for play. The problem with W-sitting is that it may cause a loss of hip external rotation, which interrupts the typical process of bone remodeling. The child also misses out on functional opportunities to develop balance reactions. While W-sitting was traditionally not recommended, it is now thought to be somewhat acceptable provided the child gets plenty of time in other positions to balance out the less ideal elements of W-sitting.

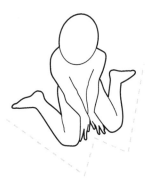

Figure 3.4.1 Child W-sitting.

For older children and adolescents with hemiplegia, it is also very important to not spend prolonged time in one position, usually sitting—a particular challenge given the not uncommon overuse of electronic devices.

Appendix 3 (online) includes information on various positions, including long sitting, side sitting, tailor sitting, prone positioning, and standing. It is important to look for a lot of opportunities during the day to incorporate different positioning—for example, while playing, reading, watching TV, or using electronic devices.

ii) Orthoses
An orthosis (also termed "brace" or "splint") is a device designed to hold specific body parts in position in order to modify their structure and/or function. One of the goals of orthoses is to achieve muscle stretch for a longer duration.

Night splints, such as ankle-foot orthoses (AFOs), which cover the ankle joint and foot, plus knee immobilizers,[*] may also be used to achieve stretching at night. Wearing an AFO plus a knee immobilizer on the affected leg allows stretching of the calf muscles (both the one-joint soleus and the two-joint gastrocnemius; see Table 2.4.2). Night splints are worn to tolerance during sleep. Orthoses are discussed in section 3.6.

iii) Casting

Casting consists of applying a plaster of paris or a fiberglass cast; for example, a below-knee cast to stretch the tight gastrocnemius and/or soleus muscles (calf muscles) to hold the muscle in a position of maximum stretch. Fiberglass casts are lighter and allow weight-bearing. Serial casting is the application, removal, and reapplication of stretching casts (e.g., weekly, for several weeks, typically three to six weeks) to gain ROM with each subsequent casting until the desired ROM is achieved.

iv) Active movement

Active movement is exactly what it sounds like. The child or adolescent needs to get plenty of active movement through the entire ROM of the joints. They can remove orthoses if they are hindering doing a task and replace them during downtime for a prolonged muscle stretch. This gives them a combination of active movement that may not be in the "best" position, and static stretch in the ideal position.

The approach used in physical therapy and many of the treatments are also used in occupational therapy, addressed next.

> I am very conscious of enabling Ally rather than disabling her, but there have been times when I got it wrong. Ally is extremely independent, but she does have a tendency to get other people to do things for her that she doesn't like doing. Her friend, Neasa, can often be seen tying Ally's zip or putting on her AFO. I think we need to find the balance between making things easier for Ally while encouraging independence.

---

[*] A knee immobilizer consists of a soft knee wrap, rigid aluminum struts, and straps to adjust the fit. As the name suggests, it prevents the knee from moving.

Occupational therapy

Occupational therapists use everyday activities (occupations) to promote health, well-being, and independence throughout an individual's life.[199] They work with children and adolescents to build confidence and independence through:

- Completing meaningful tasks to maximize independent movement, strength, and coordination
- Compensating or modifying activities or the environment to enable successful task completion
- Recommending or providing equipment (e.g., orthoses, wheelchairs, bathing equipment) and/or technology that can increase independence when performing activities

Basically, the above are in priority order: 1) try to build or remediate skill, 2) compensate or modify task to meet the individual's skill, 3) use equipment to support function.

Areas covered in occupational therapy (OT) include, but are not limited to:

- Daily living skills such as dressing, feeding, grooming, and bathing
- Fine motor skills such as writing, using scissors, and manipulating toys
- Cognitive skills such as sticking to a schedule, learning to play a new game, and following step-by-step directions
- Visual motor skills and visual perceptual skills such as using eye movement to explore and interact with the environment
- Participation in the day-to-day activities that motivate the person, such as play, sport, crafts, and vocational skills

Some occupational therapists—certified hand therapists—also specialize in upper limb involvement.

Occupational therapists can be especially important as the child grows, when daily activities and independent living skills become more demanding and potentially more difficult to complete. Below are some areas an occupational therapist may address with individuals who have hemiplegia.

a) Stretching and strengthening

As with physical therapy, occupational therapy also contains elements of stretching and strengthening. These may be included to directly help with an occupational therapy activity. (See the section on physical therapy above for more details on stretching and strengthening.)

b) Orthoses

Occupational therapists play a large role in assessing and identifying appropriate orthoses to enhance participation in activities of daily living (ADLs). Orthoses are discussed in more detail in section 3.6.

c) Constraint-induced movement therapy and bimanual therapy

Using both hands reflects everyday typical hand function. Constraint-induced movement therapy (CIMT) and bimanual therapy (performed with both hands) are two therapy types that encourage the use of the affected arm or hand. Naturally, an individual with hemiplegia tends to favor using their unaffected hand because it functions so well. CIMT and bimanual therapy can help maintain ROM, prevent learned disuse, and increase awareness of the presence and functionality of the affected arm and hand. Both interventions require a high level of parent and child education and engagement as practicing skills at home when not in structured therapy will optimize gains of either intervention.

CIMT involves two main components used in combination: restraint of the unaffected hand and intensive structured therapy. The restraint may be a soft restraint such as a mitten (on the unaffected hand). In an older child, a cast on the unaffected arm and hand may be used to enable longer periods of treatment. The child then participates in games and activities that require use of their affected hand.

Bimanual therapy consists of games and activities designed to improve the child's ability to use both arms or hands together (without any restraint placed on the unaffected hand). It involves a high level of repetition. This therapy helps translate to the child using their affected upper limb in everyday tasks such as carrying a lunch tray at school.

CIMT and bimanual therapy tap into the brain's neuroplasticity. There is strong evidence supporting both (green light).[14] It is recommended that CIMT and/or bimanual therapy begin as soon as a diagnosis of hemiplegia is suspected.[30] Each of these therapies has different functions so one should not be chosen over the other; it is good to do both in sequence.

d) Robot-assisted therapy

Robot-assisted therapy involves using a robotic device to support the arm in movement and task completion (see Figure 3.4.2). Research supports its use.[200]

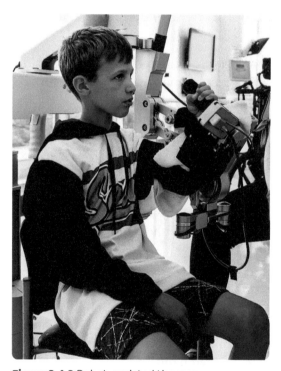

Figure 3.4.2 Robot-assisted therapy.

Table 3.4.1 shows appropriate ages for different upper limb therapies, although each of these therapies remains relevant throughout life.

Table 3.4.1 Appropriate ages for upper limb therapies

THERAPY	APPROPRIATE AGES
CIMT	3 months to 18 years
Bimanual therapy	Infancy through adolescence
Robot-assisted therapy	4 years plus; depends on size of child as there is a minimum size needed to engage with most devices

e) Activities of daily living

Occupational therapy to enhance an individual's ability to perform or assist with activities of daily living (ADLs) is goal based, and for individuals with hemiplegia, ADLs focus on performing tasks independently such as dressing, grooming, feeding, bathing, and toileting. The therapy is informed by the individual's motor abilities, cognitive abilities, and impairments. For example, occupational therapists often screen for vision impairments and use these screening results to plan ongoing treatment and adapt activities appropriately, taking into consideration how vision impairment may impact actions such as hand use. Specific ADLs focused on during occupational therapy also change depending on age:

- Young children—focus is on activities that feel like play, encouraging the child to engage and participate.
- Middle childhood to adolescence—focus is on increased engagement in family responsibilities, organized activities, and socialization such as completing weekly chores (e.g., setting the table, taking out trash) and participating in sports and recreational opportunities to begin building skills and capacity for independence in adulthood.
- Adolescence to young adult—focus is on building skills for living independently and managing adult tasks such as scheduling appointments or managing money.

Occupational therapists can also make recommendations for adaptive equipment for completing ADLs, addressed in more detail in section 3.6.

f) Building autonomy

An important part of occupational therapy is building autonomy—maximizing the capacity for the individual to be independent. Goals for independence are set based on functional and cognitive abilities. For individuals with hemiplegia, these goals may center on the ability to live independently and complete necessary home management tasks such as cooking, cleaning, and grocery shopping. They may also include skills such as money management and medication management.

When Ally was one, I met someone who recommended the book *The Brain that Changes Itself*, by Norman Doidge. It focuses on the concept of neuroplasticity, which is the ability of the brain to change its activity in response to intrinsic or extrinsic stimuli by reorganizing its structure, functions, or connections after brain injuries such as CP. The most important chapter for me was on the work completed by Edward Taub, a behavioral neuroscientist who developed a family of techniques—constraint-induced movement therapy—that has been shown to be effective in improving the rehabilitation of movement after stroke, traumatic brain injury, and CP in young children. In simple terms, it involves using the weak limb and constraining the stronger limb (in the case of CP) in order to send new messages and build new pathways in the brain.

This made sense to me scientifically and practically as there is a great body of evidence supporting the theory of neuroplasticity, and so I began a journey of finding a way to apply the technique with Ally. I started reading and researching this area to assess what was available in Ireland. At home, I began the process by putting a sock over Ally's stronger hand to prevent her from using it and simultaneously encouraging her to use her weaker hand to pick up and knock down building blocks and other items of interest to her. I can never measure the effectiveness of this intervention, but I am very confident that it *was*, in some way, effective and definitely did not cause any harm.

When Ally was two, we reached out to the neurological department of Virginia Tech in Virginia. They were running a clinical trial on the benefits of constraint-induced movement therapy for children with hemiplegic CP. We liked the content of the program and felt it was well worth taking part in the trial as we knew the importance of early intervention. We enrolled Ally in the clinical trial, and off we went with her on the first of many trips to the US for treatment.

The program included a complete assessment of Ally's condition, followed by establishing a baseline prior to one month of intensive constraint therapy with highly experienced occupational and physical therapists every weekday. A specific removable cast was made for her left (good) arm, and she had daily play therapy to build up the movement and strength in her right hand. Prior to this therapy, Ally used her right hand infrequently; thanks to the sessions, she learned a certain amount of movements that were not there previously.

This trip reignited all my feelings of guilt, and I was inconsolable for the first couple of days when I had to leave Ally with the physiotherapists. It got easier when I realized the effort they were making to ensure therapy was fun. They incorporated a substantial toolkit of games and activities that fully engaged Ally, and we could notice a bond forming between her and her therapists.

One of the therapists described the program as teaching Ally to think out the movements of her right hand as she was not subconsciously able to do it. It was described as a bit like driving a digger, where she had to be shown how the controls work and then learn how to drive it.

Again, it is difficult to measure the long-term, exact impact of this therapy, but certainly Ally was capable of doing so much more after the intervention with many more gross and fine motor skills.

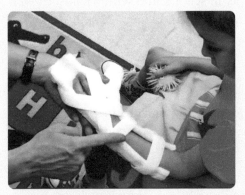

Ally with her removable cast on her strong hand.

Speech and language pathology

Speech and language pathology (SLP) is also known as speech and language therapy (SLT). Speech-language pathologists/therapists work with children, young people, and adults to support speech, language, and communication needs as well as feeding and swallowing difficulties. The following are explanations of terms:

- **Speech** refers to saying sounds accurately and in the right places in words. Speech is a motor task.
- **Language** refers to the words and symbols we use, and how we use them for communication. Language is a cognitive task.[*]
  - ○ **Receptive language** refers to understanding information from sounds, words, symbols, signs, gestures, and/or movements.
  - ○ **Expressive language** refers to the ability to communicate thoughts, wants, needs, and/or feelings through words, gestures, signs, and/or symbols.
- **Communication** occurs when a sender transmits a message, and a receiver understands the message. Communication includes speech, gestures, behaviors, eye gaze, facial expressions, and augmentative and alternative communication (AAC).[62]

Speech-language pathologists assess speech, language, and cognitive skills to determine how to improve communication. The child and adolescent may receive SLP at school, in an outpatient clinic, or both. Just as there is overlap between PT and OT, there is overlap between OT and SLP. The speech-language pathologist will work with parents, teachers, and others to identify strategies that encourage and improve the child's communication at home, in school, and with friends, as well as during activities to help develop speech and language skills.

SLP may be done individually or in a group. The following are areas of focus:

- **Language skills** allow a child to communicate in their environment, which encourages the development of cognitive skills. A speech-language pathologist will work on cognitive development

---

[*] Cognition is the mental action of acquiring knowledge and understanding through thought, experience, and the senses.

by improving language comprehension; building vocabulary; and teaching how to use words, gestures, and pictures to express thoughts, ideas, and feelings, and to know how to answer questions. Language comprehension is needed to be able to follow directions, understand the meaning of words, and understand how words go together.

- **Expressive language** allows a person to ask for what they want and need, to comment or provide information, to ask questions or ask for clarification if they don't understand, to request attention when needed, and to express feelings.
- **Oral motor skills** improve secretion management (drooling, aspiration of secretions*), which helps improve the ability to move and break down food in preparation for swallowing and for speech production.
- **Speech production** includes being able to say individual sounds accurately, with correct placement of the lips, tongue, and mouth shape, paired with adequate breath support and control of the breath stream. It also includes making the vocal folds (voice box) vibrate for some sounds and not for others. Speech production also can include sequencing of these sounds to make words, and sequencing of more than one word to make a sentence that is understood by others.
- **Social communication** includes how to take turns; how to partner with others to exchange ideas, thoughts, and jokes; and how to greet others. Social communication often impacts a person's ability to make and maintain friendships.
- **Cognitive-communication skills** include memory, attention, problem-solving, and organization. Attention to the environment, to the communication and language of others, and to what is happening in the environment is very important for cognitive development. Executive function includes many cognitive-communication skills that help the individual plan and get things done.
- **Fostering independence** helps the individual advocate for and communicate their wants and needs, as well as their feelings. It helps them develop autonomy and self-agency.

---

* Drooling is excess saliva dropping uncontrollably from the mouth. Aspiration is food or liquid entering the airway or lungs instead of the esophagus.

Delivery of therapy services

Given that the delivery of therapy services is so variable, only some broad points are addressed here. Having a lifelong condition such as hemiplegia does not mean a person will need lifelong, nonstop PT (or other therapies) or, as it is sometimes referred to, the "once a week for life" model.

Guidelines have been developed for determining the frequency of PT and OT services in a pediatric medical setting.[201] The guidelines are based on:

- The child's ability to benefit from and participate in therapy
- The parent's ability to participate in therapy sessions and follow through with activities at home
- The family's decision related to available resources (e.g., time commitment, financial resources)

Four levels of frequency of therapy are identified in the guidelines:[201]

- **Intensive:** More than three times per week—for children who are in an extremely critical period for acquiring a skill or are regressing.
- **Weekly/bimonthly:** One to two times a week to every other week—for children who need frequent therapy and are making continuous progress toward their goals.
- **Periodic:** Once a month or less—best suited to children whose rates of progress are very slow but who require the skilled services of a therapist to periodically assess a home program and adapt it.
- **Consultative:** As needed—best suited for children who have been discharged from therapy but who benefit from intermittent evaluation by a therapist.

The episodes of care (EOC) model is used for service delivery. An EOC is a period of therapy at the recommended frequency, such as listed above, followed by a therapy break. Ideally, after an EOC, the child generalizes the skills gained in therapy at home, in school, and in the community. For each EOC, the family and therapist work together to draw up goals, typically no more than two long-term and four short-term goals. Note that referring to "therapy breaks" might sound like getting therapy is the normal state of affairs for a person with CP, but living life, not receiving therapy, should be considered the normal state of affairs.

Figure 3.4.3 shows periods when different therapies may be used, interspersed with breaks in therapy, during childhood and adolescence.[202]

In addition to having formal goals, it is very important that therapists use objective measurement tools to evaluate whether therapy goals have been met. The home program, which includes practicing what the child has learned in therapy at home and incorporating it into normal life, is addressed in section 3.5.

The following are included in **Useful web resources**:

- Cincinnati Children's *Guidelines for Determining Frequency of Therapy* information leaflet for families
- Gillette Children's *Rehabilitation Therapies Episodes of Care in Childhood and Adolescence* information leaflet for families.

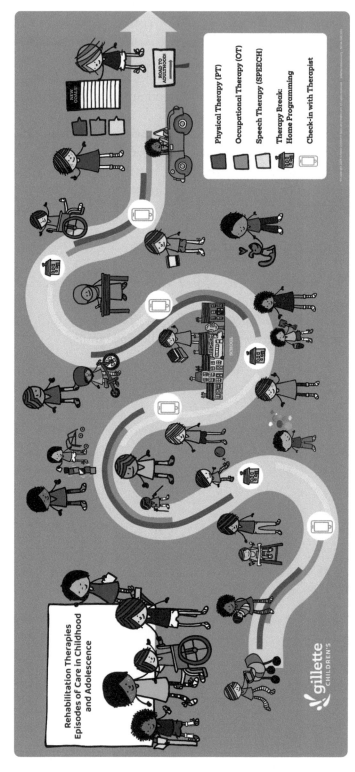

Figure 3.4.3 Episodes of care in childhood and adolescence.[202]

Getting the most out of appointments

Life with a diagnosis of hemiplegia involves many appointments, particularly in the early years. During the COVID pandemic, virtual appointments became a feature of health care delivery, and a mixture of in-person and virtual care delivery has remained in place since.

Try to ensure you are getting as much as possible from these appointments. It is useful to go with a written list of questions and to take notes after each appointment, including what you learned and what is needed to be done next. While portals to access personal medical records (where they exist) have helped reduce the need for taking notes, you may still find it useful to do some note-taking.

To get the most out of appointments on a practical level, try to ensure your child is not tired or hungry. (For that matter, make sure *you* are not tired or hungry either!)

You know your child best, and to best support their success in therapies, you should engage with the therapy team whenever you have questions, as you might see something they do not. It is also okay to request a break or a change in activity, or to ask about the purpose of an exercise. Partner with your therapists to help optimize the care being provided. Nurture the relationship with the professionals treating your child—they are your allies. You may be angry about aspects of your child's diagnosis or treatment, but avoid putting professionals on the receiving end of any misplaced anger. The expression "Don't shoot the messenger" comes to mind. You might be dissatisfied with the range of services provided to your child, for example, but remember that frontline staff are rarely the policy-makers—indeed, they may in fact agree with you. The best management of the condition is achieved when parent and child work together in partnership with the medical professionals.

Good communication between disciplines is also vital for the functioning of the multidisciplinary team. The parent and child are the constants in this relationship; thus, the parent can help support communication between the different team members. No matter how good services are, things can go wrong: for example, a referral might be forgotten, and an appointment might not get scheduled. Supporting communication between team members is particularly important when the child is getting a large part of their care in the community but has to travel to a specialist center from time to time. The parent can play an important role in the smooth coordination of care, so it is helpful to stay organized and keep medical reports together and at hand. This coordinator role may later fall to the adolescent themselves, in time, and if their development permits.

Finally, sometimes a particular medical professional is not the right match for the family. If this occurs, be sure to communicate this and try to seek an alternative to optimize the chances of success for the child or adolescent with CP.

Ally attended physio twice a week from when she was 10 months old. I would advise parents to question the physiotherapy options that are being offered to make sure they make sense for your child. There have been times when I have taken Ally to therapies that didn't suit her or that she had grown out of. As you are the parent, you do need to ensure that it makes sense to you and works for your child, and when you find something that does work, stick with it even if it is hard to fit in with everything else you may be juggling. I fully appreciated the benefits of intensive physiotherapy the summer after Ally's surgery in the US, as I could see the physical changes every day. It has reinforced my earlier and continued belief in the efficacy of early intervention and therapy.

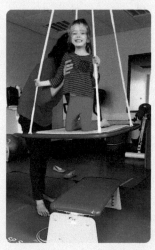
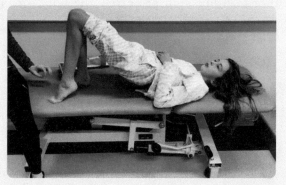

Left: Ally at physio with a local physio. Right: stretching as Ally gets older.

The home program

Spirit in motion.
Paralympian motto

Novak and colleagues defined the home program as the "therapeutic*
practice of goal-based tasks by the child, led by the parent, and supported by the therapist in the home environment."[203] In this book, we
have termed this the "homework" prescribed by therapists.

Practicing what is learned in therapy is very important, but there are
periods when the child or adolescent is not attending therapy in an
episode of care, so it makes sense to have a broader view of the home
program to include all the elements that families do at home to help
manage the condition. These are things that have to become part of
life for the child and adolescent with hemiplegia, such as stretching,
strengthening, and wearing orthoses (when prescribed).

The term "home environment" is a collective of the actual home, school,
and wherever the child spends their time. The best people to help with

---

* Recommended for reasons of health.

the child's program are those who regularly interact with the child. In addition to parents, they may be siblings, teachers, teaching assistants, grandparents, and childcare providers. They are the optimal ones to provide developmentally appropriate opportunities. Therapists are there to teach, guide, and support.

The saying "It takes a village to raise a child" emphasizes the idea that raising a child, particularly a child with a disability, is not a task that should be shouldered by parents alone. By enlisting the support of others, parents can lighten their load and create a network of individuals who are invested in the child's well-being.

Within the broader view of the home program, it is important to never forget to have fun—one of the F-words introduced in Chapter 1. This section addresses:

- **The homework prescribed by therapists**
- **Postural management**
- **Exercise and physical activity**

There are people in Ally's life who I will forever be indebted to, and we will never be able to thank them enough. When Ally came out of hospital, she remained on a breathing monitor for a year as she continued to have apnea and bradycardia. I remained out of work for 17 months, and when I did return to work, I found it almost impossible to find a childminder, especially one who could pay particular attention to Ally's needs.

Milly, my older daughter, was being minded by an amazing lady, Nora, who lives locally, but she planned to soon retire and was on her last cycle of kids. She was a little reluctant at the start to take on the task of caring for Ally and didn't really understand the consequences, but she did agree to mind her for an afternoon—and 10 years later Ally is still there!

Nora and her husband, Pat, have been an integral part of getting Ally to where she is today. They have done her physio religiously with her daily, they incorporated fun exercises with her to ensure she uses her right side, and they followed the most intricate physio plans. We never thought Ally would be able to cycle, but when she was nine years old, Nora became convinced it was a possibility and spent evening after evening until Ally took off!

If you have a Nora and Pat in your life, don't underestimate their willingness to get involved and the impact that they can make. We are eternally indebted to having them as Ally's personal physios, mentors, and friends without even asking.

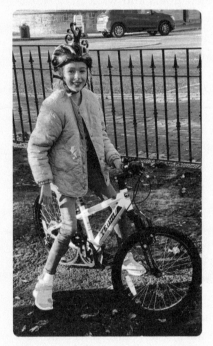

Ally on her bike.

The homework prescribed by therapists

The benefit of any therapy (PT, OT, SLP/SLT) is only partly gained in the therapy session itself. The real benefits come from regular practice at home. It's like learning how to play the piano: true learning does not happen during the weekly lesson but through consistent practice at home.

Families depend on therapists to prescribe evidence-based treatments. Therapists depend on the child or adolescent, with the support of the parent and their network, to get in the practice at home. This is a collaborative relationship. Much of what is learned in therapy has to become part of everyday life for the child or adolescent with hemiplegia in order to be effective. Working with a therapist is a partnership, and the parent and child or adolescent are partners with the therapist in the decision-making process. It is important that the parent and child or adolescent share with the therapist their goals and what may be less important to them to enable focus on what is truly valued by the team. It is recommended that you talk with your therapist and make sure you have a good understanding of the activities you'll be carrying out at home and that it is a realistic plan.

To this day, Ally is like all kids with right-side hemiplegia with her right side being much weaker than her left. I'm often asked if Ally is right-handed. Because if so, she not only has CP but also has the challenge of retraining herself to make her left hand dominant and be able to write with her left hand.

Despite all the physio and intervention, we still have to prompt Ally to use her right hand during day-to-day living. This is a noteworthy aspect of living with CP; Ally will happily sit at the dinner table and leave her right hand down by her side while eating with her left. We constantly prompt her to use "Righty" as we call it; otherwise, she would subconsciously leave it doing nothing, which we know could exacerbate her condition in the long term.

It is so important for a child to use their impacted limbs, and I strongly urge other parents to be vigilant to this aspect of CP.

Postural management

Postural management is another constant in the life of the child and adolescent with hemiplegia. "Posture" refers to the position in which a person holds their body while sitting, standing, or lying down. Good posture applies to everyone, not just individuals with CP.

For example, to maintain good posture, a person needs to have adequate strength in their trunk-stabilizing muscles and good balance reactions. This is why the typically developing child cannot sit independently until they are approximately six months old. Table 3.5.1 lists recommendations on good posture in sitting, standing, and sleeping.

Table 3.5.1 Good posture in sitting, standing, and sleeping

GOOD POSTURE IN:	ILLUSTRATION
Sitting • Feet flat on the floor, with hips, knees, and ankles at 90 degrees and both sides of the trunk straight and symmetrical. (If feet cannot reach the floor, something firm, such as a box or book, can be placed under them to ensure they are flat and that the 90-degree angle is achieved.) • Support provided at the sides, if necessary, to ensure the trunk is straight and symmetrical. • Arms close to the body and relaxed. • Head balanced on the neck (not tilted forward or backward).	
Standing • Feet flat on the floor. • Knees neither locked nor bent. • Abdominal muscles tight and buttocks tucked in. • Shoulders back and down slightly, even, and relaxed. • Head facing forward, not tilted to one side or the other. • Chin tucked and ears over the shoulders.	

Cont'd.

GOOD POSTURE IN:	ILLUSTRATION
Sleeping • Posture is midline and symmetrical (i.e., the two sides are equal). • Sleeping in a supine position (on the back) is recommended. • If lying on one side, it can be helpful to place a pillow between the legs to keep the spine in good alignment. A pillow under the top arm can also be useful to support good alignment—often the top arm is pulled down by gravity, which can result in curving of the spine or rolling to prone position (sleeping on the front) in the night.	

Exercise and physical activity

Exercise and physical activity are also constants in the life of the child and adolescent with hemiplegia. The goal of exercise and physical activity for a person with hemiplegia is the same as for their nondisabled peers. Having a physical disability does not confer any exemption from needing to exercise and stay physically active.

While exercise and physical activity are related, there are differences:

- **Exercise** is planned, structured, repetitive, and intentional movement to improve or maintain physical fitness.[204] Exercise is a subtype of physical activity. Examples of exercise include running, cycling, and attending a gym class.
- **Physical activity** is movement carried out by the skeletal muscles that requires energy expenditure; thus any movement is physical activity.[204] Physical activity varies from light to moderate to vigorous. Examples of each include:
  - Light: slow walking
  - Moderate: brisk walking, jogging, climbing stairs
  - Vigorous: fast running, fast cycling

It follows that energy expenditure is lowest while doing light physical activity and highest while doing vigorous physical activity. Recent advancements in wearable monitoring devices allow better measurement of physical activity levels in individuals with CP.[205,206]

Do children and adolescents with hemiplegia take part in enough physical activity? No. Studies have shown that children with CP walk significantly less[207] and spend more time being sedentary[208] than typically developing children. A further study[206] found that children age 3 to 12 showed a decrease in amount and intensity of physical activity with increasing GMFCS level* and increasing age. Participants at GMFCS level I showed the steepest decrease with increasing age.

Does this reduced physical activity have health consequences? Yes. Reduced physical activity has been associated with higher energy cost of walking in adolescents with mild spastic CP[209] and elevated blood pressure in children and adolescents with mild or moderate spastic CP.[210]

Do studies show exercise and physical activity are beneficial for children and adolescents with CP? Again, yes. Studies have found benefits across a range of measures, including fitness, body composition, quality of life, and happiness.[211,212,213] A physical therapy research summit sponsored by the American Physical Therapy Association emphasized the need to promote and maintain physical fitness in children with CP to improve health, reduce secondary conditions, and enhance quality of life.[214]

Verschuren and colleagues published a set of exercise and physical activity recommendations for people with CP under the following headings:[215]

- Cardiorespiratory (aerobic) exercise
- Resistance (muscle strengthening) exercise
- Daily moderate to vigorous physical activity
- Avoiding sedentary behavior (i.e., not being physically inactive)

Table 3.5.2 summarizes their recommendations, which are similar to (and based on) the World Health Organization's guidelines for nondisabled people.[216] Though these recommendations are relatively recent, the concept that "exercise is medicine" is not new.[217] Note that these are lifetime recommendations; it may take at least 8 to 16 consecutive weeks of exercise to see the benefit.[215] Also note that there is no lower

---

* Levels I and II compared with levels III to V combined.

(or upper) age limit on the exercise and physical activity recommendations for people with CP.

There is no denying these recommendations are demanding. However, research has found that typically developing infants can take up to 9,000 steps in a given day and travel the equivalent of 29 football fields.[218] It is important to be aware of the recommendations and aim to meet them as much as possible. And remember, any activity is better than no activity.

Table 3.5.2 Exercise and physical activity recommendations for people with CP

TYPE OF EXERCISE/ PHYSICAL ACTIVITY	RECOMMENDATIONS FOR PEOPLE WITH CP	COMMENTS
Cardiorespiratory (aerobic) exercise Regular, purposeful exercise that involves major muscle groups and is continuous and rhythmic in nature	3 times per week > 60% of peak heart rate* Minimum of 20 minutes per session	This is the type of exercise that gets the heart pumping and the lungs working.
Resistance (muscle strengthening) exercise	2 to 4 times per week on nonconsecutive days	Muscle strengthening is especially important because muscle weakness is a feature of spastic CP.
Daily moderate to vigorous physical activity	60 minutes ≥ 5 days per week	This is the ordinary movement of everyday life. Physical activity counts as long as it is moderate to vigorous. It is less taxing than cardiorespiratory exercise but more vigorous than gentle movement. Walking, going up stairs, and household chores are all included in this category.

* Peak heart rate can be approximated as 220 minus age. For example, at age 15, peak heart rate is 205 (220-15). Sixty percent of peak heart rate is approximately 120 beats/minute (205 x 0.6).

Cont'd.

TYPE OF EXERCISE/ PHYSICAL ACTIVITY	RECOMMENDATIONS FOR PEOPLE WITH CP	COMMENTS
Avoiding sedentary behavior (not being physically inactive)	Sit for less than 2 hours a day or break up sitting for 2 minutes every 30 to 60 minutes	A person can be physically active but still sedentary; they are separately measured. For example, if the person meets the recommendation for moderate to vigorous physical activity but sits for long periods watching TV or playing computer games, then they are physically active but sedentary. Prolonged sitting in one position, particularly with bad posture, is not good for anyone.

From Verschuren and colleagues.[215]

The Peter Harrison Centre for Disability Sport at Loughborough University in the UK has published two excellent guides specifically for people of all ages with CP. The first, *Fit for Life*, is for people with CP who are new to exercise. The second, *Fit for Sport*, is for people who want to take their athletics to a more advanced level.[219,220] The first guide contains a very useful table, "What type of exercise can I do?" listing advantages and disadvantages with adaptations and advice for each type of exercise. One of the advantages noted is that almost all can be done in the community with peers. Many children and adolescents with CP appreciate doing exercise in regular settings rather than as part of therapy. Both guides are included in **Useful web resources**.

Another resource is World Abilitysport, an international organization for the development of para sports—competitive sports specifically designed or adapted for individuals with physical, sensory, or intellectual disability.[221] Figure 3.5.1 shows World Abilitysport's list of sports and para sports for individuals with CP across GMFCS levels.

	GMFCS I 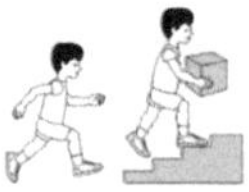	GMFCS II 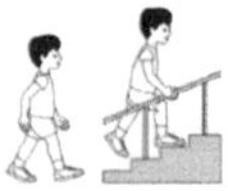
Athletics	Ambulant Athletics – Track and Field	Ambulant Athletics - Track and Field
Swimming	Unaided swimming	Unaided swimming
Football	CP 7-a-side Football	CP 7-a-side Football
Racquet Sports	Standing Badminton Standing Table-Tennis Standing Cricket	Standing Badminton Standing Table-Tennis Standing Cricket Wheelchair Tennis
Individual Sports	Taekwondo Para-Cycling (2/3 wheeler) Para Triathlon Equestrian CP Bowls Standing Archery standing Golf Para Shooting Powerlifting Seated Fencing	Taekwondo Para-Cycling (2/3 wheeler) Para Triathlon Equestrian CP Bowls Standing Archery standing Golf Para Shooting Powerlifting Seated Fencing
Team Sports	Sitting Volleyball Beach ParaVolley Ambulant CP rugby Ambulant Netball	Sitting Volleyball Beach ParaVolley Ambulant CP rugby Ambulant Netball
Winter Sports	Standing Alpine Skiing Standing Nordic Skiing Snowboarding Para Ice Hockey	Standing Alpine Skiing Standing Nordic Skiing Snowboarding Para Ice Hockey
Water Sports	Rowing Sailing Canoeing	Rowing Sailing Canoeing

Figure 3.5.1 Sports and para sports for individuals with CP across the GMFCS levels. Reproduced with kind permission from World Abilitysport. GMFCS illustrations Version 2 © Bill Reid, Kate Willoughby, Adrienne Harvey, and Kerr Graham, The Royal Children's Hospital Melbourne, Australia.

GMFCS III	GMFCS IV	GMFCS V
RaceRunning Seated Athletics - Track and Field	RaceRunning Seated Athletics - Track and Field	RaceRunning Seated Athletics – Track and Field
Unaided swimming		
Frame Football	Frame Football Powerchair Football	Powerchair Football
Wheelchair Badminton Wheelchair Tennis Seated Table Tennis Wheelchair Cricket	Wheelchair Badminton Wheelchair Tennis Seated Table Tennis Table Cricket	Table Cricket
Para-Cycling (2/3 wheeler) Seated Fencing Para Triathlon Boccia Equestrian CP Bowls Seated Archery seated Wheelchair Slalom Para Shooting Powerlifting	Para-Cycling (2/3 wheeler) Seated Fencing Boccia CP Bowls Seated Archery seated Para Shooting Powerlifting Trap Driving Wheelchair Slalom	Wheelchair Slalom Boccia Para Shooting Trap Driving
Sitting Volleyball Wheelchair Basketball Wheelchair Rugby	Sitting Volleyball Wheelchair Basketball Wheelchair Rugby	
Sitting Alpine Skiing Standing/Sitting Nordic Skiing Wheelchair Curling Para Ice Hockey	Sitting Nordic Skiing Wheelchair Curling	
Rowing Sailing Canoeing	Sailing Canoeing	Assisted Sailing

Further tips on exercise and physical activity are included in Appendix 4 (online). An appointment with a physical therapist, occupational therapist, or a recreational therapist is useful if further guidance is needed on how to create an exercise program that suits the needs and abilities of the individual.

Ally's true love is horse riding, which runs in the family as she comes from a long line of horse "addicts," including my late mum, Christine, and my sister Anne. I have taken Ally to therapeutic riding since she was four years old and believe that it really has helped her to develop her core strength and support her bilateral movement.

When she was around nine years old, Ally started getting bored of therapeutic riding and moved to mainstream riding lessons. She has since gotten her own pony, Reilly, and knows every international show jumper and dressage rider, following them religiously on YouTube. Ally is a passionate and dedicated rider, but unfortunately there are still times when the CP catches her. She recently had a bad fall, breaking seven bones in her foot and suffering a concussion. It was a setback and I have really struggled with letting Ally back in the saddle, but if I didn't, I would be taking away her true love. Ally made the decision last year that she was going to give up the jumping for the moment and concentrate on dressage, which is the art of riding and training a horse in a manner that develops obedience, flexibility, and balance. I see it as horse ballet! This decision has proven that although CP may present challenges, there are often ways around it, and we were delighted when Ally participated in the National Dressage Championships in 2023. Sometimes, irrespective of risk, if an activity is something that a kid with CP loves that also has therapeutic benefits, allowing them to do it is a no-brainer (although I would prefer if Ally adored ballet!).

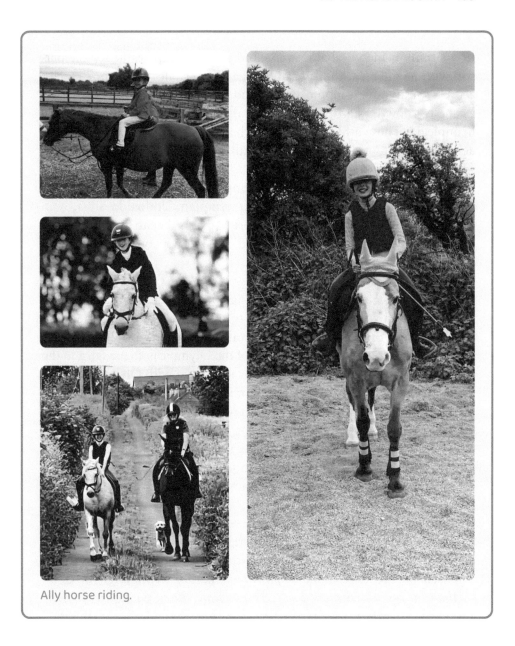

Ally horse riding.

If you think being good at exercise and sports is impossible for the person with hemiplegia, think again. Paige Van Ardale and Conor Hogan are US Paralympian alpine skiers, and Lakeisha Patterson (or Lucky as she is known) is an Australian Paralympic swimmer. All three have hemiplegia. These athletes are proof that hemiplegia is not a barrier to achieving great levels of fitness and skill.

Daniel Dias, retired Brazilian Paralympic swimmer who won multiple medals, credited fellow retired Paralympian Clodoaldo Silva, who has CP, for getting him into the sport. "I only began because I saw Clodoaldo swimming on television. I didn't know people like me could swim, could do any sport at all."[222]

Paralympians include people with a range of types and levels of disabilities. Many Paralympic athletes are able to swim, cycle, and run faster than their average nondisabled peers. For example, at the Brazil 2016 games, four Paralympic runners beat the time of the Olympic gold medalist in the men's 1,500 meters.[223] US Paralympians now train with Olympic athletes at US Olympic and Paralympic Committee training centers under the supervision of the same coaches. The guiding principle of the Paralympic movement is to keep competition as fair as possible, and classification is the cornerstone. Classification is sport specific because an individual's impairment may affect their ability to perform in different sports to a different extent. For example, in swimming:

> There are ten different sport classes for athletes with physical impairment, numbered 1-10. Athletes with different impairments compete against each other, because sport classes are allocated based on the impact the impairment has on swimming, rather than on the impairment itself. To evaluate the impact of impairments on swimming, classifiers assess all functional body structures using a point system and ask the athlete to complete a water assessment.[224]

There are currently 28 Paralympic sports sanctioned by the International Paralympic Committee: 22 summer and 6 winter sports.[224]

Summer sports:

- Para archery
- Para athletics
- Para badminton
- Blind football (for athletes with a vision impairment)
- Boccia
- Para canoe
- Para cycling
- Para equestrian
- Goalball (for athletes with a vision impairment)
- Para judo (for athletes with a vision impairment)
- Para powerlifting
- Para rowing
- Shooting para sport
- Sitting volleyball
- Para swimming
- Para table tennis
- Para tae kwon do
- Para triathlon
- Wheelchair basketball
- Wheelchair fencing
- Wheelchair rugby
- Wheelchair tennis

Winter sports:

- Para alpine skiing
- Para biathlon
- Para cross-country skiing
- Para ice hockey
- Para snowboard
- Wheelchair curling

Links to various organizations are included in **Useful web resources.**

Assistive technology

Determine that the thing can and shall be done,
and then we shall find the way.
Abraham Lincoln

Assistive technology refers to products and services designed to enhance the functional capabilities and independence of individuals with disabilities to allow them to participate.[225] This section addresses the following assistive technology* commonly used by individuals with hemiplegia:

- Orthoses
- Mobility aids
- Adaptive equipment for activities of daily living
- Adaptive recreational equipment

Assistive technology should be selected based on assessments performed by a multidisciplinary team, including professionals (e.g., physician, physical and occupational therapists, orthotist) in conjunction with the

---

* In the US, some assistive technology is referred to as "durable medical equipment" (DME) for medical insurance purposes.

individual and their family. An individual's unique health needs and the family's care and function goals help guide what assistive technology is best suited for the individual. Regular reevaluation is important, the frequency of which depends on the individual and the product.

Orthoses

An orthosis is a device designed to hold specific body parts in position in order to modify their structure and/or function. The term "orthosis" comes from the Greek word "ortho," which means "to straighten or align." Orthotics is the branch of medicine concerned with the design, manufacture, and management of orthoses. The orthotist is the professional in this specialty. The word "orthotic" is sometimes used to mean the device; "orthosis" is the more correct term, but given how alike the two terms are, their interchangeability is understandable. The terms "brace" and "splint" are also sometimes used.

Orthoses work best when a child has no contractures or bone torsions, though many children with hemiplegia may have both; then, orthoses can at least be partially effective as long as they are not too cumbersome or limiting.

Different orthoses have different functions. The goals of treatment with orthoses may include the following:[226]

* Maintain or improve ROM at a joint through a prolonged stretch
* Provide stability or support to a joint
* Improve function of a limb
* Improve balance
* Improve gait
* Provide protection
* Accommodate or minimize a joint alignment problem
* Prepare for surgery
* Facilitate positioning after surgery

There is often a trade-off or competing goals with orthoses. For example, the best orthosis for walking may not be the best for getting up and down from the floor, and using an orthosis to protect or correctly align a body part may decrease muscle strength. For this reason, if the orthosis includes the ankle joint, the child or adolescent should also spend some time out of the orthosis since it is important to maintain strength in the muscles that don't have to work when it is worn; in this case the dorsiflexors (shin muscles) and plantar flexors (calf muscles). Likewise, with upper extremity orthoses, it is of paramount importance that a balance be found between potentially competing goals. For instance, one member of the multidisciplinary team may want to see a prolonged stretch of the hand muscles and prescribe a "resting" orthosis, while another may recommend the hand remain free to encourage sensory and motor function. Reasonable balance might include only nighttime wear of the orthosis to allow time for both stretching and sensory and motor function. As a general rule, any orthosis that potentially interferes with function should be reevaluated for its true utility as it relates to the individual's goals. Additionally, different orthoses may be prescribed over the years as the child or adolescent grows and their body structure and function changes. As a result, collaborative goal-setting is important, and choosing an orthosis can involve different specialists on the multidisciplinary team.[227]

Orthoses can be custom-made (molded to a specific individual's body) or prefabricated (fit based on size and already made). Once a device has been prescribed, the individual will be evaluated and a device may be fitted the same day if it is prefabricated and readily available. A device such as a custom-made ankle-foot orthosis (AFO) requires a mold to be taken and a return visit after a few weeks for a fitting of the new device. Adjustments are made to confirm that it is comfortable and functions well. Adhering to the prescribed wear time is critical to ensure that the individual receives the full benefit of the device. After the initial fitting, further adjustments may be needed if the individual is experiencing:

- Discomfort
- Redness
- Skin breakdown
- A growth spurt
- A change in functionality
- A change in ROM

Additionally, children will likely outgrow their devices before they wear them out and may require new devices every year or so until they stop growing.

Individuals with hemiplegia may use:

a)   **Upper extremity orthoses**
b)   **Lower extremity orthoses**

a) Upper extremity orthoses

Upper extremity orthoses are used for the fingers, hands, wrists, elbows, and shoulders. They are intended to maintain ROM of the joint, to provide support, and/or to maximize positioning and function. The following upper extremity orthoses may be used in hemiplegia and are described in Table 3.6.1:

- Hand finger orthosis (HFO)
- Wrist hand finger orthosis (WHFO)
- Wrist hand orthosis (WHO)
- Elbow orthosis (EO)

Table 3.6.1 Common upper extremity orthoses for individuals with hemiplegia.

ORTHOSIS TYPE	SUBTYPE	DESCRIPTION
Hand finger orthosis (HFO)	Static	A static HFO is a device that fits in the palm of the hand and allows the fingers to wrap around it. This counteracts finger flexion contractures and prevents the pain and skin breakdown that can result from maintaining a prolonged fist position.
	Finger	The finger HFO is worn on the hand and fingers. It is made either of a rigid material to help extend and stretch the fingers or a softer material to assist with grasp, release, and positioning of the hand. These orthoses can help with functions such as pressing a button or improving grasp. (Note: This HFO includes a thumb abduction component to assist with thumb positioning.)
	Thumb abduction orthosis	A thumb abduction orthosis covers the hand and thumb. It can be made from rigid thermoplastic* or softer, flexible neoprene material. It supports the thumb joint in a functional grasp position, preventing hypermobility, and it can be useful during play activities. It also prevents the thumb from coming into the palm during fisting.
Wrist hand finger orthosis (WHFO)	Static	A static WHFO holds the wrist, hand, and fingers in one position and does not allow movement. The rigidity of the material can vary, and it may be worn at night or at rest due to its impact on the user's functionality. It is typically used to counteract or prevent painful wrist and/or finger contractures.
	Dynamic	A dynamic WHFO helps to position the wrist, hand, and fingers while allowing movement to improve overall function.

Cont'd.

ORTHOSIS TYPE	SUBTYPE	DESCRIPTION
Wrist hand orthosis (WHO)		A WHO covers only the wrist and hand (not the fingers). It can be made of a variety of materials including neoprene, nylon, thermoplastic,* or metal. A WHO helps to maintain wrist positioning while allowing finger flexion and thumb opposition (touching the tip of the thumb to the tip the fingers).
Elbow orthosis (EO)		An EO (elbow immobilizer) is worn around the elbow joint. There are a variety of options, from static EOs that maintain one position to counteract flexion contractures and protect the joint, to dynamic EOs that allow movement and can improve ROM. The image is of a static EO.

* Thermoplastic material becomes more pliable when heated and is therefore useful for making or adjusting orthoses.

Adapted from Ward and colleagues.[226] Dynamic WHFO image reproduced with kind permission from Saebo Inc.

b) Lower extremity orthoses

Lower extremity orthoses are used for the feet, ankles, knees, and hips. They are intended to maintain or improve ROM at the joint, provide support and stability, improve function and gait, and more. The following lower extremity orthoses may be used in hemiplegia and are described in Table 3.6.2.

- Foot orthosis (FO)
- Supramalleolar orthosis (SMO)
- Ankle-foot orthosis (AFO)
- Knee immobilizer (KI)
- Knee orthosis (KO)

Having well-fitting shoes is a must when wearing orthoses intended for standing or walking. If the shoes do not fit well or are worn out, the orthoses may not function correctly and may not be comfortable. In most cases, a slightly larger shoe is needed. Certain stores, including some online, allow purchase of two different-size shoes. Athletic shoes that can be zipped, laced, or fastened snugly can be a good option. Some manufacturers of athletic shoes now offer models that are specifically designed to be easy to get on and off with orthoses, such as some BILLY shoes or the Nike FlyEase. Sometimes a lift will be added to the shoes to maximize the user's alignment or to make up for a leg length difference.

Table 3.6.2 Common lower extremity orthoses for individuals with hemiplegia.

ORTHOSIS TYPE	SUBTYPE	DESCRIPTION
Foot orthosis (FO)	Functional or accommodative	FOs are semi-rigid custom-molded shoe inserts. They replace regular shoe insoles and can be left in the shoes. Accommodative FOs cushion or protect a rigid foot or a foot that lacks sensation; functional FOs provide support and help maintain proper alignment.
	University of California-Berkeley Lab (UCBL)	A UCBL orthosis, similar to the functional FO, supports, distributes pressure, and helps maintain proper foot alignment. However, the UCBL is taller and is made of more rigid plastic to provide greater support. UCBLs usually replace regular insoles and can be left in the shoes.
Supramalleolar orthosis (SMO)		A supramalleolar orthosis ("supra" means "above" and "malleolar" refers to the bony prominences of the ankle), extends just above the ankle. As with FOs and UCBLs, the SMO controls the foot. However, as the SMO also captures the ankle joint, it exerts greater control and provides additional support and stability.

Cont'd.

ORTHOSIS TYPE	SUBTYPE	DESCRIPTION
Ankle-foot orthosis (AFO) An AFO extends above the ankle joint and stops before the knee. It protects the foot, manages foot malalignments, prevents the toes from dragging during gait, provides varying levels of support and stability to the ankle and/or knee during standing and walking, and prevents the progression of ankle muscle contractures.	Articulated AFO	An articulated AFO has a hinge at the ankle joint to allow free dorsiflexion (moving the foot up). It often has a plastic posterior "stop" that blocks plantar flexion, preventing the user from moving the foot down or dragging their toes. Free dorsiflexion allows the user to easily rise to standing from the floor, transition from one position to another, and climb stairs. Articulated AFOs are also worn by adolescents and adults who would benefit from the added ROM while still preventing their toes from dragging.
	Posterior leaf spring (PLS) AFO	The PLS AFO has a calf cuff that tapers to a thinner strut behind the ankle. It prevents toes from dragging and restricts dorsiflexion, the amount of which depends on the width and stiffness of the posterior strut. Because the sides are trimmed back, it may not be the best choice for someone who requires significant ankle and/or knee support or who has severe joint contractures.
	Solid AFO (SAFO)	A SAFO is the most supportive type of AFO. It is typically made of a rigid, durable plastic and provides maximum stability for the ankle and knee. This AFO does not allow ankle movement, which can make some functional movements difficult to perform while wearing it (e.g., going up and down stairs). It is most often recommended for individuals with severe tone, muscle contractures, or bony malalignments.
	Ground reaction AFO (GRAFO) or floor reaction AFO (FRAFO)	The GRAFO is a solid AFO with an additional anterior shell. The solid ankle design provides maximum control at the ankle, and the anterior shell forces the knee to extend, helping to limit crouch gait. The GRAFO can sometimes be difficult to put on and take off because the foot has to be inserted from the rear. It is ineffective for use with knee or hip flexion contractures because the knee cannot completely straighten.

Cont'd.

ORTHOSIS TYPE	SUBTYPE	DESCRIPTION
Ankle-foot orthosis (AFO) *Cont'd*	Carbon fiber AFO	A carbon fiber AFO can be prefabricated or custom-made. It may have a posterior strut similar to a PLS AFO (top image) or an anterior shell similar to a GRAFO (bottom image). Prefabricated designs will prevent toes from dragging and provide light support while the carbon material provides energy return to the user. Custom-made carbon fiber AFOs may provide additional support for high-level activities.
	External dorsiflexion assist AFO	The prefabricated, spring-loaded external dorsiflexion assist AFO attaches to the outside of the shoe. It is best used to prevent toes from dragging in a person with minimal spasticity and adequate dorsiflexion ROM. It can be somewhat bulky and therefore potentially problematic for the person with a narrow base of support while walking.
	Nighttime AFO or stretching splint	A prefabricated nighttime AFO typically has a plastic shell, soft inner liner, and adjustable straps. It is worn just at night and is designed to help stretch the calf muscles, maintain ankle ROM, and prevent the progression of ankle muscle contractures.

Cont'd.

ORTHOSIS TYPE	SUBTYPE	DESCRIPTION
Knee immobilizer (KI)	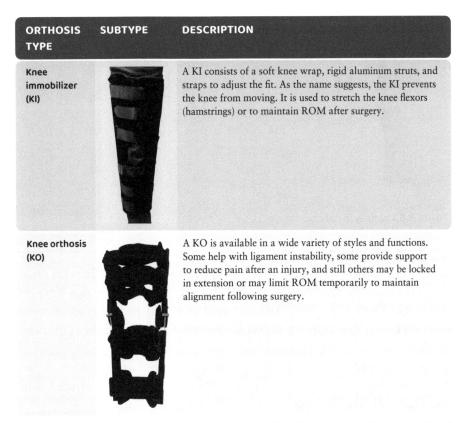	A KI consists of a soft knee wrap, rigid aluminum struts, and straps to adjust the fit. As the name suggests, the KI prevents the knee from moving. It is used to stretch the knee flexors (hamstrings) or to maintain ROM after surgery.
Knee orthosis (KO)		A KO is available in a wide variety of styles and functions. Some help with ligament instability, some provide support to reduce pain after an injury, and still others may be locked in extension or may limit ROM temporarily to maintain alignment following surgery.

Adapted from Ward and colleagues.[226] *External dorsiflexion assist AFO reproduced with kind permission from Turbo Med Orthotics.*

Research supports the use of upper limb orthoses for improved hand function (yellow light) and AFOs for improved stride length* and ankle movement.[14]

Finally, some individuals may use a functional electrical stimulation (FES) device that provides stimulation to activate the dorsiflexor muscles during gait. This is not an orthosis per se; see Figure 3.6.1. Adequate dorsiflexion ROM is necessary, and the device is best used with a steady gait. Advantages are that it is an alternative to wearing an orthosis and can be worn with any footwear. Disadvantages are its lack of water resistance and high cost. It is also often poorly tolerated in very young children and cannot be used with certain other conditions (e.g., epilepsy).

---

* Stride length is the distance covered from one heel strike to the next heel strike of the same foot. In other words, it is equal to two steps, one for each foot.

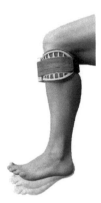

Figure 3.6.1 Walkaide functional electrical stimulation (FES) device.

Ankle-foot orthoses (AFOs) of every type have provided Ally with great support since she was two years old, but her dream is to not have to wear one. Over the years, Ally has had cuts and pressure sores from wearing her AFOs, and I do regret at times not reacting to them quicker.

An AFO should not hurt a child, and if they are causing pain, it can be a deterrent to wearing them. The shoe choice is also crucial; our discovery of Nike FlyEase shoes has been a game changer.

Sometimes the shoes recommended may not be aesthetically the best in your child's eyes. As a parent, ask yourself what makes sense; if your child is uncomfortable in an AFO, don't accept discomfort as being "normal" or "it's because they have bony feet," as I was often told. We, ourselves, would not continue to wear uncomfortable shoes, and we should not accept uncomfortable AFOs for our child. Likewise, shoes can be adapted for AFOs, and a good shoemaker can make minor adjustments, if necessary, to accommodate fashion requirements.

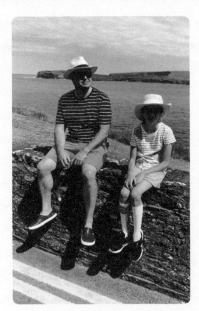
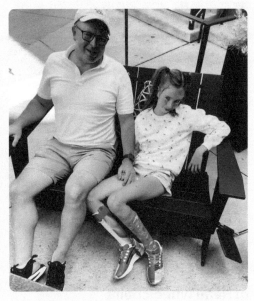

Ally with her dad and wearing her Nike FlyEase shoes.

Mobility aids

Although individuals with hemiplegia GMFCS levels I and II walk independently for the most part, those at GMFCS level II may need a mobility aid for safety and balance in some situations, and wheeled mobility for traveling long distance so as not to fatigue easily. As addressed in section 3.4, navigating high school and college campuses can involve a lot of walking, and there is a balance to be struck between independent walking and using mobility aids such as a scooter or hemi wheelchair. Mobility aids may reduce fatigue and/or pain to allow the individual to participate more in everyday life safely and with more energy available that is not spent on walking alone.

a) Scooters

Scooters are motorized mobility devices that typically have a seat and handlebars for steering, and electric-powered wheels that allow the user to navigate indoors or outdoors. See Figure 3.6.2.

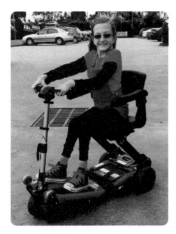

Figure 3.6.2 Motorized scooter for mobility. Reproduced with kind permission from Mounties Care.

b) Hemi wheelchairs

Hemi wheelchairs are specifically designed for individuals with limited mobility on one side of their body. The seat is typically lower than on the standard wheelchair to allow the user to put their feet down if desired to move themselves forward. They may also have systems that connect the two wheels allowing them to be moved and directed by one hand instead of two. They may be manual or power.

Adaptive equipment for activities of daily living

The following may help with activities of daily living. An appointment with an occupational therapist is useful if people need guidance:

- Adaptive shoes with Velcro, zipper closures as opposed to laces, to allow for easier fastening
- Clothing with magnetic zippers*/zipper pulls† to allow for easier dressing.

---

* Uses magnets instead of traditional interlocking teeth or coils to fasten two sides of a garment together. They typically have strips of magnets embedded along the edges of the fabric, which attract each other to create a secure closure when brought together.

† A small, usually metallic or plastic attachment that can be put on the slider of a zipper, making it easier to open and close.

There are also many "one-handed techniques" that allow for shoe tying and dressing that don't include equipment.

The following are examples of equipment that may help with food preparation and eating:

- Adaptive cutting board to help secure a food item to allow for cutting with one hand. See Figure 3.6.3.

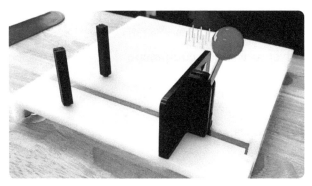

Figure 3.6.3 Adaptive cutting board. Reproduced with kind permission from Rehab-Store.com

- Adaptive silverware to allow the weak hand to assist with eating. See Figure 3.6.4.

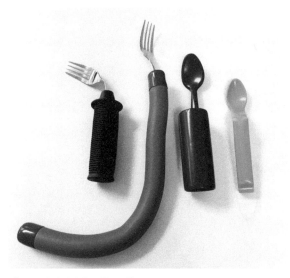

Figure 3.6.4 Adaptive silverware.

Adaptive recreational equipment

A variety of adaptive recreational equipment is available to make participation in various recreational or leisure pursuits possible or just easier. An appointment with a recreational therapist, physical therapist, or occupational therapist is useful if people need guidance. Examples of such equipment include:

a) Adaptive cycles
b) Adaptive workout equipment
c) Hiking aids
d) Other outdoor and adventure sports equipment
e) Technology options
f) Adaptive art and crafts equipment
g) Reading stands
h) Adaptive equipment for games

a) Adaptive cycles

Adaptive cycles come in many configurations, but for the individual with hemiplegia, a tricycle provides more stability because it more easily compensates for balance challenges. The adaptive steering column allows the stronger hand and arm to do more of the steering, and placing the hand brake on the strong side is fairly easy for a cycle technician to do. See Figure 3.6.5.

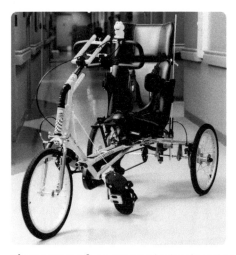

Figure 3.6.5 A foot-powered adaptive tricycle.

The following accessories may be helpful:

- Footplates (sometimes called shoe holders) with straps to keep the feet on the pedals (shown in Figure 3.6.5)
- Leg calipers (braces attached to the pedals) to keep the leg in the correct position
- Pulleys (strings attached to the front of the pedals) to adjust the rider's dorsiflexion (shown in Figure 3.6.5)
- Electric assist to compensate for endurance or rides of long duration (dependent on responsibility of rider)
- Caregiver steering control to help in circumstances when braking or turning is more difficult (on sidewalks, near traffic, down declines)

b) Adaptive workout equipment

Weight-lifting exercises may be done safely with adaptive equipment such as a wrist cuff grip to hold a free weight. They can also be done with a regular wrist weight that goes around the wrist or by using resistance bands. See Figure 3.6.6.

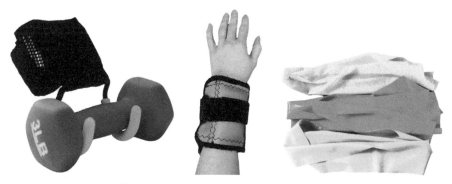

Figure 3.6.6 Wrist cuff grip to hold a free weight (left), wrist weight (middle), and resistance bands (right).

c) Hiking aids

Many individuals with hemiplegia can use hiking poles to correct for their balance challenges on uneven terrain. If the involved arm cannot hold a hiking pole or another walking aid, a track chair can allow participation. A track chair is an all-terrain wheelchair that can safely navigate outdoor spaces when mobility problems make it otherwise unsafe to enjoy the activity. Some large parks and recreational facilities have these chairs available to borrow while at the park or beach, for example.

d) Other outdoor and adventure sports equipment

Adaptive equipment is available for many other outdoor and adventure sports, including:

- Snow skiing (e.g., outriggers)
- Waterskiing (e.g., arm sling handles, shoulder wraps, sit skis)
- Golf (e.g., adaptive club grips and golf carts)
- Kayaking (e.g., angled oars, outriggers, trolling motors)
- Surfing (e.g., specialized systems)
- Horseback riding (e.g., high back saddles for balance)

See Figure 3.6.7.

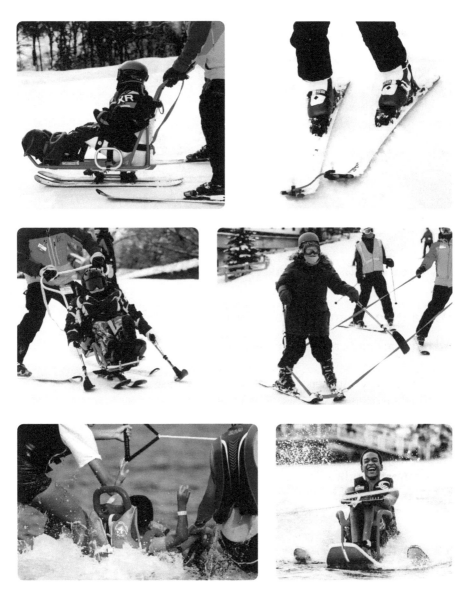

Figure 3.6.7 Adaptive snow skiing and waterskiing with various levels of assistance and support.

e) Technology options

An adaptive joystick and adaptive color-coded keyboard with large keys and letters can help with computer use (see Figure 3.6.8).

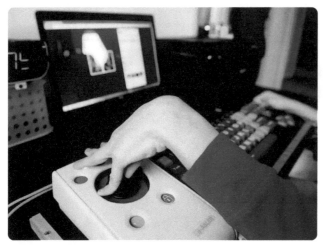

Figure 3.6.8 Adaptive joystick and keyboard.

f) Adaptive art and crafts equipment

Adaptive art and crafts equipment may include:

- Single-extremity scissors with a stability base
- Single-extremity scissors
- Easy-grip scissors
- Universal cuff (can be used for many purposes; here to hold a writing utensil)
- Foam grip aid to assist weak grip
- Paintbrush holder that may prevent fatigue
- Glue dots, paper clamps, easels, and egg-shaped palm crayons

See Figure 3.6.9.

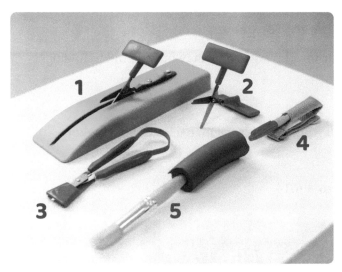

Figure 3.6.9 1) Single-extremity scissors with stability base;
2) Single-extremity scissors; **3)** Easy-grip scissors; **4)** Universal cuff;
5) Foam grip aid.

g) Reading stands

A table-top book stand allows for page turning (see Figure 3.6.10).

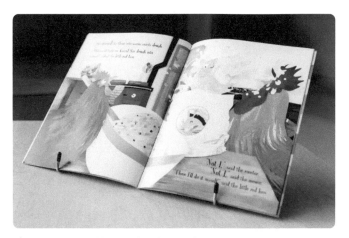

Figure 3.6.10 Table-top book stand.

h) Adaptive equipment for games

Adaptive equipment for playing games may include the following:

- Card shuffler
- Card holder
- Adaptive switch for use with a regular soap bubble-maker
- Dice popper

See Figures 3.6.11 to 3.6.14.

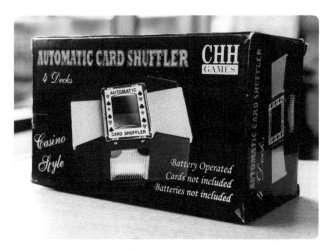

Figure 3.6.11 Card shuffler.

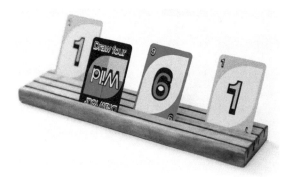

Figure 3.6.12 Card holder.

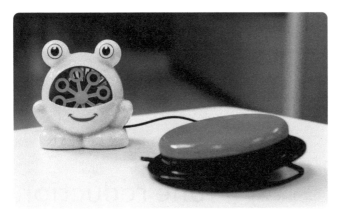

Figure 3.6.13 Adaptive switch for use with a regular soap bubble-maker.

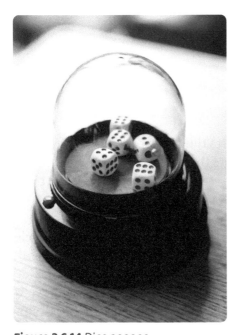

Figure 3.6.14 Dice popper.

Tone reduction

The good physician treats the disease; the great physician
treats the patient who has the disease.

Sir William Osler

Abnormal muscle tone is addressed in section 2.6. To recap: Muscle
tone is the resting tension in a person's muscles. A range of "normal"
muscle tone exists. Tone is considered "abnormal" when it falls outside
the range of normal or typical. Abnormal muscle tone occurs in all types
of CP. Spasticity is the main type of high tone in hemiplegia, but dystonia may also occur. Data from the Australian CP register shows that 16
percent of individuals with spastic hemiplegia* have co-occurring dyskinesia, while 1 percent have co-occurring hypotonia, and it is believed
that the true prevalence of co-occurring motor types is higher.[4]

Spasticity is defined as an abnormal increase in muscle tone or stiffness of muscle that can interfere with movement and speech, and be
associated with discomfort or pain.[22] Another definition highlights
the velocity-dependent nature of the condition.[104] Dystonia, a type of

---

* For those who acquired CP in the pre- or perinatal period only; also includes monoplegia.

dyskinesia, is characterized by involuntary (unintended) muscle contractions that cause slow repetitive movements or abnormal postures that can sometimes be painful.[39]

Tone reduction is a high priority in the early years. However, tone reduction is only one part of the integrated treatment of hemiplegia by the multidisciplinary team. It is usually performed in conjunction with other treatments such as PT, OT, serial casting, and orthoses. When tone reduction is included with other treatments, the effects of each treatment may be amplified—the combination of treatments may be more effective than any one treatment on its own.

Reducing spasticity helps reduce the harmful effects of high tone on skeletal growth. It also helps reduce stiffness and increases the overall ROM of joints. Increasing the ROM a person can move through facilitates strengthening, working on motor control, balance, and other functional goals. It can also improve a person's tolerance for wearing orthoses.

Table 3.7.1 explains tone reduction treatments commonly used in individuals with hemiplegia.

The AACPDM (American Academy for Cerebral Palsy and Developmental Medicine) has published a care pathway, "Cerebral Palsy and Dystonia"; a link to it is included in **Useful web resources.**

Table 3.7.1 Tone reduction treatments

TREATMENT	TONE TYPE	AREA OF EFFECT **Generalized** = treatment affects a large region of the body. **Focal** = treatment has an effect on a local area (e.g., a single muscle)	DURATION OF EFFECT
Oral medications (medications taken by mouth)	Spasticity	Generalized	Temporary
Botulinum neurotoxin A (BoNT-A) injection	Spasticity*	Focal: injected into muscles	Temporary
Phenol injection	Spasticity	Focal: injected around nerves that control spastic muscles	Temporary
Intrathecal baclofen (ITB)	Spasticity and dystonia	Generalized	Temporary
Selective dorsal rhizotomy (SDR)	Spasticity	Generalized	Permanent

* Botulinum neurotoxin A (BoNT-A) may sometimes be used to treat pain caused by dystonia in some individuals with hemiplegia.

Many medical centers have special team evaluations for spasticity treatment planning because of its complexity and significance in CP. At Gillette Children's, for example, a spasticity evaluation for improving gait function or for improving hand function involves several professionals together at a spasticity evaluation clinic or upper extremity tone clinic. The team includes professionals from physical medicine and rehabilitation (PM&R), orthopedics, and neurosurgery. The specialists see the child together, not individually, and come to a consensus on the best spasticity treatment for the child to improve gait or hand use. The spasticity evaluation for improving hand function includes a detailed OT evaluation and may also include upper extremity motion analysis. The spasticity evaluation for improving gait function includes a gait analysis and functional PT assessment completed as part of the (typically) two-day evaluation. Spasticity clinics at other facilities may include additional team members from other specialties, including neurology and developmental pediatrics.

Different medical centers have different protocols for how they perform each tone-reducing treatment.

As with all treatments for hemiplegia, clear goals for tone reduction and assessment of outcome are required. Because the child has to adjust to their new, relaxed muscles, they may initially experience perceived weakness or temporary loss of function. Though the use of tone reduction treatment peaks in early childhood, it can continue into adolescence and adulthood.

We now look at the different tone reduction treatments in more detail.

Oral medications

Oral medications (those taken by mouth) are used to achieve generalized tone reduction. There are several oral medications physicians may prescribe to reduce high tone[228] including:

- Baclofen
- Diazepam
- Dantrolene
- Tizanidine

These medications may have different brand names in different countries. They act on different sites in the body, with different effects on the muscles, brain, or spinal cord.[228]

The challenge of treatment with oral medications is balancing their side effects with their efficacy; benefits are greater for some people than for others. The medications are sometimes used in combination or in conjunction with focal spasticity reduction measures such as BoNT-A. They can also be used episodically to reduce muscle spasms after orthopedic surgery, for instance.

Research supports use of diazepam (green light) and dantrolene and tizanidine (yellow light) for reduced spasticity. Research supports use of oral baclofen for reduced spasticity (yellow light).[14]

Botulinum neurotoxin A injection

Botulinum neurotoxin A (BoNT-A), as a medication, is injected directly into the muscle and acts by blocking the release of a chemical called acetylcholine at the neuromuscular junction (where the nerve meets the muscle). Botulinum neurotoxin* is produced by the bacteria that causes botulism, a lethal form of food poisoning. However, as a medication, the purified toxin is delivered at a much smaller dose. There are seven different types of botulinum neurotoxin, from A to G. Type A is the main form used to reduce spasticity.[229]

The effects of BoNT-A become apparent approximately three to seven days after injection and last for approximately three to six months.[230] The age at which treatment with BoNT-A begins varies among medical centers, with peak use between two and six years of age.[230] Protocols for use of BoNT-A (e.g., dosage and frequency of injection) also are different.[231] The effects of BoNT-A diminish with time. The original nerves regain their ability to release acetylcholine, but conflicting evidence exists on its long-term effect on the muscle itself.[229,230]

Several muscles may be treated in one session, although there is a limit to the total body dose of BoNT-A that can be safely given at one time.[229] Depending on the age of the individual and the number of muscles being injected, anesthesia may be required. Typically, no overnight hospital stay is necessary.

As with any injection, there may be some pain associated with the needle puncturing the skin and the delivery of the medicine. Different centers use different methods to manage pain; these may include distraction techniques (e.g., watching a video), topical or oral medication, nitrous oxide (laughing gas), or general anesthesia. Some children may experience stress and anxiety from repeated episodes of injection. One limiting factor of this treatment is the possibility of diminishing effect with repeat injections, or it may stop being effective entirely.[229]

The simultaneous use of BoNT-A and strength training has been found to be successful at reducing spasticity, improving strength, and achieving

---

* A poison that acts on the nervous system.

functional goals over and above treatment with BoNT-A alone.[232] This is an example of combined treatments working better together.

While there is strong evidence supporting BoNT-A treatment,[14,233,234] concerns are being raised. BoNT-A is regarded as a temporary treatment for reducing spasticity, but important questions have been asked about its long-term effects, including muscle weakness, muscle atrophy (wastage), changes in the muscle structure, and atrophy of the underlying bone.[3,230,235–241] Some studies suggest there may be permanent changes. For example, Multani and colleagues reported that human volunteers and experimental animals show muscle atrophy for at least 12 months after BoNT-A treatment.[230] They added that "muscle atrophy was accompanied by loss of contractile elements in muscle and replacement with fat and connective tissue," and that it was not currently known if these changes are reversible. They concluded that there is a need to use BoNT-A "more thoughtfully, less frequently and with greatly enhanced monitoring of the effects on injected muscle for both short-term and long-term benefits and harms."[230]

Ally had Botox treatment at the start of one summer, followed by really intensive physio. We did see an improvement, but I cannot stand over its efficacy as I don't know the long-term benefits. I do believe that everything is worth a try as long as it makes sense and you can justify the benefits in your own mind.

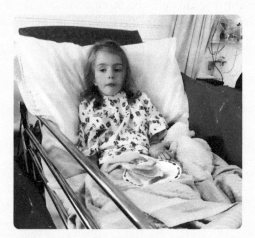

Ally after her Botox procedure.

Phenol injection

Phenol is another medication delivered by injection. It was used as a treatment for spasticity for many decades before the advent of BoNT-A. Phenol is injected directly around the motor nerve,* causing a breakdown of the insulation around the nerve, which prevents it from sending messages to the muscle. (Note that phenol is injected around the nerve, whereas BoNT-A is injected into the muscle.) Treatment with phenol is normally done under general anesthesia to minimize both discomfort for the patient and movement during the injection process. Usually, two to four muscle groups are injected in a single session.

Side effects of phenol may include paresthesia (a pins-and-needles or burning sensation if sensory nerves are affected instead of just the motor nerves) and weakness. The paresthesia may last a few weeks and is treated with gabapentin. The weakness usually resolves within two to four weeks. Again, no overnight hospital stay is typically necessary.

The effects of phenol generally last 3 to 12 months. Repeated injections can lead to a cumulative effect, meaning longer than one year,[229] but this is not common.

The use of phenol differs around the world. It has become less popular for a number of reasons, including the advent of BoNT-A.[229] Sometimes it is used in conjunction with BoNT-A because it allows more muscles to be treated without exceeding the dosage recommendations for either medication.[203] Some centers may use other alcohols in addition to phenol.

There is only one study of phenol use in CP,[14] which points to the lack of research evidence, but clinical expertise supports its use.

---

* A nerve that sends signals away from the brain and spinal cord to a muscle; contrast with a sensory nerve, which sends signals (about temperature, pain, touch, etc.) from all parts of the body to the spinal cord and brain.

Intrathecal baclofen

Intrathecal baclofen (ITB) is another method for delivering the medication baclofen as a tone-reducing treatment for both spasticity and dystonia. It is generally better at reducing tone in the lower extremities than the upper extremities.[242]

The following is an explanation of each term:

- **Intrathecal:** "Intra" means "within," and the "theca" is the sheath enclosing the spinal cord. The intrathecal area is the fluid-filled space surrounding the spinal cord; cerebrospinal fluid flows through this area, bathing and protecting the spinal cord.
- **Baclofen:** The name of the medication.

With ITB, a pump stores and delivers baclofen directly to the cerebrospinal fluid in the intrathecal space. Implanting an ITB pump is a surgical procedure. The pump is filled with baclofen and inserted under the skin and its soft tissue layer, typically in the abdomen. A catheter (a narrow, flexible tube) is connected to the pump and routed under the skin and its soft tissue layer to the patient's back. Surgeons make an incision to thread and position the tip of the catheter in the intrathecal space, where it delivers the baclofen directly to the cerebrospinal fluid. The pump is programmed to slowly release baclofen either in a consistent dose or in bursts of medication over a 24-hour period, depending on which method best helps the individual's high tone.[243] See Figure 3.7.1.

Delivering baclofen directly into the cerebrospinal fluid is much more effective and requires a much lower dose (about one-thousandth of the oral dose). It can help avoid or minimize side effects that individuals may experience when taking oral baclofen such as dizziness and drowsiness.

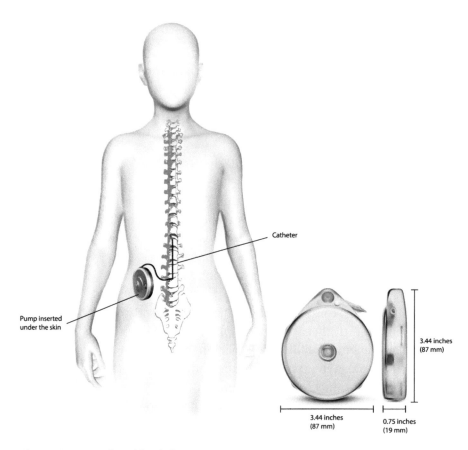

Catheter

Pump inserted under the skin

3.44 inches (87 mm)

3.44 inches (87 mm)

0.75 inches (19 mm)

Figure 3.7.1 Intrathecal baclofen.

Implanting an ITB pump usually requires a hospital stay, typically five to seven days. It is important for the patient to lie flat for up to three days afterwards to allow the surgical site to heal and avoid spinal fluid from leaking. The patient wears an abdominal binder for six to eight weeks afterward to support the pump and prevent swelling.[243] The pump has to be refilled with baclofen about every three to four months, on average, in an outpatient clinic. The pump runs on a battery that has limited life, requiring the pump to be surgically removed and replaced after about seven years. This can usually be done with an overnight hospital stay.

Research supports the use of ITB for reduced spasticity and/or dystonia and other outcomes (green and yellow lights).[14]

Selective dorsal rhizotomy

Selective dorsal rhizotomy (SDR) is a neurosurgical procedure that reduces spasticity by selectively cutting abnormal sensory nerve rootlets[*] in the spinal cord. SDR reduces spasticity only, not other types of high tone. It is an irreversible tone-reducing treatment. The following is an explanation of each word in the full term:

- **Selective:** Only certain abnormal nerve rootlets are cut.
- **Dorsal:** "Dorsal" refers to the sensory nerve rootlets. (They are termed "dorsal" because they are located toward the back of the body. The motor nerve rootlets are termed "ventral" because they are toward the front.)
- **Rhizotomy:** "Rhizo" means "root," and "otomy" means "to cut into."

Putting it all together, "selective dorsal rhizotomy" means that certain abnormal, sensory nerve rootlets are cut to diminish the overactive reflex loop causing spasticity.

SDR involves removing the back of the vertebrae (the lamina) to access the spinal cord. This is called a "laminectomy." During the operation, the sensory (dorsal) nerve roots are dissected into their individual rootlets. The rootlets are then individually electrically stimulated to determine whether they trigger a normal or abnormal (spastic) response. If a rootlet triggers an abnormal response, it is cut. If not, it is left alone. The percentage of rootlets cut varies among medical centers.[244] At Gillette Children's, the percentage of rootlets cut during SDR is lower than what is typically reported in the literature. If too high a percentage of rootlets are cut, there is greater risk of inducing weakness.

While SDR is more commonly performed in children with spastic diplegia, and studies support its use for reduced spasticity and improved gait (green light),[14] it can also be performed on children with hemiplegia who meet selection criteria.

More information on SDR is included in Appendix 5 (online).

---

[*] Think of a stick of string cheese, or a telephone cable with many smaller wires together in it. The nerve root is the whole cheese stick, or the whole telephone cable, and the smaller cheese strings or wires within the cable are the rootlets.

Choosing the tone-reducing treatment

No one treatment meets every child's needs, which is why a range of tone-reducing treatments exist. Tone reduction to manage spasticity (and dystonia, if present) is tailored to the individual child's needs. Which treatment will be recommended depends on many factors, including age, GMFCS level, degree to which the tone interferes with function, and type of high tone. A child may receive different treatments as they grow. Though the use of tone reduction peaks in early childhood, it can continue into adolescence and adulthood.

Some tone-reducing treatments are available only at specialist centers. To be able to choose the most appropriate treatment for each individual child, access to the specialist center is needed to supplement what is available locally.

Finally, note that as with all areas in the management and treatment of CP, best practice may change as more research emerges.

Orthopedic surgery

He jests at scars that never felt a wound.
William Shakespeare

Single-event multilevel surgery (SEMLS) involves multiple orthopedic surgical procedures performed during a single operation. The goals are for the surgeon to identify and correct all the muscle and bone problems in the same surgery to avoid multiple hospital admissions, repeated anesthesia, and multiple rehabilitations. SEMLS is now considered best practice for orthopedic surgery in CP.[129]

This section addresses both upper limb and lower limb orthopedic surgery in children and adolescents with hemiplegia GMFCS levels I and II. SEMLS is more frequently needed for the lower rather than the upper limb. It may be possible to combine upper and lower limb orthopedic surgery, but several factors must be considered, including:

- Optimum timing for each does not always coincide.
- Following surgery, function takes time to recover. A reduction in function (albeit temporary) in both the arm and leg on the affected side could leave the child or adolescent unsafe for navigating their

environment with greater postoperative care and rehabilitation challenges (e.g., if both upper and lower limb are in casts).

- Treatment needs to be coordinated if two areas of the body are operated on. Surgeons in CP usually specialize in either upper or lower limb surgery, not both, so different specialists need to be coordinated. This is possible at some specialist centers but is not always logistically possible. An example of where coordinating treatment is necessary is that arm swing is an integral part of gait, and elbow contracture can contribute to abnormal gait in the individual with hemiplegia.
- Similar coordination is needed for rehabilitation, as occupational therapists largely look after the upper limb while physical therapists look after the lower limb.

Orthopedic surgery can involve soft tissue and bone surgery.

Soft tissue surgery can include:

- **Tendon release:** Severing the tendon of a contracted muscle to allow for a greater range of motion of the joint. Once the tendon is severed, the function of the muscle is markedly diminished, which therefore decreases the problematic pull of the muscle.
- **Tendon transfer:** Reattaching the tendon at a different point to change the function of the muscle. For example, a muscle that behaved as a joint flexor, when transferred, could become a joint extensor. The goal is to improve the balance of muscles around a joint.
- **Muscle and/or tendon lengthening:** Lengthening the muscle and/or tendon, though not releasing the tendon entirely, allowing for continued action of that muscle.
- **Muscle recession:** Dividing the sheet of tissue where the muscle ends and the tendon begins. This is most commonly done in the calf, with the sheet of tissue of the gastrocnemius being separated from a similar sheet for the soleus (as they come together at their common Achilles tendon) and only the gastrocnemius tissue (the two-joint muscle) being divided.

It is important to note that with tendon release or muscle and/or tendon lengthening surgery, variable degrees of weakness occur, and with further growth, the contracture may recur.

Bone surgery can include:

- **Osteotomy:** Surgical cutting of a bone
- **Fusion:** Permanently joining two or more bones to eliminate joint movement and provide stability, also termed "arthrodesis"

Upper limb orthopedic surgery

The goals of upper limb orthopedic surgery include improving upper limb function and positioning to facilitate gait and enhance self-image or ease of daily cares.* For example, surgery may improve reach, grasp, release, or pinch, all of which help with functional tasks. It's important that the individual, family, and the multidisciplinary team agree on realistic goals, taking into account the child's present level of function, and understanding that while surgery may improve it, it will not restore full hand function.

Evaluation for upper limb surgery at Gillette Children's includes the following:

- Medical history
- Physical examination, which involves both a motor and sensory evaluation including, for example, active and passive range of motion, presence of spasticity, dystonia, contractures, selective motor control, muscle strength, and sensory deficits
- Functional questionnaire (e.g., House upper limb functional use scale)
- Parent-reported functional questionnaires for children (self-reported by older individuals where possible)
- Evaluation of arm and hand movement, which can be done by videotaping and then review; for example:
  - The SHUEE or Melbourne videotape assessment.†

---

* Daily activities such as dressing, feeding, toileting, and cutting nails, completed by the individual themselves, or supported by a caregiver.

† The SHUEE (Shriners Hospital Upper Extremity Evaluation) videotapes upper extremity function (e.g., position, grasp, and release). The Melbourne videotape assessment is similar.

- o Motion analysis: two-dimensional* video combined with electromyography (EMG) in real time. EMG measures the activity
  of muscles. Measurement is taken while the child performs functional tasks. This is normally completed in a motion analysis
  laboratory.†
- X-rays of the joints or limbs, sometimes to assess growth plate status

Once a full evaluation is done, a customized treatment plan is developed.
Several surgical procedures are commonly necessary for the affected
upper limb, and they are normally carried out together in a SEMLS.

Typical procedures at the shoulder, elbow, forearm, wrist, hand, thumb,
or finger level may include:

- Soft tissue surgery (tendon release, tendon transfer, muscle lengthening)
- Bone or joint (osteotomy or fusion)
- Neurectomy (severing of a nerve, partial or complete)

Common upper limb abnormalities and their appropriate surgeries
include:

- Elbow flexion: surgical lengthening or release of elbow flexor muscles
- Forearm pronation: surgical release of pronator teres muscle
- Wrist flexion:
  - o Surgical release or lengthening of wrist flexor muscles
  - o Tendon transfers of wrist flexor muscles to wrist extension
  - o Wrist fusion (usually adult with fixed contracture)
- Thumb in palm and finger flexion: surgical lengthening or release of
  muscles, with possible tendon transfer

Rehabilitation after surgery may involve casting, orthoses/splinting,
and therapy to maximize results.

A comparison of the preoperative and postoperative scores on the
House upper limb functional use scale in 85 individuals with hemiplegia who had upper limb surgery showed an average improvement of 2.7
functional levels.[245] For example, this would mean that hand function

---

* Front and side views.

† Note that upper extremity motion analysis varies among centers.

improved from a good passive assist (can hold object and stabilize it for use by other hand) into hand function as a good active assist (can actively grasp object and manipulate it). Smitherman and colleagues reported satisfaction with both functional and cosmetic outcomes in children with hemiplegia who had SEMLS.[246] Van Heest and colleagues reported that tendon transfers, especially for wrist extension, can be beneficial in improving upper extremity joint positioning in children with spastic hemiplegia. However, residual impairment in hand function can persist.[247]

Subsequent surgery to address changes with growth and development may be necessary if changes occur over time.

Lower limb orthopedic surgery

There are two main peaks in the management of the musculoskeletal problems affecting gait. The first occurs in early childhood, when tone reduction (in conjunction with other treatments such as PT and orthoses) is very important. The second occurs in later childhood (at approximately 8 to 12 years) when orthopedic surgery may be needed to address the secondary problems—the muscle and bone problems that have developed.[193]

Delaying orthopedic surgery allows motor patterns to mature, and by this stage the gains from tone reduction have largely been achieved. Delaying orthopedic surgery is also important because it helps avoid the unpredictable outcomes of early surgery.[229] Orthopedic surgery becomes necessary when the muscle and bone problems (the secondary problems) can no longer be adequately managed by more conservative means, and they are having a significant adverse effect on gait and function.

We now address:

a) **Three-dimensional gait analysis**
b) **Lower limb single-event multilevel surgery (SEMLS)**

a) Three-dimensional gait analysis

Lower limb SEMLS in hemiplegia is guided by computerized three-dimensional (3D) gait analysis,[74,248] which provides detailed information about a person's manner of walking and how far it deviates from typical walking. Computerized 3D gait analysis uses complex technology, some of it the same as what is used in the movie industry, such as in animations and video games. Gait analysis allows treatment to be individualized (i.e., tailored to each individual child), which is important because two children with hemiplegia may walk in a similar manner, but the mechanisms behind their walking may differ. Analyzing those mechanisms allows treatment to be tailored to each individual child. This is why gait analysis prior to SEMLS is so important.

Gait analysis is done for two main reasons:

- To identify all gait deviations and create a problem list. A treatment plan to meet the family's and surgeon's goals can then be devised. This is an example of data-driven decision-making in medicine.[*]
- To help measure the effectiveness of treatment—in other words, to assess the outcome of treatment. This allows for a critical appraisal of the decision-making process and the postoperative period (including rehabilitation) for the individual.

Analyzing gait is a complex process involving many technologies. The precise elements of gait analysis vary slightly between institutions. Gait analysis at Gillette Children's includes the following elements:[†]

- Medical history
- X-rays
- Parent-reported functional questionnaires for children (self-reported for older individuals where possible)
- Two-dimensional video
- Standardized physical examination

---

* Multiple variables are evaluated using multiple measurement tools within gait analysis.

† Some of these elements are also used at other times in the management of hemiplegia, outside of formal gait analysis.

- 3D computerized motion analysis*
  - Kinematics: 3D measurement of motion (movement)
  - Kinetics: 3D measurement of forces and mechanisms that cause motion
- Electromyography (EMG): measurement of the activity of muscles
- Pedobarography: measurement of the pressure distribution under the feet
- Energy expenditure: measurement of the energy used during walking

"Gait analysis," means including 3D computerized motion analysis. It does not mean merely observing gait or gait analysis done with simpler technologies. We acknowledge gait analysis is not universally available.

The key part of gait analysis is 3D computerized motion analysis, which measures gait in three planes simultaneously (hence the term "3D"). The three anatomical planes are illustrated in Figure 3.8.1. They are:

- From back or front: the coronal plane
- From the side: the sagittal plane
- From top or bottom: the transverse plane

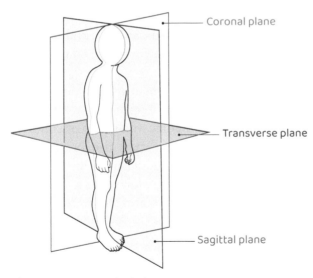

Coronal plane

Transverse plane

Sagittal plane

Figure 3.8.1 Anatomical planes.

---

* 3D computerized motion analysis is the broader term because it includes other forms of motion besides gait, such as upper body motion. However, the terms "3D computerized motion analysis" and "3D computerized gait analysis" can be used interchangeably.

The list of gait deviations is derived from the elements of gait analysis listed above. The information from all these sources provides a complete picture of a person's gait problems. Each source provides critical and unique information. When combined, data from one source can explain findings and/or complement data from another source. Comparing the gait of the individual with CP to a group of individuals with typical gait is very useful because it reveals how far the person's gait deviates from typical gait, as well as which joints are principally affected.

Once all the gait analysis data is collected, a team of professionals interprets all the pieces of data. This may include physicians, physical therapists, and engineers, all of whom have specialized training in this area. The team identifies gait deviations from the gait analysis data, then creates a problem list from which a treatment plan can be devised. It is important to note that gait analysis provides only data; the *interpretation* of that data (i.e., to determine the gait deviations, problem list, and treatment plan) is done by the team of professionals. The family will typically meet their physician at a separate appointment to discuss the results.

Repeat gait analysis after treatment is done to assess the treatment outcome. This closed-loop approach (plan, treat, evaluate) is very important for each individual because it objectively assesses whether the decisions and treatment (data interpretation, treatment plan, SEMLS, and rehabilitation) were effective and provides a new baseline for future comparison.

This closed-loop leads to continuous improvement in the standard of treatment offered by a treatment center over the long term. For example, gait analysis can be used to evaluate the outcome of a group of children who had a particular procedure. Gait analysis may also be repeated many years after a procedure to evaluate the long-term outcome of that particular procedure. These evaluations inform practice at a center. In addition, shared learning and research lead to treatment improvements on a national and international level.

Reasons for referral for gait analysis vary between centers, but a referral is usually made when a person reaches a plateau in their progress and previous treatments are no longer effective. The age at which gait analysis is recommended varies, but it is usually recommended for children above three years of age, when gait is stable. Before age three, children are often too small, they are less able to tolerate the equipment and duration of the testing, and their walking pattern is still changing as it matures. When gait is changing, outcomes are less predictable. The ability to cooperate is also a consideration and is variable. It may remain challenging even in slightly older children.

Further information on gait analysis is included in Appendix 6 (online).

b) Lower limb single-event multilevel surgery (SEMLS)

The four gait patterns[*] observed in individuals with hemiplegia are addressed in section 2.9 (see Table 2.9.3). The number of procedures performed during orthopedic surgery in hemiplegia depend on the gait group number. Typically, they are:

- 0 to 1 procedure for gait pattern group I
- 1 procedure for gait pattern group II
- 3 to 4 procedures for gait pattern group III
- 5 to 7 procedures for gait pattern group IV

Before gait analysis was common, orthopedic surgery for children with CP typically involved carrying out single procedures on a yearly basis followed by intensive rehabilitation. Mercer Rang, an English-born orthopedic surgeon who practiced in Toronto, coined the phrase "birthday syndrome" to refer to this type of orthopedic surgery: the child had an operation each year, followed by rehabilitation for the rest of the year.[249] Thankfully, orthopedic surgery for CP has progressed significantly since those days.

As we have seen, many muscles span more than one joint. Thus, for example, a procedure at the ankle also affects the knee. A procedure at the knee also affects the hip and foot. This is another reason why SEMLS has replaced the "birthday syndrome" approach.

The overall goal of SEMLS is to improve or maintain gait over the long term. Secondary goals may include improvements in gait efficiency,[†]

---

[*] Note these are the *gait patterns* addressed in section 2.9, *not GMFCS levels*.

[†] Gait efficiency can be measured by how much energy is consumed during walking. Think of energy expenditure during walking like the fuel efficiency of a car: a more efficient car will consume less fuel while traveling a set distance.

appearance, gross motor function, independence, and quality of life.[250] Improving gait efficiency might mean that the person doesn't tire as easily while walking, and improving the appearance of walking can have huge effects on self-esteem, particularly during adolescence.

Most care centers have patient education material that describes the different operations and what the individual and family can expect. Gillette Children's has developed a booklet, *All about Your Single-Event Multilevel Surgery (SEMLS)*, that explains possible procedures carried out as part of SEMLS. A link is included in **Useful web resources**.

The following are common **soft tissue surgical** procedures:

- Psoas lengthening
- Adductor lengthening
- Hamstring lengthening
- Rectus femoris transfer
- Calf muscle (gastrocnemius) lengthening/recession
- Achilles tendon Z-lengthening
- Tibialis anterior split transfer
- Posterior tibialis lengthening
- Posterior tibialis split transfer

The following are common **bone surgical** procedures:

- Pelvic osteotomy
- Proximal femoral osteotomy
- Distal femoral extension osteotomy
- Tibial tubercle/patella tendon advancement
- Tibial derotation osteotomy
- Various foot osteotomies and foot arthrodeses

The expectations and goals of the surgeon and the family (both the parent and the child or adolescent) must be aligned and are part of shared decision-making in medical care. A recently developed outcome measure, the Gait Outcomes Assessment List (GOAL) questionnaire (two versions: one for the parent and one for the individual), evaluates family priorities in conjunction with gait-specific functional mobility outcomes.[188,189,190,191] It was developed with direct input from children with CP and their parents. Assessing priorities and goals on an item-by-item basis is useful because it can help the surgeon (or any care provider) understand the family's priorities and expectations and open a discussion about what can or cannot be achieved through surgery and subsequent rehabilitation. Ultimately, this results in a mutual understanding and alignment of goals for the proposed surgery.

Although SEMLS is evidence-based best practice, Vuillermin and colleagues have noted that many orthopedic surgeons still perform single-level surgery because of differences in surgical philosophy as well as the limited availability of 3D gait analysis.[251]

SEMLS is usually followed by an intensive rehabilitation program to gain the maximum benefit from the surgery. The ultimate outcome is the result of the entire "package": the gait analysis–guided surgery planning, the surgical technique, and the postoperative rehabilitation. Family support systems also come into play. Most centers will consider SEMLS only if the child, with their family, is capable of completing the rehabilitation program. As with any orthopedic surgery, the better the rehabilitation, the better the outcome is likely to be.

The hospital stay for SEMLS is about two to four days. Though rehabilitation may begin with a hospital physical therapist, it is usually continued with the child's community physical therapist. Communication between hospital and community physical therapists is very important to ensure a smooth handover of care. Although there is no consensus on optimal rehabilitation post-SEMLS,[252,253] work is being done to achieve this, and protocols have recently been developed.[253,254] Each person who undergoes SEMLS will receive a detailed rehabilitation program; the program will vary depending on the procedures carried out during the surgery. Information on rehabilitation after SEMLS at Gillette Children's is included in Appendix 7 (online).

If implants (plates and/or screws inserted during surgery) are used in SEMLS, they may need to be removed approximately one year after surgery. The recovery from implant removal is minimal and often the procedure does not require a hospital stay or any additional rehabilitation.

Following SEMLS, it typically takes nine months to a year for the child to return to their presurgical level of function (or longer, depending on age and other factors). Thus, full recovery following SEMLS can take up to one year, and the full benefit of surgery may not be seen for up to two years. Recovery is often longer in adolescents and adults compared to children. Short-term outcome, after SEMLS including gait analysis, is generally assessed when recovery is complete or nearly so (again, generally about one year after surgery).

Though SEMLS is a major undertaking, it should not be seen as an end point. It is just a treatment along the journey to adulthood for the child or adolescent with hemiplegia. SEMLS cannot alter the primary problems (the underlying cause of impaired bone and muscle growth), and a gradual recurrence of some muscle and bone problems may occur post-SEMLS. Until the body reaches skeletal maturity, it is important to keep muscle growth at pace with continuing bone growth through activity, episodes of physical therapy, and consultation to update the home program. Puberty is a period of very active bone growth, so stretching and strengthening are as important in the years after SEMLS as they are in the years before.

Overall, there is good evidence supporting SEMLS.[252,255,256,257] Schranz and colleagues found that children with hemiplegia benefit from SEMLS and maintain gait improvements over the long term (the last evaluation was 10 years post-SEMLS).[256]

It must be emphasized that SEMLS reduces, but does not eliminate, the possible need for further surgeries. Schranz and colleagues reported that further surgery was required for 36 percent of children with hemiplegia.[256] Dreher and colleagues suggested the term "SEMLS" might be misleading because of the possibility of further surgery; they suggested removing "single-event" from the term and using "multilevel surgery (MLS)" for the initial surgery.[258] Regardless of the term used, the initial surgery is designed to correct muscle and bone problems in one surgical event. If further muscle and bone problems arise during subsequent adolescent growth, then further surgery may be required.

Finally, one surgery that may be required outside of SEMLS is to address limb-length discrepancy. Limb-length discrepancy is usually treated when the difference in length is greater than 2.5 centimeters (1 inch)[138] and is best done before skeletal growth is complete; thus, the timing of this surgery is very important. The aim is to arrive at skeletal maturity (i.e., when bone growth is complete) with the length of the two lower limbs equal or nearly so. The procedure is called "epiphysiodesis," describing where a growth plate (epiphysis, see Figure 2.7.1) in a long bone of the longer limb (the longer leg) is intentionally interfered with to slow or stop its growth and to allow the shorter limb to catch up. Planning this surgery involves measuring remaining growth in both limbs, balancing remaining growth with current difference in limb lengths, and then extrapolating to the future to plan the correct time to do the surgery. Note that equalizing limb length through use of an external fixator[*] to promote growth of the affected, shorter leg is not recommended for individuals with spastic CP.[259,260]

Ally had SEML surgery in Minnesota in July 2023 when she was 11 years old. It was a difficult decision to agree to the surgery, but we had great recommendations and support from other parents who had taken this road, and the medical team was incredibly reassuring.

We were immediately struck by the professionalism of the hospital staff. It was wonderful for Ally to see other kids with similar issues to hers, and to see them at various stages before and after surgery.

Ally was in hospital for three days and had the following procedures:

1. Right os calcis lengthening
2. Right first cuneiform plantarflexion osteotomy
3. Right calcaneal tuberosity medialization
4. Right tibial derotational osteotomy
5. Right Baumenn gastrocnemius lengthening

After the surgery, we stayed in Minnesota for two weeks while Ally recovered. The hospital managed pain relief and her comfort really well, and happily we found lovely accommodation nearby.

Ally used a wheelchair for eight weeks post-surgery, and so we had to navigate two airports and two planes home to Ireland during that period. We returned to Minnesota in September 2023 (eight weeks after

---

[*] An external fixator in limb lengthening surgery is a device attached to the outside of the limb to gradually extend bone segments, aiding in bone regeneration and ultimately increasing limb length.

surgery) to get the cast removed and to begin the intense and hugely impressive program of rehabilitation physiotherapy over the course of a further two weeks.

It was an unbelievable surgery and has really improved Ally's foot and gait. It was a significant day for us when Ally cycled for the first time since having the surgery; she was totally convinced that she was on an electric bike as it was so easy to cycle! It was the first time in her life that her leg was at the correct angle to make turning the pedal easy. I think that says it all; if you can make turning the pedal easier for a child with CP, you will have achieved a lot!

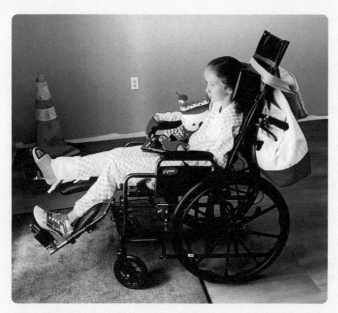

Ally in her wheelchair post-surgery.

Managing associated problems

The purpose of life is to live it,
to taste experience to the utmost,
to reach out eagerly and without fear
for newer and richer experience.
Eleanor Roosevelt

Hemiplegia affects the upper and lower limbs of one side of the body, and the upper limb is usually more affected than the lower limb. We saw in sections 2.1 and 2.10 that a proportion of children with hemiplegia (all GMFCS levels) had some associated problems. The management of each of these challenges needs to be addressed as part of the multidisciplinary care of the child and adolescent with hemiplegia. These problems, if present and unaddressed or inadequately addressed, may reduce participation far more than their limb problems.

- **Speech, language and communication, and feeding:** The management of speech, language and communication, and feeding was addressed in section 3.4.
- **Sensation:** Sensory problems are primary problems and are more difficult to remediate. Early intervention that taps into neuroplasticity

can help. A study by Peterson and colleagues found that stereognosis (inability to identify an object by feeling it) remained unchanged following operative and nonoperative treatments.[261] However, Auld and colleagues found that a single session of mirror-based tactile and motor training improved tactile perception.[262] Similarly, positive results with sensation training were reported in a further study.[263]

- **Vision:** For those with vision challenges, an early referral to a pediatric ophthalmologist and regular follow-up is important. Pediatric ophthalmologists specialize in concerns related to vision and eye health for children. These specialists are medical doctors. An optometrist can evaluate for some concerns with vision, but they are not trained to do surgery on the eyes. Vision development is rapid from birth to age six, but visual acuity (sharpness) can continue to change throughout life. If any concerns are noted, annual follow-up with pediatric ophthalmology is recommended.

- **Hearing:** Early screening for hearing loss should be done, as hearing loss can impact the development of speech, language, and communication, and cognition. Hearing loss can be difficult to evaluate in an individual with cognitive problems; however, specialized testing is available for those unable to recognize and reliably respond to sounds. Early referral to an audiologist, an otolaryngologist (a physician specializing in ear, nose, and throat, or ENT), and a speech-language pathologist is recommended if there is any hearing loss. Regular follow-up will be necessary. As with vision, once hearing problems are identified, supports can be determined for the child to enjoy maximum participation.

- **Epilepsy:** For those with epilepsy, regular and routine evaluation and follow-up with pediatric neurology is imperative as untreated epilepsy has the potential to slow or cause regression in development. Furthermore, although seizures are often thought of as being obvious abnormal movements that persist and are therefore unmistakable as epilepsy, seizures can be very quiet and challenging to identify, or even occur without any outward signs. Close surveillance by neurology specialists is required if there are any concerns related to seizure activity. Intervening to address seizure activity can allow the child to make significant gains in their development once the abnormal brain activity has been stopped. More information on epilepsy management is included in Appendix 8 (online).

- **Pain:** Because pain is prevalent in CP, the presence of pain should be closely monitored and addressed throughout childhood and adolescence. Early recognition of pain is important because pain in children with CP significantly reduces quality of life and is connected to mental health.[150] When pain is severe and prolonged, involving a specialist in pain should be considered. Pain specialists focus on alleviating pain using a multimodal approach, frequently combining nonmedication modalities with medications to maximize relief and improve comfort. It is important to support children with language about pain (e.g., how to describe pain) and how to advocate for their needs, not just accept that their pain is normal.

- **Nutrition and hydration:** Good nutrition and hydration are as important for the child and adolescent with hemiplegia as they are for their peers. No special diet is needed so long as they are eating a nutritious, balanced diet. Parents are encouraged to get advice on this if necessary; the whole family might benefit. One area affected by nutrition is bone health. As shown in section 2.7, there is some evidence of lower bone mineral density in ambulatory children (and adults) with CP GMFCS level II.[264] To promote optimum bone health throughout life, good nutrition, ensuring no deficiencies in calcium and vitamin D, and physical activity, especially weight-bearing or impact activities, can help promote good bone health.[265] It is also worth noting that some medications, for example, antiseizure medications and steroids, may contribute to lower bone mineral density. Weight management is also important; it's important for everyone, but even more so for people with hemiplegia because muscle strength is already compromised, and excess weight can limit walking.[266] Good eating habits start early in life, and children are much more likely to have good habits if their parents do. The influence of parents can have an impact long after the child has left home. It is never too late to recognize unhealthy eating habits and make the decision to change.

- **Constipation:** Constipation should be closely monitored throughout childhood and adolescence and addressed if present. It can contribute to pain and can complicate toilet training and contribute to urinary incontinence.

- **Sleep:** Because one-third of ambulatory children with CP have disturbed sleep[147] and sleep is required for good daytime function and development, sleep quality should be closely monitored throughout childhood and adolescence, and any problems should be addressed. A healthy nighttime routine is encouraged to promote good sleep. This includes limiting screen time (no screens 60 minutes before bedtime) and keeping screens and other distractions out of the bedroom. Choosing a regular bedtime that allows for adequate sleep through the night, and sticking to it nightly, promotes healthy sleep patterns. These efforts are collectively referred to as "sleep hygiene." If the child is having trouble falling asleep or staying asleep despite good sleep hygiene, their physician should be consulted.

- **Cognition:** One-third of children with hemiplegia have some level of intellectual challenge,[79] so close attention should be paid to how well the child is learning from very early in life. By the time the child is preparing to move into kindergarten, elementary, or primary school, definitive neuropsychological testing* may be considered. This formal evaluation of the brain's processing of information allows the child, the family, and the school team to identify where there may be challenges in learning, and to gain understanding of how the child learns best. This allows for the teaching team to adapt the learning environment to maximize the child's ability for success. Adequate support in school needs to be addressed both from a cognitive and social perspective. The earlier challenges can be identified, the sooner the child can receive support services to maximize their function. The wider aspects of education are addressed in section 3.11.

- **Sexual relationships:** This is an area where both the family and professional team can support the adolescent with CP. Despite data showing that young adults with CP may experience problems with sexual relationships, 90 percent reported not having discussed the topic with health care professionals.[155] Health care professionals need to be proactive to inform young people with CP about sexual relationships to prevent sexual difficulties and to treat problems if they arise.[155]

- **Mental and behavioral health:** Mental and behavioral health symptoms and disorders are common in children and adolescents with CP.[158,159,160] Evaluations for mental and behavioral health should be incorporated into multidisciplinary assessments for individuals with CP, and appropriate treatments prescribed. Treatments for mental and behavioral health disorders are similar to those for typically developing children and adolescents and may include behavioral

---

* Neuropsychological testing helps evaluate broad areas of cognitive function; for example, intelligence, language, visuospatial function, executive function, attention, memory and processing speed. These areas frequently work in collaboration for efficient cognitive functioning.

therapy, psychotherapy, and medications.[163] Parenting programs that help parents manage challenging behavior may be of help. There is evidence supporting the Stepping Stones Triple P program for improving child behavior and reducing parental stress (green light).[14] This program, specifically for parents of preadolescent children who have a disability, is available online, and a link to its website is included in **Useful web resources.**

Alternative and complementary treatments

It is possible in medicine, even when you intend to do good, to do harm instead. That is why science thrives on actively encouraging criticism rather than stifling it.

Richard Dawkins

Alternative (as a substitute) and complementary (in addition to) treatments are treatments that are not part of current standard conventional medical or rehabilitation treatments and care.[267]

Parents want only the best for their children, and for a number of reasons they may consider alternative and complementary treatments. These reasons can include:

- Hearing about a treatment option in the media (Internet, radio, TV, newspapers, magazines) or from well-meaning family and friends
- Wanting to try all treatment options in case the one they haven't tried is the one that works
- Wanting to complement or increase the effectiveness of present treatment

- Wanting to relieve symptoms (such as pain)
- Believing their child can do better

Often, alternative and complementary treatments are expensive. If the parent-professional relationship is good, parents should be able to discuss them with the medical professionals who treat their child. Both parents and professionals should be guided by the best research evidence available, which is the very principle that has guided the writing of this book.

Table 3.10.1 lists a number of common alternative and complementary treatments.

Table 3.10.1 Alternative and complementary treatments

TREATMENT	DESCRIPTION	EVIDENCE (OR LACK OF) SUPPORTING TREATMENT IN CP
Hyperbaric oxygen	The person inhales 100 percent oxygen in a pressurized hyperbaric chamber. The theory behind its use in CP is that there are inactive cells among the damaged brain cells that have the potential to recover.	Strong recommendation against its use for all purposes (red light).[*][14]
Massage	Involves applying pressure to muscles, generally using the hands, to relieve pain and tension.	Green light for improved passage of stool frequency. Yellow light for other purposes.[14]
Osteopathy (including cranial sacral osteopathy)	Treatment through the manipulation and massage of the skeleton and muscles. Cranial sacral osteopathy focuses on the cranium (bones of the skull) and sacrum (the five fused vertebrae that connect the spine to the pelvis).	Strong recommendation against its use (red light) for improved gross motor function. Yellow light for reduced constipation and improved sleep.[14]
Acupuncture	Thin needles are inserted into the skin at specific points.	Yellow light for improved gross motor function and reduced spasticity.[14]

* See section 3.3 for explanation of traffic light system.[14]   *Cont'd.*

TREATMENT	DESCRIPTION	EVIDENCE (OR LACK OF) SUPPORTING TREATMENT IN CP
Reflexology	Massage based on the theory that there are reflex points on the feet, hands, and head linked to every part of the body.	Yellow light for reduced spasticity, improved gross motor function, and reduced constipation.[14]
Yoga	A practice that includes specific body postures, breath control and meditation.	Yellow light for multiple outcomes.[14]

Novak and colleagues' summary of the state of the evidence as of 2019 for interventions for children with CP (including further alternative and complementary treatments)[14] is included in **Useful web resources.**

A Canadian study looked at the extent to which adolescents with CP across all five GMFCS levels had used alternative and complementary treatments in the previous year. The most commonly used were massage (15 percent), hyperbaric oxygen (10 percent), and osteopathy (6 percent), but most of those surveyed (73 percent) did not currently use any.[267]

Graham noted that many parents delay or refuse conventional treatments because they have unrealistic expectations of other unproven treatments. For example, although Australia has an efficient hip surveillance program, the most common cause of a dislocated hip in a child with CP is delayed intervention because they have heard that stem cell treatment* may cure the child.[268]

Parents cannot afford to abandon conventional treatments with their evidence base for any unproven treatment, nor should they delay care that is currently available for their child, anticipating that a better option is "around the corner." As treatments are studied and when they are identified as potentially helpful, good physicians will be aware of the developing research and will share with families if any new options are on the horizon.

---

* An alternative treatment that may potentially replace damaged nerve cells and support remaining ones in the brain.

Community integration, education, independence, and transition

The Child is Father of the Man.

William Wordsworth

Going through the normal changes of puberty, graduating from high school, choosing the next life stage, leaving home, assuming responsibility for one's own health care, and transitioning from the familiar and more organized setting of children's health services to the unfamiliar and more fragmented adult services—putting it all together, there is a lot going on packed into a short amount of time in the life of a child and adolescent with hemiplegia.

A study of older adolescents with CP (age 18 to 20) defined success in life as being happy. Three key psychosocial factors related to this success were being believed in, believing in oneself, and being accepted by others (a sense of belonging).[269] The seeds of these factors are sown early in life, and parents do the sowing—through supporting community integration, education, independence, and transition.

Drs. Rosenbaum and Rosenbloom give some excellent advice to parents to take the long view when it comes to the life of the child with CP and supporting them into adulthood:[8]

> *We encourage [parents] to take a long-term view of their child's journey through childhood. We remind them that the adult world imposes on all children the expectation (at least in school) that they try to perform in a wide range of areas. Adults expect children to learn and hopefully demonstrate skills in many activities—be they social, physical, intellectual, artistic—that are much more demanding than what the adults ever expect of themselves, or even perform, on a day-to-day basis ... [Parents] can help their children weather the childhood years with these many and varied demands (demands which often challenge many children without disabilities) ... in the course of their developing years, to develop competencies, interests, and a sense of self-confidence despite their "disabilities," because after the childhood years they will have many more opportunities to find their niche in life.*

Community integration

The diagnosis of CP typically occurs early in life when the nuclear family—parents and siblings—play a large part in the infant's life. However, as the child grows, their social circle expands. It is important for all children, regardless of disability, to be integrated into their communities. In section 1.8, we addressed the ICF framework, which provides an understanding of how a health condition affects individuals across various levels and their interconnectedness. This framework underscores the importance of considering the broader context in which a person with a disability exists, aiming for their full participation in the community. Both environmental and personal factors exert influence at every level within the framework.

When a child is diagnosed with a disability, especially one that is unpredictable, the parents can spend a lot of time at appointments and really trying to "fix" their child. That was highlighted in a movie I watched a number of years ago, *Wonder*, about a boy who has a rare facial abnormality, and the parents spend a lot of time and attention on him.

While this attention is often warranted when you have a child affected by a disability, I feel that parents have to be careful to remember their other children who also have their own emotional needs and unique challenges. It is often easy to rely too much on the unaffected sibling or not recognize, without any malintent, if they are struggling, too. They often spend a lot of time listening to their sibling's development stories as well as waiting in the car outside physio clinics. Even though those experiences will likely help them to be empathetic and patient adults, they too are children and need significant support.

It is important to also accept the disability as a parent, and even though we do everything in our power to support our children, we will not necessarily fix them. Their disability is part of who they are, but does not define them; we all must live with it while remembering the importance of everyone else in the family.

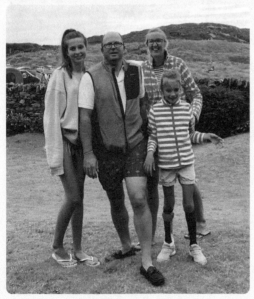

Our family (right to left) Milly, Alec, Ally, and Eimear.

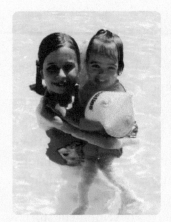

Milly and her sister Ally.

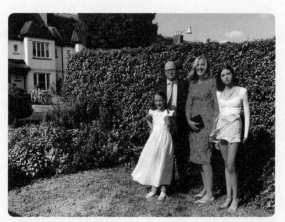

Ally's communion day.

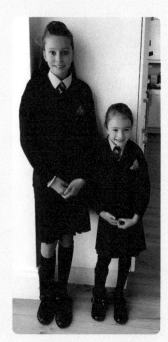

Milly with Ally on her first day at school.

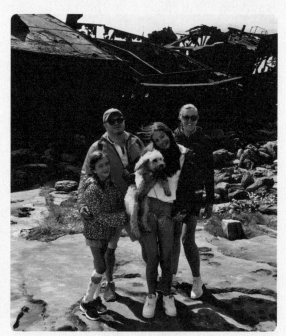

Our family on holiday.

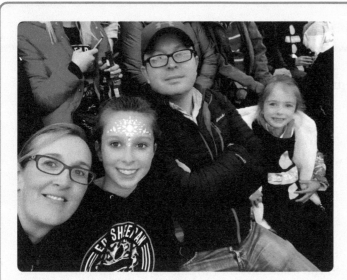

Our family at an Ed Sheeran concert.

It is important to recognize that having a disability does not define a person, whether they are a child, adolescent, or adult. The family's perception and treatment of a child with a disability are critical, as they set the tone for how others, including extended family, friends, and teachers, will view and interact with the child. It is essential for the family to avoid perceiving the child as more limited than they actually are and, rather, foster an environment that encourages the child's full potential. A simple way to check yourself on this is to think about how you, the parent, assign chores and responsibilities to a typically developing child and then modify that task as needed and assign it to the child with CP. This supports their active role in the family and later independence.

Self-determination refers to a person's ability to act as their own primary decision-maker. Independent of cognitive level, young adults with disabilities who demonstrate increased levels of self-determination have been found to fare better across multiple life categories, including employment, access to health care and other benefits, financial independence, and independent living.[270] It is also useful to instill an aptitude for self-advocacy—the ability to represent oneself or one's views or interests.

I think it is extremely difficult to tell your child that they have cerebral palsy. We have always tried to be very honest and open with Ally from a young age and speak about it openly, but it is often challenging when confronted with questions from the public, so having a stock answer is helpful.

People regularly ask Ally what is "wrong" with her leg. She sometimes struggles with this, as do we, which contributes to Ally's reluctance to wear her AFO. Some parents we know choose not to use the term "cerebral palsy" and just say their child is affected by a stiff leg, etc.

I don't believe there is a right way or wrong way of dealing with this, or if there is, I'm not aware of it. I do wish that I had received support on how to deal with the questions and ultimately help Ally do so too. Recently, she has come to me saying she is struggling with the questions being asked at school about her leg and her need for an AFO.

As social beings, humans require social connections for optimal mental health and well-being throughout their lives. Building strong social connections is crucial, and any factors that enhance social connectedness are valuable. Engaging in exercise and physical activities can be an excellent means to promote community integration. These activities can be pursued with the family and alongside nondisabled friends in informal settings rather than in therapy settings. In fact, the child's need for physical exercise can motivate the entire family to become more active. Choosing activities that are enjoyable for both the child and the family increases the likelihood that everyone will stick with it.

Tom Shakespeare, a prominent disability rights activist in the UK, argues that social barriers often pose more significant challenges than the impairments themselves. These barriers include lack of access and negative attitudes.

Education

Damiano considered physical activity to be very important in CP—titling a paper "Activity, Activity, Activity: Rethinking Our Physical Therapy Approach to Cerebral Palsy."[271] A further mantra could be "Education,

Education, Education." A person with a physical challenge is less likely to choose employment in a role requiring significant physical prowess; they will more likely rely on other skills. It is important to maximize the child's intellectual abilities to maximize their opportunities for employment and their participation in all aspects of life. A good education is important for every child—indeed, education is included in the United Nations Convention on the Rights of the Child.[272]And a good education is needed to open doors to different careers. Today, the range of career options available to people with hemiplegia is large; their disability places only a small limit on their choice.

Given that teachers have such a profound influence on the lives of their students, parents should speak with their child's teacher to ensure they understand both the child's abilities and their challenges. This is not a one-off conversation—as the child progresses through school, teachers change. If the student has multiple teachers, talking with a key staff member may work best.

We saw in section 2.1 that most children with hemiplegia across all GMFCS levels have no intellectual problems; however, 22 percent have mild or probable problems, and 11 percent have moderate to severe intellectual problems.[79] Careful planning at each stage of school is needed to maximize the school experience of children and adolescents with intellectual problems. This will ensure sufficient accommodations are made to ease transitions and optimize the child's opportunity for a good school experience and education.

Health care professionals can be a good resource for planning ahead and problem-solving if or when challenges arise. Practicing skills that might be needed in the next phase of life at home with time, supervision, and someone with whom to problem-solve is highly beneficial, both for activity completion and to boost the child's self-confidence. One example is practicing dressing skills for changing in the locker room.

Regrettably, school bullying continues to affect significant numbers of children and adolescents, and those with disabilities are at higher risk.[273] One study found that children and adolescents with CP experienced bullying and social exclusion at school.[161] Strategies suggested by the children and adolescents to help improve social inclusion at school include:[274]

- Creating awareness of their disability by disclosing their condition to peers and teachers (with the suggestion that health care professionals could help with this)
- Being vocal about incidents of bullying and exclusion (to peers, teachers, and parents)
- Building quality friendships as an effective peer support network

They also emphasized the importance of teachers paying close attention to the needs of students with disabilities. A student teacher who has mild CP created the following excellent tip sheet for teachers of students with mild CP.[275] (A link to the full paper is included in **Useful web resources.**)

- There are varying forms of CP. CP can involve just physical symptoms, but it may be accompanied by intellectual or learning disabilities.
- Many students have surgery when young and may be in casts or use wheelchairs following surgery and will need extra support during this time.
- Students may become fatigued due to the extra physical strain involved in carrying out everyday tasks, such as writing, walking, or playing at recess.
- Most students experience pain at some point in the day, although they will be used to it and may not mention it.
- Most students with CP want to be treated like other students, so they may not ask for help when they need it.
- Most students with mild CP do not want attention drawn to them because of their disability.
- Teachers should be attentive to students' hesitation to participate in physical activities they may feel uncomfortable with.
- Teachers should intervene when young children ask questions that appear insensitive or call children with CP inappropriate names.
- When students talk about their CP, do not express sympathy; it is a part of who they are.

Social support for children struggling to connect with their peers may be available through the child's school team. Assertively pursuing these connections for the child who is struggling is imperative so that they may feel integrated into their social school environment. Social engagement goals could also be built into occupational and speech therapy.

Change is the one constant in life. Transitions are a big step for any child, and they keep coming: from home to daycare, to preschool, to elementary school, middle school, high school, and on to college, higher education, or work. Transitions can be more challenging for the child with CP because of, for example, difficulties with mobility or difficulties participating in some activities at school.

Independence

When does adolescence actually begin? The World Health Organization defines adolescence as the period between 10 and 19 years of age. The great majority of adolescents are, therefore, included in the age-based definition of the child adopted by the UN Convention on the Rights of the Child, which defines a child as a person under age 18.[272] Adolescence can thus be viewed as that vaguely defined period between childhood and adulthood. The adolescent is gaining independence from the parent but is not yet there.

For children with moderate to severe intellectual problems, independence in adulthood may not be a realistic goal. Questions such as legal guardianship, supported living arrangements, and shared decision-making will need to be considered. For where independence is a realistic goal, there are points to consider.

Parents play a huge role in the life of their child, and assuming the child achieves independence, a much smaller role in the life of their adult son or daughter. At some point in adolescence, we parents must try to facilitate this change. This is a change for both the parent and the adolescent, and it ideally happens gradually, over time. Indeed, increasing independence ought to begin early in childhood: we need to be preparing for this separation from the cradle.

The parent has to learn to cut the cord at the end of adolescence, but the adolescent also has to be ready for the cord to be cut: it is a two-way process. As with exercise and good eating habits, the foundations for becoming an independent adult are laid early in childhood.

Leaving the security of home is daunting for any adolescent, and they need to be equipped with the skills to look after themselves. The adolescent with hemiplegia also needs to be able to manage their own health care as much as possible. Health care for the person with hemiplegia usually changes from pediatric to adult services at the end of adolescence, which is another daunting change. It can be a big challenge for an adolescent to lose the services from professionals that they have effectively grown up with.

Being able to practice independence in a safe environment is important. For example, the adolescent can start running their own medical appointments with a parent there as a safety net and support, or complete chores or cook at home with the parent there to help if something goes wrong. In the age of increasingly digital communication, it can be helpful for the adolescent to be involved in phone conversations that they will be responsible for as they age. Using a speaker phone to include the young person when scheduling appointments or resolving issues with, for example, payment of services can be helpful. Initially the adolescent can listen, but over time, the parent can listen and coach. Practicing these skills at home, in a familiar environment, and learning from mistakes in a safe setting makes the transition to their highest level of independence less difficult, less scary, and more successful. Occupational therapy is a great resource in this area.

Thomason and Graham made the very interesting point that the decision to proceed with SEMLS for younger children is largely made by parents, but adolescents must be given the freedom to make their own informed decisions about surgery and rehabilitation.[276] They added that an adolescent who feels they have been forced into SEMLS against their will or without their full consent is likely to be resentful and may develop depression and struggle with rehabilitation. Indeed, this advice may be applicable to other areas in the life of the adolescent.

It's important to remember that the road to independence starts early in life. Then, the child is too young to participate in education around diagnosis, cause, and expectations for the future. However, families need to actively pass on this education to the child at age-appropriate times in their life to prepare them for living with their condition in adulthood. Too often, older children, adolescents, and adults have little understanding of their condition, which can hamper their involvement in management of their condition and independence.

Transition

Health care transition is defined as the planned process and skill-building to empower adolescents and their families to navigate an adult model of health care. It is more than simply changing medical professionals (termed "transfer").

Pediatric services for CP care are usually much better resourced than adult services and are better at following up with the individual. With adult services for CP care, it is usually up to the individual and family to do more proactive service procuring. Adult services are often much more reactionary rather than proactive.

Transition involves three steps: preparing, transferring, and integrating into adult services. That is, just because a file has been transferred does not mean the individual has successfully integrated into an adult service provider.

Helping children and adolescents with hemiplegia to become as independent as possible is the overall goal, which is why the focus on that transition must start early (from about the age of 12)—although supporting their independence really starts from birth. Transition doesn't involve just health care; it also involves other areas such as education, finance, insurance coverage, and guardianship planning. It is very important that the individual with CP is involved.

Figure 3.11.1 is a comprehensive look at some important transition questions the individual needs to ask: Where will I live? Who is my care team? How will I pay for things? What will I do?

Figure 3.11.2 shows a typical form that can be used for preparing an individual for transition to adult services.

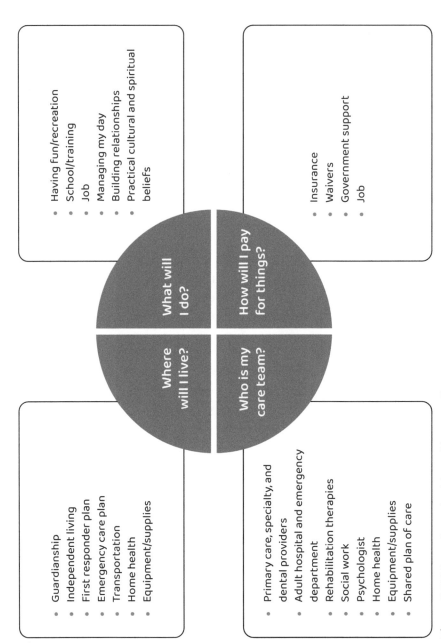

What will I do?
- Having fun/recreation
- School/training
- Job
- Managing my day
- Building relationships
- Practical cultural and spiritual beliefs

How will I pay for things?
- Insurance
- Waivers
- Government support
- Job

Where will I live?
- Guardianship
- Independent living
- First responder plan
- Emergency care plan
- Transportation
- Home health
- Equipment/supplies

Who is my care team?
- Primary care, specialty, and dental providers
- Adult hospital and emergency department
- Rehabilitation therapies
- Social work
- Psychologist
- Home health
- Equipment/supplies
- Shared plan of care

Figure 3.11.1 Some important transition questions.

Transition Readiness Assessment Questionnaire (TRAQ)

Patient Name: _____ Date of Birth: ___/___/___Today's Date ___/___/___ (MRN#_____)

Directions to Youth and Young Adults: Please check the box that best describes *your* skill level in the following areas that are important for transition to adult health care. There is no right or wrong answer and your answers will remain confidential and private.
Directions to Caregivers/Parents: If your youth or young adult is unable to complete the tasks below on their own, please check the box that best describes *your* skill level. **Check here** if you are a parent/caregiver completing this form. [ ]

	No, I do not know how	No, but I want to learn	No, but I am learning to do this	Yes, I have started doing this	Yes, I always do this when I need to
Managing Medications					
1. Do you fill a prescription if you need to?					
2. Do you know what to do if you are having a bad reaction to your medications?					
3. Do you reorder medications before they run out?					
4. Do you explain any medications (name and dose) you are taking to healthcare providers?					
5. Do you speak with the pharmacist about drug interactions or other concerns related to your medications?					
Appointment Keeping					
6. Do you call the doctor's office to make an appointment?					
7. Do you follow-up on referrals for tests or check-ups or labs?					
8. Do you arrange for your ride to medical appointments?					
9. Do you call the doctor about unusual changes in your health (for example: allergic reactions)?					
Tracking Health Issues					
10. Do you fill out the medical history form, including a list of your allergies?					
11. Do you keep a calendar or list of medical and other appointments?					
12. Do you tell the doctor or nurse what you are feeling?					
13. Do you contact the doctor when you have a health concern?					
14. Do you make or help make medical decisions pertaining to your health?					
15. Do you attend your medical appointment or part of your appointment by yourself?					
Talking with Providers					
16. Do you ask questions of your nurse or doctor about your health or health care?					
17. Do you answer questions that are asked by the doctor, nurse, or clinic staff?					
18. Do you ask your doctor or nurse to explain things more clearly if you do not understand their instructions to you?					
19. Do you tell the doctor or nurse whether you followed their advice or recommendations?					
20. Do you explain your health history to your healthcare providers (including past surgeries, allergies, and medications)?					

Please circle how you feel about the following statements

	Not at all important	Not too important	Somewhat important	Important	Very Important
How important is it to you to manage your own health care?	1	2	3	4	5
How confident do you feel about your ability to manage your own health care?	1	2	3	4	5

© Wood, Reiss, & Livingood, McBee, Johnson, 2020

Figure 3.11.2 Transition Readiness Assessment Questionnaire. Reproduced with kind permission from Dr. David L. Wood.

Following are some pointers for transition for the individual with CP:

- Try to get help from your pediatric care team (and possibly others) to connect with the best health professionals to care for you in adulthood.
- You might find it useful to make a summary of your CP and relevant medical history with someone who knows your experience, such as a parent or health professional. When meeting new health professionals, it is helpful to have a short (one- to two-minute) summary of your health care journey to date that can help guide the conversation, or, if easier, a one-page written summary (written by you) to hand to a new health professional. Keep a copy for yourself, and take both copies to the appointment. This summary should include your diagnosis, associated problems, history of treatments, current challenges, and more. This information is very helpful to the new health professional to better help you.
- Find out about the roles of different health professionals and how they might help you.
- Be open and honest and tell the new health professionals everything. You are the expert on your health. The more information you give them the better they can meet your needs.
- If you notice any changes in your condition or any problems such as pain, visit your primary care provider or a PM&R specialist* for advice. Don't wait and see.
- Learning how to advocate for yourself is important in health, just as it is in other parts of your life. Being prepared to advocate for your needs and make decisions about your health can give you more control over your quality of life. To help you advocate, you might practice; for example, you could explain your CP and medical history to someone you trust. Remember to stay calm and polite but assert yourself to get the support or information you need.
- Make a list of all the things you need to keep yourself healthy, such as being physically active, eating well, socializing, taking part in hobbies, working, and resting. By thinking about these, you can start to understand what positively and negatively affects your CP and find a good balance between your condition and lifestyle.

---

* PM&R aims to enhance and restore functional ability and quality of life among those with physical disabilities.

Got Transition is a US federally funded national resource center for health care transition. Its aim is to improve transition from pediatric to adult health care through the use of evidence-driven strategies for health professionals, adolescents, young adults, and their families. The website has a lot of useful guidance.

In its *Lifespan Journal Digest*, the American Academy of Cerebral Palsy and Developmental Medicine routinely spotlights recent studies focused on lifespan issues, including the transition to adult care and aging with a disability.

Links to both these resources are included in **Useful web resources.**

Key points Chapter 3

- It is important to understand what best practice in the medical care of individuals with hemiplegia looks like. Best practice currently includes family-centered care and person-centered care, a multidisciplinary team approach, evidence-based medicine and shared decision-making, data-driven decision-making, specialist centers, early intervention, setting goals, and measurement tools and measuring outcome.

- While a lot of attention is given to development of hand function, movement and posture and secondary musculoskeletal problems, for some individuals with hemiplegia, difficulties with communication or learning may pose bigger barriers to participation.

- Naturally, an individual with hemiplegia tends to favor using their unaffected hand because it functions so well. Both constraint-induced movement therapy (CIMT) and bimanual therapy are recommended to encourage and promote the use of the affected upper limb.

- Monitoring musculoskeletal development is a constant throughout childhood and adolescence.

- Hip and spine surveillance (monitoring) are important and should start early in life.

- Treatment of musculoskeletal concerns in both the upper and lower limb in hemiplegia generally begins at diagnosis with physical and occupational therapies. Over time, orthoses and casting may be added, and tone reduction may be considered as well.

- Despite best efforts, the development of some muscle and bone problems is largely inevitable in individuals with hemiplegia. Depending on the degree to which they impact function and participation, orthopedic surgery may be recommended. Single-event multilevel surgery (SEMLS)—a single operation to address all muscle and bone problems at once is often used. SEMLS is more frequently required for the lower rather than the upper limb. If SEMLS is required for both, they may be carried out together, but they are generally carried out separately for a number of reasons, including the optimum timing for both may not coincide.

- The home program (including exercise and physical activity) is a constant in the life of the child and adolescent with hemiplegia.

Chapter 4

The adult with spastic hemiplegia

Section 4.1 Introduction 269

Section 4.2 Aging in the typical population 274

Section 4.3 Aging with spastic hemiplegia 278

Section 4.4 Management and treatment of spastic hemiplegia
in adulthood 290

Key points Chapter 4 301

Introduction

I don't think motor neurone disease can be an advantage to anyone,
but it was less of a disadvantage to me than to other people,
because it did not stop me doing what I wanted.
Stephen Hawking

CP is diagnosed in childhood and is a lifelong condition. It is often thought of as a children's condition, but it is not. People with CP who walk during childhood tend to have a relatively normal life expectancy.[277] If one considers a normal life span to be 80 years, that means for every child and adolescent with CP there are approximately three adults with the condition.

The World Health Organization (WHO) defines an adult as a person older than 19 years of age.[278] But what does being an adult really mean?

While everybody's path in life is different, one description of being an adult includes the following accomplishments:[279]

Completing formal education, entering the labor force, living independently, having romantic relationships and sexual experiences, getting married and having children, establishing peer and family relationships, participating in recreation/leisure, driving a car, and enjoying group social encounters.

Preparing our children to become independent adults is the ultimate goal of most parents—and that's a realistic goal for the parents of the majority of children with hemiplegia. However, while this chapter focuses on the majority, it is important to remember that a small minority of adults with hemiplegia have moderate to severe intellectual problems, and therefore they will likely need supported living arrangements, legal guardianship, and support with decision-making.

As a person with hemiplegia reaches adulthood and skeletal growth has ceased, a certain stabilization of the musculoskeletal aspects of the condition occurs. The rate of change of the condition is slower in adulthood, assuming the adult remains physically active.

People with hemiplegia may, however, develop secondary conditions in adulthood. Some of these are consistent with typical aging, but some may be unique. Each may influence body systems in more complex ways because of the interactions with CP itself.

The Centers for Disease Control and Prevention (CDC) explain secondary conditions as follows:[280]

As a result of having a specific type of disability, such as a spinal cord injury … other physical or mental health conditions can occur. Some of these other health conditions are also called secondary conditions …

The specific secondary conditions that may develop depend on the primary condition. For example, eye problems are secondary conditions that may develop from having diabetes; osteoarthritis is a secondary condition that may develop from having hemiplegia.

This chapter addresses the secondary conditions associated with hemiplegia. Note that the secondary conditions referred to here are general health conditions and separate from the secondary musculoskeletal problems that develop as a result of the primary brain injury in CP, addressed in Chapters 2 and 3.

The development of secondary conditions is not inevitable. Good management can help prevent or minimize their development. Though they are addressed in this chapter on adulthood, some secondary conditions may appear earlier in life.

In childhood and adolescence, growth is the major challenge for the person with hemiplegia. In adulthood, typical aging becomes the main challenge. Though there are far more adults than children with CP, most of the efforts of health care professionals are directed at children and adolescents.

Meeting the needs of young people with CP is absolutely essential, but given that CP is a lifelong condition and further issues may arise with age, the medical establishment must better address the lack of service provision for adults with CP. To that end, currently, a clinical practice guideline for adults with CP is being developed. Once published, the guideline will, hopefully, pave the way for better service provision for adults with CP.

In addition to the challenge of reduced service provisions, there are significant personal, societal, and economic costs associated with suboptimal health. For example, as addressed in section 4.3, adults with hemiplegia are underemployed.

If the moral argument for improving service provision and, thus, quality of life for adults with hemiplegia is not sufficiently persuasive, then perhaps the economic argument will be. Novak and colleagues in 2016 reported that care, loss of income, and tax revenue losses for individuals with CP cost the Australian and American economies $87 billion per year.[281] That cost has likely increased.

Much of the limited research in CP to date has focused on children. An analysis of National Institutes of Health (NIH)[*] funding for CP research from 2001 to 2013 found that only 4 percent of available funding went toward studies of CP in adulthood.[282] As well, as was noted earlier in

---

[*] The NIH is the primary US body responsible for health research.

this book, funding generally for CP research is very low relative to the prevalence of the condition and its impact across the life span.

While research on CP in adulthood is considerably less than in childhood, it has been growing over time, as shown by the increase in the annual number of studies from a search using the terms "cerebral palsy" and "adult." See Figure 4.1.1.

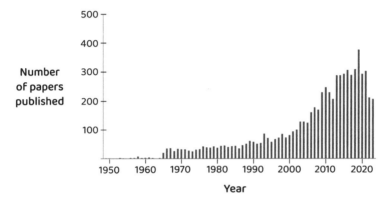

Figure 4.1.1 Number of studies on CP in adulthood per year (PubMed).*

More research is needed to fully understand how CP changes in adulthood and what can be done to prevent or minimize the problems that arise as adults with CP age. Because "adults" range in age from 19 to 80-plus years, they are not a homogenous group. It is necessary to have a better sense of how health care challenges evolve across the decades. Longitudinal research studies for adults with CP as they age would offer valuable information.

A 2008 workshop to define the challenges of treating and preventing secondary conditions in adults with CP concluded with this very worthy goal:[283]

> *The same sense of responsibility and compassion that motivated the research that led to such advances as increasing the survival rates of very low birth weight infants must now be applied to developing the best means of caring for children with CP as they reach adulthood ... The medical and research communities have*

---

* A free online database of medical and life sciences research articles.

helped these individuals survive. It is now our responsibility to help them thrive and live productive lives, as uninhibited as possible by the chronic pain and secondary conditions associated with CP.

USEFUL WEB RESOURCES

Aging in the typical population

Send me a postcard, drop me a line
Stating point of view
Indicate precisely what you mean to say
Yours sincerely, wasting away
Give me your answer, fill in a form
Mine for evermore
Will you still need me, will you still feed me
When I'm sixty-four.
The Beatles

The *Oxford English Dictionary* defines aging as "the process of growing old." But that doesn't give us much information. The fact that decline occurs with age is obvious from observing those around us and from seeing how the performance of elite athletes declines relatively early in life. Before addressing aging in adults with CP, let us first look at aging in the typical population.

Examples of the decline that may occur with age include sarcopenia (loss of skeletal muscle mass and strength), joint pain, osteoarthritis, osteoporosis, falls, and low-trauma fractures (easily acquired bone breaks). Many conditions become more prevalent as people age, including cardiovascular disease, cancer, respiratory disease, and diabetes. These conditions are termed "noncommunicable diseases" (NCDs).

Some of the above can be considered part of "normal" aging (e.g., sarcopenia), but most are diagnosable medical conditions. Diagnosable medical conditions occur in the typical population, but they are not "normal." This section addresses sarcopenia, osteoporosis, and NCDs in more detail.

Sarcopenia

Sarcopenia is the loss of skeletal muscle mass and strength.[284] Typically developing adults achieve peak muscle mass by their early 40s, which progressively declines and results in as much as 50 percent loss by the time they are in their 80s. As we saw earlier, muscle strength is related to muscle size. Losing muscle mass has consequences for maintaining the level of function we need to carry out activities of daily living as we age; for example, lifting and carrying objects or even just getting up from a chair. By performing simple muscle strengthening exercises, adults can offset the natural loss of muscle mass that commonly occurs with age.

Protein is required for muscle growth. Older people are less efficient than younger people at extracting protein from food, which means older people need to be especially vigilant about meeting their daily protein needs.[285] For adults over age 65, an average daily intake of at least 1 to 1.2 grams of protein per kilogram of body weight is recommended.[*286]

Osteoporosis

Bone fractures as a result of falls are closely linked to osteoporosis (addressed in sections 2.7 and 3.9). The risk of falling increases with age due to factors such as decreasing muscle strength and balance. Maintaining muscle strength and balance is therefore very important

---

* For example, a person over 65 weighing 57 kg (126 lb) requires 60 g (just over 2 oz) of protein per day.

for preventing falls. The consequences of a fall can lead to further complications—for example, a broken leg may lead to much-reduced activity, or a broken wrist may lead to difficulties with self-care. Either may lead to reduced independence. Fear of falling can be another consequence, which may lead to self-imposed restrictions on activity.[287]

The AACPDM (American Academy for Cerebral Palsy and Developmental Medicine) has published a care pathway, "Osteoporosis in Cerebral Palsy," and a link to it is included in **Useful web resources.**

Noncommunicable diseases

A noncommunicable disease (NCD) is a medical condition not caused by an infectious agent.* NCDs, also known as chronic diseases, tend to be of long duration. The World Health Organization reported that NCDs are the cause of over three-quarters of all deaths globally. The following four conditions account for over 80 percent of all deaths due to NCDs:[288]

- Cardiovascular disease (e.g., heart attack and stroke)
- Cancer
- Respiratory disease (e.g., chronic obstructive pulmonary disease and asthma)
- Diabetes

In section 1.3, we examined the difference between causes and risk factors. NCDs share four behavioral risk factors:[288]

- Tobacco use
- Physical inactivity
- Unhealthy diet
- Excess alcohol consumption

People have control over each of these risk factors—they are lifestyle choices. However, it is important to acknowledge that socioeconomic factors can adversely affect nutrition and health. Very often, multiple

---

* A communicable disease is caused by an infectious agent such as a bacterium or virus.

combinations may be present, such as an unhealthy diet combined with physical inactivity.

Cardiometabolic risk factors ("cardio" refers to heart and "metabolic," refers to the process the body uses to turn food into energy) include:

- High levels of blood cholesterol (a type of fat in the blood)
- High levels of triglycerides (another type of fat in the blood)
- High blood pressure (also termed "hypertension")
- Insulin resistance* or diabetes
- Being overweight or obese†
- Metabolic syndrome (a person is diagnosed with metabolic syndrome if they have at least three of the five risk factors above)
- High levels of C-reactive protein (a protein in the blood; high levels are a sign of inflammation in the body)

In addition to good lifestyle choices, regular health checks with a primary care provider are important for managing our health as we age. A primary care provider will check many of the above risk factors. Most developed countries also have screening programs for many cancers, such as breast and colon cancer. Appropriate health checks and screening can lead to early identification and therefore earlier treatment of conditions.

Finally, not everything goes downhill as we age. Wisdom, sense of self, and comfort in one's own skin generally increase as we get older. Happiness appears to follow a U-shaped trajectory (also known as a "happiness curve"), declining from the optimism of youth to a slump in middle age, then rising again around age 50.[289]

---

* Insulin resistance is the body's reduced responsiveness to insulin, potentially leading to higher than normal blood sugar levels.

† Measured by body mass index (BMI) and/or central obesity. BMI is calculated by dividing a person's body mass in kilograms by the square of their body height in meters. A large waistline (≥ 40 in/102 cm for men and ≥ 35 in/89 cm for women) is a measure of central obesity. This body type is also known as "apple-shaped," as opposed to "pear-shaped," in which fat is deposited on the hips and buttocks. Apple-shaped people are known to be more at risk for cardiometabolic disease than pear-shaped people. A CDC resource on weight is included in **Useful web resources.**

Aging with spastic hemiplegia

You are never too old to set another goal or to dream a new dream.

C.S. Lewis

Adults with hemiplegia are not a homogenous group. They range in age from 20 to 80-plus years. They vary in how their condition was managed during childhood and adolescence. They also vary in personality, level of drive, determination, perseverance, and interest in self-care. This is no different from nondisabled adults or those with other primary conditions such as diabetes.

Adults with hemiplegia have had their condition since childhood, but they are also susceptible to the same challenges of aging as their nondisabled peers. For the person with hemiplegia, it is almost as if, on entering adulthood, two roads converge: the challenges of growing up with the condition meet the challenges of typical aging. The adult with hemiplegia must manage these two sets of challenges in combination. The problems of aging may occur at a younger age and with more severity in adults with CP than in those without the condition.[290]

A recent systematic review and meta-analysis* of 69 studies from 18 countries found that the prevalence of several chronic physical and mental health conditions was higher among adults with CP than those without CP.[291] However, much can be done to prevent or minimize many of the secondary conditions that can arise.

The management and treatment of hemiplegia in childhood and adolescence has improved in recent decades. This influences how today's children and adolescents will fare as tomorrow's adults. The general public's awareness of many health issues has also improved. For example, people today are much more aware of the downsides of smoking and the important contribution of physical exercise to overall health. As in childhood and adolescence, hemiplegia in adulthood affects not only the individual with the condition but also their family and those in their immediate circle.

This section addresses the following challenges of aging with hemiplegia:

- Musculoskeletal decline
- Mobility
- Falls
- Pain
- Noncommunicable diseases and risk factors
- Fatigue
- Depression and anxiety
- Participation
- Areas of unmet need

Though these challenges will be addressed separately, they are very much interdependent.

Musculoskeletal decline

Chapter 2 addressed the primary, secondary, and tertiary problems of hemiplegia. Chapter 3 addressed the optimal management of the

---

* A systematic review summarizes the results of several scientific studies on the same topic. They can be qualitative (descriptive) or quantitative (numerical). The quantitative approach is called a meta-analysis.

condition in childhood and adolescence. The aim is to arrive at adulthood (when bone growth ceases) with the best possible musculoskeletal alignment. If correction of the muscle and bone deformities is not addressed (or not fully addressed) during childhood and adolescence, they may persist into adulthood.[292] These muscle and bone problems may cause further decline in upper arm function and mobility as well as pain, fatigue, and other problems in adulthood. As people age, further coping responses (tertiary problems) may develop to compensate for decreased muscle strength and deterioration in balance. However, as we will see in the next section, orthopedic surgery to address muscle and bone problems is still possible in adulthood.

The conditions that occur in typically aging adults can have even greater implications for adults with hemiplegia. For example:

- **Sarcopenia** (loss of skeletal muscle mass and strength): For individuals with hemiplegia, muscle mass and strength have been challenges since childhood. In adulthood, these individuals acquire the added challenge of loss of muscle mass and strength due to aging. Hip and knee extension strength was found to be considerably lower (less than 75 percent of normal) among adolescents and young adults with spastic CP (GMFCS levels I and II, 57 percent unilateral, both lower limbs tested).[293] Maximum plantar flexor strength was found to be approximately 50 percent less in young adults with spastic CP (average age 25, GMFCS levels I and II, 61 percent unilateral) than in typically developing young adults, and approximately 35 percent less than in typically developing adults above age 70.[294]
- **Osteoarthritis**: The prevalence of osteoarthritis among middle-age adults with CP (GMFCS levels I to III, 27 percent hemiplegia) was 33 percent.[295] In another study, the age-adjusted prevalence of arthritis was found to be significantly greater among adults with CP than among those without CP: 31 percent versus 17 percent.[296] Individuals with hemiplegia have to watch for overuse syndrome—overuse of the uninvolved side.
- **Osteoporosis or osteopenia**: The prevalence of osteoporosis or osteopenia among middle-age adults with CP GMFCS levels I to III was 32 percent.[295] Adults with CP had a higher incidence of osteoporosis compared with adults without CP.[297]

- **Fractures:** Adults with CP (no breakdown by type) had a higher prevalence of fractures compared with adults without CP; 6 percent versus 3 percent.[298]

Mobility

Retaining the ability to walk (independently or using mobility aids) for at least household distances is important for independence. A systematic review and meta-analysis found that 56 percent of adults with CP experienced a perceived decline in walking over time.[299] Those with hemiplegia have lower rates of decline, and decline at a later age on average, compared with those with diplegia or quadriplegia.[300] Elsewhere it has been noted that individuals at GMFCS levels I and II are at lower risk of gait deterioration and generally continue to walk in their 60s.[301]

People who engage in regular physical activity were found to be at lower risk of experiencing decline in mobility. Deterioration in gait was strongly associated with inactivity.[300] In other words, mobility and physical activity are intricately linked. This emphasizes how important it is to remain physically active throughout adulthood.

Falls

Earlier we saw that balance is affected in hemiplegia. Although adults with CP may have become somewhat used to falling (and are more aware of situations where they are at risk of falling and how to protect themselves when falling), it tends to be more socially uncomfortable when a fall occurs. In addition, for reasons of physics, an adult is more likely to be injured from a fall than a child. Citing from a number of studies on falls:

- Fall frequency in ambulatory adults with CP was two- to threefold higher than in adults without CP (GMFCS levels I to III, 37 percent unilateral).[302] Fall frequency was lowest among those with hemiplegia compared to other CP subtypes.[302]
- Eighty-nine percent of adults with hemiplegia reported at least 1 fall in the past year, with 26 percent experiencing more than 10 falls.[303]

- Of 34 adults with CP (GMFCS levels I to III, 29 percent unilateral), 33 reported at least 1 fall in the past 12 months, with an estimated range of 0 to 200. Only 6 of the 34 participants were classified as infrequent/nonfallers (fell two times or less).[304]

Falls occur naturally with aging, but they usually occur later in life in adults who do not have a disability and who have better overall health and fitness. The incidence of falls is higher for people with CP at younger ages[305,306] and may be more common if they do not use mobility aids.

Psychological effects of falls include embarrassment and loss of confidence.[302] Additionally, the fear of falling is a real concern in adulthood when responsibilities and activities change. For example, when pregnant and/or caring for an infant, the fear of falling is great due to the increased consequences.

Pain

A systematic review and meta-analysis reported a pain prevalence of 65 percent among adults with CP, though studies report different prevalence depending on their definition of pain.[299] Studies report higher levels of pain among adults with CP compared with the general population: 28 percent versus 15 percent[307] and 44 percent versus 28 percent.[296] Adults with hemiplegia reported pain in the back (47 percent), neck (41 percent), foot/ankle (38 percent), shoulder (39 percent), knee (38 percent), hip (34 percent), arm (31 percent), head (24 percent), and other (4 percent).[307]

Pain is a major determinant of quality of life and affects physical and mental functioning. It leads to reduced productivity and concentration.[279] Pain may lead to problems with sleep, which causes fatigue, which can further exacerbate pain.

Pain negatively impacts activity, mental health, and employment in adults with CP.[308,309,310] CP alone does not predict reduced quality of life. However, adults with CP who have pain have reduced quality of life, and increased prevalence of pain with age coincides with decline in quality of life from childhood to adulthood.[311,312]

Noncommunicable diseases and risk factors

Recall that noncommunicable diseases (NCDs) are medical conditions that are not caused by infectious agents, and they are generally chronic conditions. A systematic review and meta-analysis reported the prevalence of several chronic conditions among ambulatory adults with CP: obesity (20 percent), hypercholesterolemia (high cholesterol, 26 percent), and hypertension (high blood pressure, 10 percent).[291]

A study by Cremer and colleagues of adults in the US with CP GMFCS levels I to III (demographic details in Table 4.3.1) reported chronic condition prevalence by gender as shown in Figure 4.3.1.[295] The prevalence of chronic conditions was higher among women than men for five of the seven conditions. It is worth noting that prevalence rates may vary by country.

Table 4.3.1 Demographics of adults in the Cremer study

	WOMEN	MEN
Number of participants	112	94
Average age (years)	50	48
Body mass index (BMI) kg/m²	31	27
% obese (BMI>30)	44	18
% smokers	14	16

Data from Cremer and colleagues.[295]

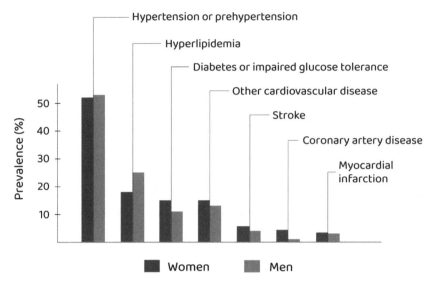

Figure 4.3.1 Prevalence (percent) of chronic conditions in adults with CP GMFCS levels I to III, by gender. Data from Cremer and colleagues.[295] **Hypertension** is a condition characterized by high blood pressure. **Prehypertension** is a condition characterized by blood pressure levels that are elevated but not yet classified as hypertension. **Hyperlipidemia** is a condition characterized by high levels of fats in the blood. **Impaired glucose tolerance** refers to a prediabetes condition where blood sugars are higher than normal but not high enough for a diabetes diagnosis. **Myocardial infarction** is also known as heart attack.

Multimorbidity is defined as the presence of two or more chronic conditions.[291] The prevalence of multimorbidity was significantly higher among obese than nonobese adults with CP GMFCS levels I to III (76 percent versus 54 percent).[295]

Using data from 2002 to 2010, Peterson and colleagues reported the age-adjusted prevalence of eight chronic conditions among adults in the US with and without CP.[296] (See Figure 4.3.2.) The prevalence of the eight chronic conditions was higher among adults with CP. It's understandable why adults with CP might have a higher burden of joint pain and arthritis, but the remaining conditions do not have a direct link to the condition. However, as we will see, lower levels of activity due to CP lead to lower fitness. Since people who are less active and less fit have a higher incidence of diabetes, hypertension, and cardiovascular disease, it makes sense that CP puts people at increased risk of these conditions.

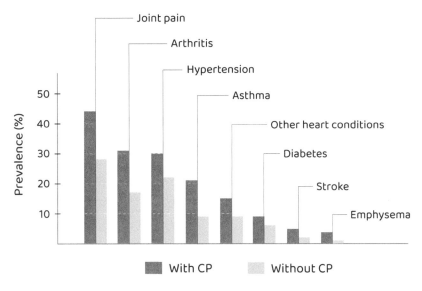

Figure 4.3.2 Age-adjusted prevalence of chronic conditions in adults with and without CP. Data from Peterson and colleagues.[296] **Age-adjusted** refers to a data standardization method to account for differences in ages allowing for more accurate comparison. **Emphysema** is a condition in which the air sacs of the lungs are damaged and enlarged, causing breathlessness.

There is ample evidence to suggest that the burden of NCDs and their risk factors are higher among ambulatory adults with CP compared with the general population.[291]

Fatigue

Fatigue describes feeling exhausted, tired, weak, or lacking energy.[313] A study found that adults with CP (38 percent hemiplegia) had significantly more physical fatigue, but not more mental fatigue, than the general population.[313] The strongest predictors associated with fatigue included bodily pain, deterioration of functional skills, and low life satisfaction. However young adults with unilateral CP were less fatigued than those with bilateral CP.[314] One study emphasized the importance of physical activity and good weight management to both prevent and treat fatigue in adults with CP.[315]

Depression and anxiety

Depression is a common and serious mood disorder. It can affect how a person feels and thinks, and it influences activities such as sleeping, eating, and working.[316] For a depression diagnosis, the symptoms must be present for at least two weeks.[316] A UK study found that only adults with CP and without intellectual disability have a higher risk of developing depression than adults who do not have CP.[317] However, a US study found no such difference between adults with CP and the general population (where the rate of depression in both groups was 20 percent).[318]

Occasional anxiety is normal; however, anxiety disorders are more than just occasional worry or fear. There are several types of anxiety disorders, each with distinct symptoms and triggers.[319] The same UK study found that only adults with CP and without intellectual disability were found to have a higher risk of developing anxiety than adults who do not have CP.[317]

Participation

Participation is one of the three levels of human functioning identified in the ICF (addressed in section 1.8). Participation restrictions are problems an individual may experience in their involvement in life situations. Employment, relationships, and having children are indicators of participation in society.

A Dutch study of individuals with CP without intellectual disability found that individuals at GMFCS levels I and II achieved autonomy in adulthood in most participation domains (leisure, transportation, finances, education and employment, housing, and intimate relationships). However, with regard to intimate relationships, they had slightly less experience (approximately 80 percent of individuals) than age-matched peers (approximately 90 percent).[320] A Swedish study of 1,888 adults with CP, age 16 to 78, however, reported different results for participation.[321] See Table 4.3.2.

Table 4.3.2 Participation for adults with CP GMFCS levels I and II

AREA OF LIFE	GMFCS LEVEL I (%)	GMFCS LEVEL II (%)
Having no partner	77	82
Housing		
Independent	40	41
With parents	51	39
Assisted living	7	18
Other	2	3
Personal assistance		
None	98	80
>160 hours per week	1	6
Occupation		
Mainstream education	39	18
Special education	5	9
Competitive employment	27	18
Supported employment	4	3
Activity center	14	39
No occupation	11	14
For all the above, the proportion full time	71	52

Data from Pettersson and Rodby-Bousquet.[321]

While there are no comparable figures for the typical population, the levels of participation can be assumed to be lower. For example, a high percentage of those with CP GMFCS levels I and II did not have a partner, and this applied across all age groups.

Employment is important for many reasons, including financial independence, social interaction, self-esteem, and sense of self, but it may also have implications for future health care and retirement costs. Very often, the barriers to employment are small and require only simple accommodations—a high percentage (59 percent) of accommodations cost absolutely nothing to make while the rest typically cost only $500 per employee.[322] Indeed, research shows that companies that embrace employees with disabilities clearly see the results in their bottom line. They have higher productivity levels and lower staff turnover rates, are twice as likely to outperform their peers in shareholder returns, and create larger returns on investment.[322]

A US study found that women with CP who were surveyed about their desire to have children (30 percent) or had experienced pregnancy (20 percent) exhibited significantly higher functional levels, including mobility, manual dexterity, and communication ability.[323] A higher rate of cesarean section (50 percent), preterm births (12 percent), low birth weight infants (16 percent), and very low birth weight infants (7 percent) were reported by women with CP compared with national statistics.[323] The authors concluded that in addition to the need to discuss and support the desire of women with CP to have sexual relationships and experience pregnancy, there is a need to investigate preterm and low birth weight infants born to women with CP.

Finally, higher general self-efficacy* was found to be related to better participation.[324]

Clearly, participation in society is very important and more research is needed, particularly in the area of participation restrictions.

Areas of unmet need

The greatest area of unmet need reported by young adults with CP was information about their condition† (79 percent), followed by mobility (66 percent) and health care (66 percent).[325] The authors suggested that while parents may receive information, they might not be communicating it adequately to their children, leaving them with unanswered questions. Furthermore, a person's questions about CP might change over time as their needs change during adolescence and adulthood.

---

* The belief in your ability to plan and carry out actions to achieve desired outcomes.

† For example: complications, consequences, causes of CP.

Other studies have reported a similar lack of information during the transition to adulthood,[326,327] underscoring the need for a book like this one, as well as more research on adults with CP.

———

Finally, while the most recent definition of CP is very useful, it may not sufficiently alert us to the secondary conditions that may arise in adulthood. As O'Brien and colleagues explained, the definition was developed to be used in childhood—it was not intended to imply that progressive problems might not appear in adult life.[328]

Management and treatment of spastic hemiplegia in adulthood

People do not decide their futures, they decide their habits and their habits decide their futures.

F. M. Alexander

This section addresses the management and treatment of hemiplegia in adulthood, specifically:

- Health services for adults with CP
- Treatments
- The home program
- General pointers

Health services for adults with CP

The general consensus in the literature is that services for adults with CP are extremely limited. Multidisciplinary care teams in place for children and adolescents with CP largely do not exist for adults at a time when their needs are becoming ever more complex. This disparity has been observed in many countries, including Norway,[168] the US,[279] the Netherlands,[329] Ireland,[330] Germany,[331] and Canada.[332] Scandinavian countries are known for their well-developed social health systems, yet other than Sweden,[321] they too experience this fall-off in services. It is very unfortunate that care for people with CP becomes fragmented just as they enter adulthood.

In their 2009 report following a workshop to define the challenges of treating and preventing secondary complications in adults with CP, Tosi and colleagues noted that pediatric facilities are starting to extend their mandate to include adults.[283] They cited Gillette's model of life-time care.* Gillette provides lifelong specialty care to adolescents and adults who have conditions that began in childhood. This specialization means that even though Gillette is a lifetime care provider, it does not treat lifelong conditions that develop after early childhood.

For the adult with CP, three different components of health need monitoring:[333]

- Acute health problems (e.g., infections)
- Lifestyle health risks
- Secondary conditions

As has been shown, there is strong evidence that adults with hemiplegia encounter more and earlier health problems than their typically aging peers, and these problems affect a broad range of areas spanning all ICF levels. But much can still be done to prevent, minimize, or deal with these challenges. However, because of limited specialist health services for adults with CP, they must take great personal responsibility for their own health and well-being.

It has been reported in the literature that health care professionals often blame their CP diagnosis for just about all the symptoms and problems that develop in adulthood.[334,335] Rosenbaum noted: "We hear too many stories from adults with cerebral palsy whose abdominal pain, for example, was assumed to be 'part of (your) cerebral palsy,' when in fact they had treatable Crohn's or gall bladder disease."[335] It is important to

---

* The Gillette adult clinic is a lifelong outpatient clinic for those age 16 and older who have conditions that began in childhood. It includes access to an inpatient unit for adults age 18 to 40. Specialists may provide care to adults whom they previously treated as children.

ensure that the cause of a health problem is not wrongly attributed to CP when there may be another cause.

Sometimes, changes with aging versus new neurological changes are difficult to separate, especially in adults with CP who are older than 40 years, but it is important to determine the cause.[336] New neurological changes might include a decreased level of alertness or cognitive functioning, decreased ability to communicate, weakness, or numbness, including paresthesia (pins-and-needles sensation.) For example, cervical myelopathy should be considered with new neurological changes. Cervical myelopathy refers to the symptoms related to spinal cord compression (myelopathy) in the neck (cervical) region. Symptoms may include weakness, numbness, loss of fine motor skills, and bladder issues. In addition, dual diagnoses (for example, multiple sclerosis* or even genetic conditions) should also be considered with functional decline.[336]

All adults—those with and without disabilities—should attend regular health screenings (e.g., for cancers, bone health, and sexually transmitted infections) and have an annual medical checkup with their primary care provider. Research has found that many adults with CP do not receive adequate health checks and screening.[283,337,338]

Addressing medical caregivers, Murphy succinctly summarized the situation: "It should be a humbling revelation to all caregivers that this population of adults is almost certainly under-studied, under-screened, and under-diagnosed."[334] (Note that "underdiagnosis" here refers to other conditions, not CP.)

Because of their higher risk of osteoporosis, people with hemiplegia need to be attentive to bone health. It is recommended that adults with CP have at least an annual bone health assessment (including medical history, lifestyle review, nutrition, and, as needed, evaluation for any concerning changes in bone health, such as new fractures or medications that affect bone health) with appropriate blood testing and imaging. DXA scans† may be used for surveillance every three to five years.[339]

---

* A chronic autoimmune disease of the central nervous system where the immune system mistakenly attacks the myelin, the protective covering of axons, leading to interruption in the transmission of nerve impulses. See Figure 1.2.2.

† A test that measures bone mineral density.

Good nutrition, ensuring no deficiencies in calcium and vitamin D, and physical activity, especially weight-bearing or impact activities, can help promote good bone health.[265]

Despite these concerns, this optimistic opinion is heartening: "Much improvement in specialty health care for adults with CP has occurred over the past three decades. Surely the best is yet to come."[334]

Treatments

The goals of treatment or intervention for adults with CP are inclusion and participation in major life areas.[279] Objectives include minimizing problems with body functions and structure, preventing secondary conditions, and optimizing activities and participation.

The different treatments for hemiplegia are reviewed in Chapter 3. Here, we focus on what these treatments look like in adulthood. When planning any treatment, it is important to set SMART goals, as discussed in section 3.2. Note that the goal for a particular treatment may be different in adulthood than in childhood.

a) Physical therapy and occupational therapy

Physical therapy (PT) and occupational therapy (OT) remain very relevant in adulthood and are usually delivered as an episode of care (EOC).* Rosenbaum and colleagues described the focus of therapy for adults with CP as helping individuals in areas including employment, relationships, and childbearing. They added that adults with CP may require specific focused surveillance and intervention for pain, joint wear and tear, and general mobility in addition to fitness and recreational activities.[164]

In adulthood, the focus of therapy shifts to guidance and education more than intervention, but both are used as required. Therapists at the Gillette adult clinic provided the following examples of EOCs for adults with CP. In these examples the therapist is acting as an educator in prevention and giving guidance rather than providing intervention.

---

* A period of therapy (at the appropriate frequency) followed by a therapy break.

- Instruction in balance, gait, strength-training exercises, and the home program. As addressed in Chapter 3, with hemiplegia, particular attention needs to be paid to more weight-bearing on the weaker lower limb and to symmetrical walking to prevent overuse syndrome and osteoarthritis with aging.
- Fall assessment to determine the reasons for falls and offer instruction in balance and strengthening exercises for fall prevention. They can also offer guidance on appropriate mobility aids or orthoses and footwear to prevent falls.
- Pain education and instruction in ways to decrease pain: certain therapists have advanced training in pain management. Many research studies show pain education can greatly decrease chronic pain.[340,341]
- Advice on gentle postural exercises and possible affordable adaptations (e.g., changing the angle of a keyboard or the height of chair or desk for optimal posture).
- Instruction in preservation and strengthening exercises to help prevent overuse injuries; for example, when using a manual wheelchair. (Power-assist wheelchairs can also help prevent overuse injuries.)
- Recommendations for home and environmental adaptations (such as adding handrails, removing throw rugs, or improving lighting).
- Mobility assessment and training on ways to continue to be as independent as possible throughout the day in the home, at work, and in the community.
- Equipment provision: for example, a walker or other gait aid to maintain safe walking and prevent falls, a manual or power-assist wheelchair for long distances, or bathroom equipment for safe showering.
- Driving assessment: driving specialists can assess driving ability, including determining if behind-the-wheel and car adaptations are needed to allow independent driving.

The following are useful pointers on mobility:[342]

- Mobility aids are "tools," and people might benefit from having a variety of options available. For example, an individual may use a walker or wheelchair occasionally for longer distances, in certain environments, or when feeling fatigued. They may choose to use a mobility aid in a way that suits their needs; the decision to use one does not have to be "all or nothing." Part-time use may help with participation.

- A crutch is not a "crutch"—mobility aids are tools that can help the person participate more in everyday life.
- Deciding to use a mobility aid can be a positive rather than a negative step, allowing for greater participation and less pain and fatigue. A wheelchair or motorized scooter can help a person with CP conserve energy, which they can then use to engage with peers or become more involved at school or at work. O'Brien and colleagues noted that:[328]

  [The] decision to become a regular wheelchair user is often a positive step, not a negative one. People in this situation typically report not only reductions in pain and fatigue, but also associated improvements in initiative and self-esteem, consequent upon a decision to elect to use a wheelchair, rather than to struggle on painfully and awkwardly, trying to walk.

- A mobility aid can help prevent falls, excessive sway through the trunk, or overreliance on one limb at the expense of the other. It may help lessen age-related musculoskeletal changes and pain over time.
- Those for whom walking demands a lot of extra energy may sometimes lie awake at night imagining where they will have to walk the next day, expending mental energy as well as physical energy on walking.
- The design of mobility aids has improved over time. Wheelchair design and function, for example, has greatly improved in recent years: modern wheelchairs are smaller, faster, and better designed. There are also sports wheelchairs available.
- Mobility aids can include the use of balance dogs (or service dogs), which are dogs trained to wear a particular harness or handle. The dog and harness can serve as a gait aid or for other tasks as needed. These dogs also know how to brace their backs so that if the person falls or is on the floor they can push off the dog to stand up. There's a lot of work involved in caring for a dog, but they can also serve as an emotional support animal and are often perceived as more socially acceptable than a gait aid. Dogs are also great icebreakers for getting to know other people. A video about a student and her balance dog is included in **Useful web resources**.

b) Tone reduction

Tone reduction may include oral medications, botulinum neurotoxin A (BoNT-A) injection, phenol injection, intrathecal baclofen (ITB), and selective dorsal rhizotomy (SDR). BoNT-A has been shown to be effective in improving spasticity among adults with CP, but there have been mixed results for other functional outcomes.[343]

c) Orthopedic surgery

Adults may have orthopedic surgery to address individual or multiple musculoskeletal problems. Orthopedic surgery to address degenerative joint disease with possible joint replacement can be performed as an isolated procedure or as part of multilevel surgery.

Rehabilitation after surgery (of any type) is more prolonged in adults than in children because adults heal more slowly and their lives are generally more independent with more responsibilities. Children are already dependent on their parents: after SEMLS, they return home to an environment where their needs are already being met by others. This isn't the case for the adult. Since rehabilitation takes considerable time, once the initial rehabilitation is over, the adult may be trying to juggle further rehabilitation with work, caring for family, and other responsibilities.

Significant challenges for independent adults following multilevel surgery include loss of independence, loss of ability to care for others (such as children or elderly parents), and loss of income. Can the adult even "go home"? If going home is not an option (because, for example, there is no one to care for them), where do they go? They can't go to a rehab facility right away because they are non-weight-bearing. A nursing home is often the answer, but this is far from ideal because the adult generally has little in common with typical nursing home residents. Transitional care units (or short-term care facilities) are an option: these are typically set up for people whose medical needs are too intense for home but not intense enough for an acute hospital setting.

Thomason and Graham reported that rehabilitation after multilevel surgery can be an "order of magnitude" more difficult for adolescents and adults than it is for younger children, and that adolescents and adults are more prone to anxiety, depression, and functional regression.[344]

In addition to the age-dependent difference in rehabilitation time, rehabilitation for the same procedure (e.g., knee replacement surgery) can take longer for adults with CP than for their nondisabled peers. This is important to note because adults with CP may expect a rehabilitation period similar to that of their nondisabled peers.

As for outcome, total hip replacement was found to be safe and effective in selected individuals with CP with severe degenerative arthritis.[301] Long-term follow-up studies have shown pain relief of more than 90 percent and improved function with time even in adults as young as 30. Wear and tear to the replacement hip joint was found to be minimal.[301]

Because research funding is limited, very few outcome studies on adults with CP exist. Medical professionals treating adults with CP must rely more on their clinical skill and experience rather than the results of research studies.

The home program

This section needs to be read in conjunction with section 3.5, which details the home program for the adolescent with CP. That information applies equally to the adult with CP. The following are some points specific to adults.

During childhood and adolescence, prolonged stretching is needed to achieve the daily hours of stretch required to keep muscle growth at pace with bone growth until bone growth ceases at around age 20. In adulthood, stretching is recommended for the same reasons as for non-disabled adults: to keep muscles flexible, maintain joint range of motion (ROM), and avoid injury. Even nondisabled people do not fully stretch out their muscles while going about their normal daily lives. A study of adults with CP found that decreased hip flexion ROM may contribute to an increased risk for low back pain.[318] Stretching exercises two to three times per week are recommended for both nondisabled people and those with CP.

The WHO notes that "participation in regular physical activity reduces the risk of coronary heart disease and stroke, diabetes, hypertension, colon cancer, breast cancer, and depression. Additionally, physical activity is a key determinant of energy expenditure and thus is fundamental to energy balance and weight control."[216] Consistently strong evidence demonstrates that people with CP participate in less physical activity and spend more time engaged in sedentary behavior than their nondisabled peers throughout the life span.[338] Studies have shown that:

- Adults with CP who reported preserved mobility throughout adulthood attribute it to regular physical activity, participation, and maintenance of strength, balance, and overall fitness.[345]
- Adults with CP who engaged in regular physical activity were at lower risk of decline in mobility. Deterioration in gait was strongly associated with inactivity.[300]

Details of the exercise and physical activity requirements for people with CP, as recommended by Verschuren and colleagues, are included in Table 3.5.2 and are summarized below.[215] The first four are the same as in childhood and adolescence; the fifth is an addition to the list for adults:

- Cardiorespiratory (aerobic) exercise
- Resistance (muscle strengthening) exercise
- Daily moderate to vigorous physical activity
- Avoiding sedentary behavior
- Neuromotor exercise (training balance, agility, and coordination)

The last, neuromotor exercise, is important for all adults, not just those with CP.[216,346] It is particularly important for avoiding falls, which we know can be a problem for adults with CP. A therapist can recommend suitable neuromotor exercises.

General pointers

These pointers assume autonomy is possible but it is recognized that this is not always the case.

- Try to understand your condition as much as possible, as well as the possible changes that may occur with aging. In a sense, forewarned is forearmed.
- Because services for adults with CP are, unfortunately, extremely limited, you are encouraged to build your own team. Do not wait for services for adults with CP to improve. As noted in Chapter 3, it is important to recognize that you, the person with the condition, are the most vital member of your team. You are responsible for putting your own care team in place. Find and connect with a center that provides services to adults with CP. There may not be one in your area, but take the time to research the best options available. An adult physical medicine and rehabilitation (PM&R) specialist will be able to help you prevent problems and deal with those that may arise. Try to find a good local primary care provider or general practitioner who understands CP for routine general health checks. Find a physical therapist and/or occupational therapist (again, preferably one who has experience working with people with CP) who will be able to support you if, and when, you need it.
- Get a copy of the clinical practice guideline for adults with CP when it becomes available. (It will be available online through the Cerebral Palsy Foundation.)
- Completing and maintaining an exercise and physical activity program is a crucial aspect of self-care. It is something each person must do for themselves. The benefits of exercise and physical activity accrue at so many levels, from preserving function to cardiometabolic health to preventing secondary conditions. Think of exercise and physical activity as a powerful medication that is available for free. (How many more people would "take" it if they thought of it this way?) The concept of "exercise is medicine" has been recognized since ancient times.
- Getting adequate rest is important. Walking is more demanding for an adult with CP than for a nondisabled adult. Additionally, the amount of exercise and physical activity required demands a lot of energy. It's important to achieve the right balance between activity and rest.

- A healthy diet is important for all adults—nondisabled and those with a disability. This includes adequate hydration. Get dietary advice from a specialist if you need it. Excess weight is not good for anyone, but it is especially taxing for a person with CP. Weight management is important not only for reducing the risk of NCDs but also for better musculoskeletal health and to help maintain walking. Because of their smaller and weaker muscles, people with CP cannot afford to be carrying excess weight. Keeping track of your BMI and central obesity is important. Try to keep your BMI in the healthy range and your waist circumference within recommended limits; all you need is a weighing scale and a measuring tape. It is worth monitoring both metrics because some people with a "normal" BMI can still have an unhealthy level of body fat. Finally, regarding diet, keep in mind that older adults require more protein. Read food labels and be mindful of the amount of protein in what you're eating. It can take some effort to achieve the recommended protein intake.

- Prevent, prevent, prevent. Think of aging with CP like taking care of your teeth. Brushing and flossing every day and visiting the dentist or hygienist regularly are the best ways to prevent tooth decay, but problems may still arise, and when they do, a dentist can help address them. The outcome may not be perfect, but problems can be dealt with. Take the same approach to the management of aging with CP. Be aware of the problems that may arise and work hard to prevent or minimize them. Time spent preventing problems is generally much more effective than time spent dealing with problems. However, if problems do arise, medical professionals can help.

- We each "own" our health. We may be able to get people to clean our house, pack for a move, walk our pets, and perform many more of life's chores, but we cannot get people to do our walking, cycling, or swimming for us. We must own our fitness, BMI, and cardiovascular health. We can call in experts to help, and they may provide valuable guidance, but they do not own our health.

- All adults should strive to maintain participation in society as they age. Try to add friends as you age; our peer groups tend to diminish later in life.

- Finally, as C.S. Lewis put it, remember: "You are never too old to set another goal or to dream a new dream."

Key points Chapter 4

- CP is diagnosed in infancy and is a lifelong condition. It is often thought of as a children's condition, but it is not. If one considers a normal life span, for every child and adolescent with CP there are approximately three adults with the condition.

- As a person with hemiplegia reaches adulthood and skeletal growth has ceased, a certain stabilization of the musculoskeletal aspects of the condition occurs. The rate of change of the condition is slower in adulthood, assuming the adult remains physically active. People with hemiplegia may, however, develop secondary conditions in adulthood. Some are consistent with typical aging, some may be unique. Each may influence body systems in more complex ways because of the interactions with CP itself.

- Examples of the decline that may occur with typical aging include sarcopenia, joint pain, osteoarthritis, osteoporosis, falls, and low-trauma fractures. Many conditions become more prevalent as people age, including cardiovascular disease, cancer, respiratory disease, and diabetes. These conditions are termed "noncommunicable diseases."

- Adults with hemiplegia have had their condition since childhood, but they are also susceptible to the same challenges of typical aging. For the person with hemiplegia, it is almost as if, on entering adulthood, two roads converge: the challenges of growing up with the condition meet the challenges of typical aging. The adult with hemiplegia must manage these two sets of challenges in combination. The problems of aging may occur at a younger age and with more severity in adults with CP than in those without the condition.

- The prevalence of several chronic physical and mental health conditions has been found to be higher among adults with CP than those without CP. However, much can be done to prevent or minimize many of the secondary conditions that can arise.

Chapter 5

Living with spastic hemiplegia

> We read to know we are not alone.
>
> C.S. Lewis

In this chapter, people share stories of living with spastic hemiplegia.

Kelly, mother of six-year-old Leo, from Minnesota, US

We never anticipated this. My pregnancy was very normal—no illness, a normal level of life stress, no falls, nothing that would lead me to think Leo would have any differences relative to his two siblings. Leo's birth was even the most uneventful of all three of our children because he actually came out as planned on his scheduled C-section date without any complications. I had had a very traumatic birth experience with his older brother five years prior, which led to an emergency C-section, and then another C-section for his sister three and a half years later, even though she tried to come on her own. Leo was the one who stuck with the plan and let us do what was needed to keep us both as safe as possible during delivery.

He was also a very normal baby. It was maybe harder to get him on a schedule, but it often is for a third child with so much going on in a growing family. It wasn't until he was around five or six months old that I started to notice some things: he seemed slouchier and not really interested in rolling or moving too much, and he was starting to grab for things, but always with his right hand, never his left. I looked back on his siblings' five- and six-month milestone pictures that showed them both sitting up straight, and videos that showed them more mobile. But Leo was super happy and sleeping and eating well, so I didn't get too worked up about it.

I brought up my observations at our six-month wellness check with the pediatrician. Initially, she didn't show concern and explained that it can be normal for a baby to favor one side. She advised us to give it a little more time but said that if we felt there was anything we wanted to check out further, she would give a referral for Leo to be seen by other specialists. As he was still pretty young and with no real obvious reasons for delays, we all hoped he would catch up by the next visit. The plan was to check in again at nine months.

We didn't wait that long. Just one month later, when Leo was seven months old, I called our pediatrician to say that we were now obsessively watching him and he for sure was not even trying to use his left hand. I also noticed that his left leg wasn't really kicking when he was lying on his back or putting his feet in the water. This seemed different from his siblings, and I wanted to know why. With no hesitation, the pediatrician wrote the referral for physical therapy and neurology.

I understood the relationship between what we were noticing with Leo and the referral to physical therapy, but "neurology" was a big new word for me that I didn't correlate to our concerns. Our pediatrician explained that they could be looking for something brain related, which had not been on my radar. It was then I began to worry.

I called to make the neurology appointment on May 25, 2018, and was told by the scheduler, who was very pleasant and calm, that we couldn't get in until August 26. I thought, WHAT? That felt like having to wait 10 years considering the rapid pace of change in babies. The thought of having to wait three months to have someone see what was going on with Leo simultaneously broke my heart and made me furious. When I asked the scheduler what I was supposed to do in the meantime, she found earlier availability with a nurse practitioner of neurology for June 18. I took that appointment while also still hanging onto the August date with the neurologist, just in case.

The day finally came, and the nurse practitioner asked a lot of questions about my pregnancy and when we first noticed changes with Leo. She completed a physical exam of him and determined that his reflexes weren't where they should be and that he had higher tone in his limbs. She recommended an MRI as a next step.

It was at this appointment with the nurse practitioner that I first heard the words "cerebral palsy," which caught me completely off guard.

I got the sense that the possibility of CP was told to a lot of families because she immediately explained that it was not an official diagnosis, but that she wanted me to be aware. In my uneducated mind at the time, my first thoughts were about extreme lack of mobility and confinement to a wheelchair. I soon learned that CP is a spectrum with the impacts being varied.

As I got in the car to drive home, I became completely overwhelmed with the confirmation that something did actually seem wrong with my baby. I sobbed most of the way home, releasing weeks of emotions that I had been suppressing.

The MRI was scheduled about a month later. Leo was sedated for it and very groggy after the 90-minute procedure. We weren't allowed in the room with him. Afterwards, we took him home and waited for about a week for the results. Our hope was that the MRI would provide some answers, of course: if it showed nothing of concern, we knew Leo would have to have other tests to try to find answers.

When the nurse practitioner called, she said the MRI was successful in that it showed something even if what it showed was hard to comprehend. She explained that Leo had what appeared to be an old brain bleed on his right frontal lobe, which accounted for his left side weakness. The likely explanation for the bleed was that Leo had had a perinatal stroke. While this result was very surprising to us, we felt lucky to have this answer when Leo was just nine months old.

Out of precaution, we met with a pediatric neurosurgeon to make sure the brain bleed was contained and that there were no areas of concern. The doctor gave us the good news that there didn't seem to be any reason to operate as all the images pointed toward an old and contained injury. It was then that we felt like we could move ahead.

Finally, the August 26 appointment that I had kept became an opportunity to meet with both a physical medicine and rehabilitation doctor and the neurologist together. This was a full body and brain appointment with the doctors collaborating to determine the cause of Leo's delays. One of my favorite lines from one of the doctors was, "We are going to make Leo be the best Leo he can be." That has become my mission as his mom and number-one advocate.

Shortly after that appointment, we began meeting with our school district's resources, including a special ed teacher. It was with this group that I learned how amazing and critical early intervention is for the child and the family. This team of a teacher, physical therapist, and occupational therapist started coming to our home weekly to see Leo and work with us. It was comfortable and helpful to do adaptive work in our home setting that would be realistic for us to continue after they left. We also began seeing a private physical therapist, which led to Leo being fitted with an ankle-foot orthosis on his left leg and foot, and a supramalleolar orthosis on his right foot to help with stability.

What no one could tell me in those early stages of his diagnosis was what to expect for Leo down the road. Would he walk? Would he talk? Would he have any other complications or issues? Looking back, I understand why they couldn't say much with certainty. It would take some time to figure out what impact Leo's brain injury would have on his development. But because the injury occurred as early as it did, Leo had the best possible chance of rewiring his brain to accomplish what he wasn't able to do at that point. With that knowledge, we stuck with the plan of PT and the services from the school.

March is CP Awareness month, and I decided that was the appropriate time to share our story with others. My goal was twofold. First, I didn't want to hide what we were going through because it was a real part of Leo's and our family's story. He was doing well and I was proud of him and us. Second, I knew that sharing could both help others and be a way for us to learn about more resources. It was the right decision: the support we received from everyone was overwhelming. Some shared their own stories with CP or what their children had dealt with and were in the process of overcoming. I was able to gain great perspective and comfort in knowing we weren't alone. Others recommended services and organizations that could help. Those suggestions have turned into critical opportunities for Leo and our family. I'm glad we did share our story and I encourage others to do the same. There is no reason to navigate this road alone.

Leo's journey has mostly been on an upward trajectory. We started Botox injections in his left arm and hand to reduce spasticity, which seemed to work well for him, and it encouraged him to move and keep making progress. He had the injections about every four to six months for a few years. He accomplished walking at 26 months. He started with a gait trainer to help him build stability and balance, but after some time he ditched it and walked on his own. When he was four and a half, we did serial casting on his left ankle to help him get a better stretch. I had the mentality of "Let's do as much as we can now, early, so that he has a better shot at doing less later." I don't know if my thinking was right, but now that Leo is six, physically bigger and stronger, and understands more, I can say I'm glad we did what we did when he was younger.

There are some difficulties. He has a hard time being at doctors' offices because he understands that there could be something uncomfortable involved. Transitions from one environment to another and being with unfamiliar people can be hurdles for him. We're learning more about how to help him prepare and get through that. The early intervention has been key. We have been so lucky to get help as early as we did. I feel so lucky that we live in a community that has great resources for Leo.

Leo is now a very happy kindergartner even though the adjustment to more structure and expectations has not been easy. He has come a long way with speech, independence, and social skills, but he has a lot still to work on. I hope he will continue to be accepted by his peers, to learn, and to keep his happy disposition as he is faced with the challenges of CP that will never go away. He is more like other kids than he is different. I'm in awe of him every day, knowing how much he has had to overcome to get to this point. I know he is meant to do something great and will continue to make us extremely proud. I'm here to support him, advocate for him, and make Leo the best Leo he can be.

Mark, father of six-year-old Elliot,
from London, England

It's difficult to know where to start when talking about such a defining thing in my life. Elliot was born after a very long and tough labor for my partner, Sian. Almost as soon as he was born, the alarm bells started ringing when the nurse noticed that something was wrong, and he was whisked away from us to intensive care.

He was having a series of life-threatening seizures, and the brilliant staff in intensive care worked tirelessly to save him. Eventually, he came through and started to recover, but we didn't know what the cause of the seizures was. Later scans showed that he had had a stroke and that the damage had been extensive, which resulted in him being diagnosed with cerebral palsy. Initially this diagnosis was frightening and hard to take; our minds automatically went to imagining the most severe cases of what can be a devastating disability.

As Elliot developed, it became clear he had a weakness on his left side, and his left hand was largely immobile. We took him to baby classes in the first few months of his life, and I remember the moment so clearly when I noticed that all the other babies in the group were able to sit up unaided, but Elliot still needed support.

We were not given any support or guidance after Elliot was born, but Sian was very driven to find help and funding for him. We worked very hard with him in the early days with standing supports and weekly therapy at a London-based charity for children with cerebral palsy.

Elliot has a real drive to overcome his difficulties and there have been many proud moments—like the first time he walked unaided. Now six years old, he is making us very proud at school by keeping up with his peers. Still, there are many obstacles and difficult moments to overcome. He must wear a splint when walking as he's very unsteady and has frequent falls. He requires one-to-one support at school and has difficulty processing information; he was recently assessed as having a developmental age of a four-year-old.

For me, the most difficult aspect of dealing with Elliot's disability has not been the physical challenges but the difficulties he has with communication and his mood swings we often have to deal with. There is still a lot of uncertainty about his development and whether as an adult he will be able to live independently, but we know the only way to deal with these fears is by living one day at a time and staying focused on the positives.

Elliot has a habit of repeatedly proving us wrong about our deepest held fears. He is a beautiful and engaging little boy and, most encouragingly, he is steadily developing—but at his own pace and on his own terms.

Maria, mother of seven-year-old Sophie, from Ireland

Sophie was born in October 2016. When we got the first indication that Sophie may have suffered a form of brain damage resulting from a brain bleed, I was a little worried, but by no means extremely alarmed. She was 14 months old and such a happy, smiley, bright little thing, so I felt whatever her problems were they would be minor in nature and she would overcome them.

Prior to this, Sophie had missed some important milestones in terms of motor skills and speech, but I had thought that these would come in "their own time" as everyone was advising, and the public health checks and hospital appointments did not note anything out of the ordinary. Looking back, I should have been far more aware, but I suppose that's hindsight. We did not know at the time that Sophie had right hemiplegic cerebral palsy.

After an initial referral by our family doctor to a lovely physiotherapist at the hospital, Sophie was immediately further referred to the neurology team. We will never forget that first appointment when, after having been asked a lot of questions about the pregnancy, we were told by one of the consultant's team that Sophie might not ever walk or talk. We left that appointment devastated, to say the least. We just could not believe what we were being told about our little girl.

Subsequent appointments followed quickly with the neurology team, accompanied by a lot of tests and a CT scan. We met with a wonderful consultant in March 2018 at the large hospital near where we live; she gave us the diagnosis and was so reassuring and full of optimism for Sophie that it really helped us at the time. We accepted the diagnosis there and then, took the positives out of that appointment with the consultant, and moved on immediately to discussing treatment and therapies that would help. I remember we were commended as parents for accepting the diagnosis and moving straight on to the plan of action, but to us that just seemed the only logical thing to do, and I think the attitude of the consultant really helped us with that.

The next step was to get into the early intervention program for children with disabilities. Sophie was put forward for this by the medical team but, to our disbelief, was turned down. Our helpful consultant stepped in and pushed the matter, Sophie's case was reviewed, and she was accepted onto the program. Still, months passed by and Sophie was getting no services, which was a huge blow for us. Our positive attitude started to diminish quickly and was replaced with frustrations with the inadequacy of the so-called early intervention program. Sophie needed help badly with speech, occupational therapy, and physiotherapy. She had been diagnosed in March 2018 and we found ourselves preparing for Christmas, still with no services for her. This situation of having little or no services continued, and then COVID came along and exacerbated it.

However, while waiting for the services, the impossible happened as family members pulled together to fill the gap. Sophie's auntie, godmother, big sister, nephews, and nieces collectively used every spare minute of their time to work with Sophie along with what we were doing as parents. In return, Sophie remained determined and hardly ever complained. With the family's help over a five-month period, Sophie learned how to go from sitting to kneeling, and then over six more months, from kneeling to standing. The physical strength it took her to get up from the ground to a standing position was incredible. As her mother, I knew one day Sophie would walk. We did not want a walker. We knew Sophie would do it on her own.

While we continued to wait for physio and all the other services, I started to ask around for other options and was lucky to find a brilliant private physiotherapist near where we lived. She provided services well beyond neurodevelopmental therapy; she gave us hope, helped us advocate for Sophie, and above all, kept us sane. Sophie immediately bonded with this kind woman, and it was during one of the therapy sessions with her that Sophie took her first steps. We, mum and therapist, hugged each other and were elated. Sophie was two years and four months old and had defied the odds that were overwhelmingly stacked against her. It was onwards and upwards.

While Sophie had gained motor function in her right leg, her right hand was still badly impacted, as were her communication skills. Again, the family stepped up to help. We really wanted to maximize opportunities for Sophie before she hit the three-year milestone. Where we live in Ireland, we had no CIMT,* no casts and for the most part, no occupational therapist to even advise us what to do. So we pulled Sophie's sleeve over her left hand and tied a knot in the sleeve to limit her to using her right hand during mealtimes and when playing with her toys. Sophie got on with it, never complaining, always smiling and laughing. It was hard to know if this was the right thing to do as we didn't really have anyone to ask, but I think it has had a lasting impact on her right-hand functionality.

Sophie has autism, which is likely linked to the brain damage, and her communication and social skills are still a major challenge. She is definitely a people person. She loves people and most people she meets love her, which is a huge bonus. Her eye contact is amazing. And while I may be biased in my opinion, she is a very beautiful little girl with long black hair and huge blue eyes, so she melts the hearts of many. Her vocabulary is building up each year, and she definitely knows how to get her point across!

We have often heard some medical professionals say that the years zero to three are when the brain is most plastic and when most lasting change can be made with therapy. And that after six years of age, neuroplasticity is limited. This always stressed us a lot in the context of the

---

* Involves restraint of the unaffected hand combined with intensive structured therapy.

ongoing waiting list situation. Naturally, early intervention is essential for our children. However, our advice to other parents is, don't live by this or let it dishearten you. In Sophie's seventh year on this planet, she has moved onto new skill sets. She has learned to run for the first time, she has learned to jump up and down with both feet, she manages the stairs to bed by herself, and she walks the dog. She is doing things that people never thought she would. She has never needed surgery to achieve these skills; she has achieved them through pure determination, stretching, and by being provided with lots of opportunity for activities. We find that going on holidays as a family is important; this is when Sophie excels the most and learns new skills. While some health professionals say she is only mimicking, she is now learning to count, match letters to words, and even do spelling, thanks to her fantastic school environment. The sky is the limit for this little girl.

It took several years and a change of management in the early intervention program for Sophie to get what she was entitled to. Sophie is very lucky to now be in the care of a fantastic team: all of whom are very capable, motivated, and dedicated individuals. Sophie's new speech therapist has been incredible in helping with increased speech and interaction (Sophie was able to ask Santa for what she wanted for Christmas for the first time this year!). Her new occupational therapist is working relentlessly, which has resulted in really promising improvements in Sophie's right-hand awareness and function with her new upper limb clinic. But most of all, Sophie's physiotherapist, who we met just over a year ago, is an amazing human being, believes so much in Sophie and has been instrumental in her recent achievements: her beautifully symmetrical stance and full range of movement.

The future is so bright.

That first hospital consultant who was so helpful said to us at the time, "You need to be Sophie's advocate. You need to be her voice." That is advice we follow to this day. Our own advice to other parents facing similar challenges is to work only with those who see the potential in your child. Surround yourself by great people—great therapists who believe in your child completely. We have met many along the way who want to limit our child, who talk her abilities down, who don't see the potential, and that is reflected in their therapies. It is important to quickly recognize and move away from those types of therapists and medical professionals and for you to find and stick with the good ones. There are, of course, ups and downs and downright frightening experiences (too many stories to mention), but never stop moving forward. Celebrate all the big and little wins. Sophie has surpassed and continues to surprise those in the profession, despite her right hemiplegia GMFCS level II, which is often very difficult to spot. She will never stop improving and learning.

As for us parents, while we would have preferred for Sophie not to have had to deal with these challenges, we feel we are blessed with having a very real perspective on life, and we never stress the little things anymore.

Moriom, mother of 15-year-old Dulal, from Bangladesh

Moriom

I had two children, but my husband and I desired another baby. I did not realize I was pregnant until I noticed my belly growing, and others confirmed my suspicions. At three months, my belly appeared unusually large, and I felt movements on both sides, which puzzled me. Being concerned, we visited a doctor who recommended an ultrasound. To our surprise, the ultrasound revealed I was carrying twins.

As my pregnancy progressed to six months, I experienced swollen limbs and pain. Consulting the doctor again, I discovered that the baby on the right side was healthy, but the baby on the left was lying beneath the other and not doing well. The doctor prescribed medication and warned me that if my water broke, the baby would be at risk of death. Although the doctor advised taking the medication for the entire duration of the pregnancy, I could only manage a couple of weeks.

One evening, around seven months into the pregnancy, my water broke. We immediately set out in a van to find help. Initially, we visited a midwife, who suggested attempting a normal delivery. However, my family disagreed with this plan due to my previous cesarean delivery and the premature stage of the pregnancy. Then we were sent to see a gynecologist at the hospital, where I waited while lying on a bed, enduring continuous water breakage, my clothes and hair soaked.

Nurses sporadically visited me to check my blood pressure, but no doctor came. We later discovered that the doctor was unavailable, but nobody informed us. It wasn't until 2 a.m. that another gynecologist finally arrived and initiated surgery. To my horror, they began the procedure without ensuring I was fully anesthetized. The incision in my belly caused intense pain, but they proceeded. When the doctor pulled out my larger baby, I lost consciousness.

When I awoke after the delivery, I noticed one of my babies was crying incessantly and appeared smaller, while the other baby was calm and slightly larger. My little one weighed only around 1 kilogram (2.2 pounds), and the doctor advised us to take the babies to Ma o Shishu Hospital (Mother & Child Hospital). However, the hospital authorities directed us to Sirajganj, an urban district. We pleaded with them to keep my children at that hospital, fearing the journey to Sirajganj might endanger their lives. After much persuasion, they agreed to provide treatment for my children. My smaller baby had a tube inserted through his nose as he couldn't consume breast milk. We spent six days in that hospital before finally taking the twins home.

We named my tiny baby Dulal and the larger one Alal. On Dulal's eighth day of life, he began retching and choking as if his life were hanging by a thread. My father-in-law brought in a kabiraj (traditional healer) who tried traditional medicine, but it didn't work. In desperation, my elder sister fed him cooked milk, and gradually, he started recovering.

Dulal continued to struggle. At one year old, he hadn't learned to sit, unlike other babies who could roll and sit up by then. Alal, on the other hand, learned to sit at five months and started crawling at eight months. Concerned, I tried supporting Dulal with pillows, but he couldn't maintain the sitting position and would frequently fall back.

I have endured gossip and rumors within the village due to having a disabled child. People sometimes referred to Dulal as a "cripple," which deeply saddened me. I couldn't eat or sleep well. Some even blamed me for my child's disability. In response, I would say that Allah gave him to me, and only Allah knows best.

When Dulal turned two, I learned about a medical camp for disabled children organized by an organization called CSF Global. We attended the camp, where they informed us that Dulal had experienced brain trauma. They demonstrated some exercises that would help his condition. I was skeptical about the benefits of the exercises as I didn't fully understand what his condition was or how exercises could help. When Dulal turned three, a neighbor suggested visiting a disability clinic in Bogra, another district. The doctors at the clinic also recommended exercises for Dulal, but I remained unconvinced of their effectiveness.

One day, I heard about the Centre for the Rehabilitation of the Paralysed (CRP), a tertiary-level rehabilitation center in Dhaka. We learned that CRP admits children like Dulal and provides appropriate treatment. When Dulal turned six, we admitted him to CRP for a 14-day stay. There, he received various therapies throughout the day. They taught us how to help him perform daily activities independently and provided exercises for his limbs and speech therapy. Although they advised us to take Dulal to CRP at least twice a month, financial constraints and family responsibilities made it challenging.

Gradually, I began to grasp the importance of exercises for Dulal's development. I started practicing the exercises with Dulal that I learned from CRP at home two or three times a day. Then a staff member from CSF Global visited our house and encouraged us to enroll Dulal in a free therapy program at the Shishu Shorgo (Children's Heaven) center in our subdistrict. There he received three hours of therapy sessions, five days a week. Along with therapy, they provided him with nutritious foods.

A community therapist at the center taught me how to assist Dulal with various activities such as crawling, sitting on the toilet, four-point kneeling, and standing with assistance. Before this treatment started, Dulal still couldn't sit or roll. Imagine my surprise when, one day after therapy, I couldn't find him on the bed where I had left him and discovered him sitting next to the bed by himself. That filled me with joy and renewed hope that Dulal would be able to do everything independently one day. Through consistent practice at the center and at home, Dulal learned to sit cross-legged, crawl, use the toilet independently, and stand without my assistance. By the grace of Allah, he eventually started walking on his own and exploring the house and surroundings. The entire family rejoiced at Dulal's progress, and I felt happiness deep within me.

Unfortunately, after my daughter got married, I couldn't continue taking Dulal to Shishu Shorgo due to lack of support at home, and consequently, his progress halted after four years of treatment. Now he can walk with a limp, but not as smoothly as a typical child. If we had continued attending Shishu Shorgo for a few more months or years, I believe he would have developed even better walking abilities.

Raising a child with a disability has made me stronger and more courageous than any other woman in my village. I am prepared to face life's challenges. I am content with Dulal's current condition, and my only wish is for Allah to grant him the strength to lead a fulfilling life. My son is intelligent and understands everything. He even reminds us not to waste electricity, water, or money. He expresses his sadness at being confined to home and unable to work. I often wonder if I had followed the advice I received from CSF Global about Dulal's exercises when he was only two years old, his condition might be better. I wish that I had the knowledge to understand that exercises were the key to giving Dulal the best chance at life. Whenever I encounter a child in a similar situation, I urge their parents to seek support from Shishu Shorgo. I share with them that my child learned to perform all functions after attending the program.

Dulal

I feel a lack of strength in my right hand and leg. I eat adequately, but my strength doesn't improve. I've heard that it's because of something in my brain. I feel bad when I see other children cutting paddy in the field, picking mangoes from trees, or going to school for studies, while I can't do any of these activities. I want to feed my cows and goats, cut grass for them, go to the village fair, and pray in congregation during Eid, but I can't do anything I want. How long can a person sit inside a home? Time doesn't pass without activities! I can't even play sports like football or cricket, which children of my age can do. All I can do is sit in a make-believe shop and play with younger children. It makes me sad that I can't play like other boys.

Sometimes, I wonder why this happened to me and not to others. I pray and cry for divine help to find a cure, but it doesn't work. Children often call me "crippled" or "disabled," especially when I misbehave or get into arguments. They also tell me that I won't be able to marry anyone. I laugh at them. I've accepted it, and it doesn't make me feel bad anymore.

I've been taken to many places for my treatment. I've received different types of treatment, including medicine and exercises. I went to the Shishu Shorgo center for four years. My therapy stopped because after my sister's marriage my mother couldn't find time to take me there. When I was doing the therapy, I was able to walk much better and my leg was straighter. However, I lost my strength soon after I stopped therapy. Now, I can walk on flat surfaces but I struggle on rough terrain, and I can't get up if I fall. The most difficult task for me now is cleaning after using the toilet. I have fallen on the ground many times while trying to clean myself.

I also used to go to school in my mother's lap and studied up to class five. My school teachers liked me very much. But after my sister's marriage, my mother couldn't find time to take me to school. I have forgotten many things I learned before. I used to write Bengali and English letters, and count from 1 to 40, all of which my sister taught me. Now I regret not continuing my studies because I could have gotten a job.

I wish I could tell other children not to say hurtful words to me. I think that if I had had more therapy as a child, I may have been able to do more. Nevertheless, I am happy with my physical condition as Allah has placed me.

Nathalie, mother of 16-year-old Lucas and 19-year-old Leo who has CP, from Georgia, US

Nathalie

I am the mother of two young men, Lucas and Leo. Leo, the older of the two, has hemiplegic cerebral palsy (spastic and dystonic), that resulted from hemorrhage and inflammation in his brain when he was born at 27 weeks. I separately asked my boys how they thought Leo's condition had affected our family over the past 19 years. It was enlightening seeing how similar their viewpoints were, and how they saw our small family.

Lucas

My brother's CP has affected our family a lot. It's complicated though.

For me, I grew up with it, so I didn't really notice it much until other people pointed it out. Then I realized that I hadn't known how fragile he is and that he couldn't do all the things I did. I remember one moment really well when I was four years old: I wondered why my brother had to go on a treadmill because he was only seven years old, and then I was shocked that he had fallen off and was hurt. I could see my au pair was really worried and crying, but my mom just took it in stride, as if this were normal, and she treated him and bandaged him and then she put him back on the treadmill the next day—with a lot more supervision.

I learned a lot from being with my brother because he has a totally different viewpoint. He has also experienced more pain than anyone I know, and frustration at not being able to do the things he wants. I admit that he is very strong; I have never had to work as hard as him to do anything. When I was eight, I remember feeling bad for him, but he was so mad even then about it. He absolutely hates any pity, so I can't feel bad for him. It is strange, because he is my big brother and I always look up to him, but I can do things he can't.

The dynamic in our family is different from others, as much as I can tell from seeing my friends and schoolmates' families. I think our family is more flexible than others. We adapt to different requirements at different times; there is no one rigid rule that will make things always work for my brother and our family. We don't have traditional roles. We must adapt, all the time. Change for us is every day.

I think my brother's CP has maybe affected our values. Tolerance, unconditional kindness, and empathy are very important to us. I can't tell if my mom passed these down to us or if we all developed them together because we grew up this way. It's so hard to imagine life differently. I think my mom holds me to a higher standard of empathy and kindness with everyone because she knows I get it. When I was little, I thought people paid more attention to my brother. But now I see we each get time together with my mom and it is totally different; we are treated differently because we are individuals. My mom gives us each a ton of attention even if we don't want it. We have dinner every night together and the only time we indirectly talk about his CP is when he complains about accommodations and his frustration with people not understanding what he needs even when he explains it.

Also, we don't have a dad in our lives like other kids do, so it makes it so much harder that my brother has CP. Sometimes I think if we had a dad role filled in our family, all the stress and work and extra worry of making sure my brother is okay wouldn't fall on one parent, and she would have more time for us both.

Leo

It's complicated. Certain things came out of me having CP that were quite good, and others that made our lives a lot harder.

The worst part was probably my scoliosis. None of the treatments out there were made for scoliosis in CP, and none of them worked. The doctors had us try things like braces that made my school life horrible, especially the Boston brace which kept me from doing things with my friends, made me lose my balance and fall when I never did before, and all to find out it did nothing at all to help with my scoliosis. I still ended up with surgery, which didn't fix everything. I still have kyphosis which keeps me from standing the way I did when I was a preteen, and I have to work intensively with a trainer on posture.

When I was little, I remember having to go to frequent therapy sessions. It involved a lot of hard work, especially at the beginning when my mom tried several kinds of AFOs before choosing a WalkAide and night stretching splints instead. At night while I was growing up, we would sing songs together while my mom helped me do stretches, which were hard at first but then just became a part of routine. And the singing was more important than the stretching. I ended up in choir for six years, likely because of this.

As far as my dad is concerned, I have a good relationship with him and I love him a lot, but he is not there on a day-to-day basis. So my CP affects him differently. He is very conscious of my need to stay healthy in the big picture. In very practical terms though, he doesn't always understand CP, despite the best of intentions. Because we don't live with him, my CP doesn't affect his everyday life the way it does ours.

Some of the good things: we became more persistent as a family and individuals. In a way, my CP changed my brother' life and my mom's life a lot. We never give up, not just for CP, but in life. Also, we always see a lot of different solutions to a problem instead of a single one.

My brother and mom can't just say they will help me. They need to have a problem-solving mindset that changes every day. When I was growing up, if I was hurting or stressed or out of balance, everything was always changing and they had to adapt. All of us developed a mindset where if something didn't work it was just time to try something else. I think my mom reads not only for her own research, because she is passionate about her job, but also because it pushes her to think differently in all other areas. Every time she reads about something, she comes up with a hundred crazy ideas and then researches how they might work. My CP is an outlet for all her curiosity.

Nathalie

Yesterday I asked Leo after dinner if he could change anything about his life, what would it be. He said, "I wish Dad lived near us." Lucas and I quietly cried at this answer, stunned into silence and amazement, yet again. My children have taught me the wonder of loving someone more and more every day, with every touch and every connection. This helps temper urgency and worry, with joy in the present moment. I can see that my sons have become amazing young men, in all their complexity and grace. Leo's CP has changed us as a family, and according to both my boys, it has made us more tolerant, adaptable, persistent, problem-solving, empathetic, and kind. But CP is a lifelong condition and there will be more challenges and more pain and more joy. I need to have faith that my children are right: that we truly never give up and that change for us will still be every day.

Emma, an adult from the UK

I was diagnosed at the age of two with cerebral palsy. I was discharged from medical services when I was 16, being told that I was the best I would ever be. As you might imagine, as a young teenager I met-aphorically hopped and skipped out of the clinic where I had spent the best parts of my childhood being poked, prodded, and made to do things I couldn't do—things that were uncomfortable and often painful. In retrospect, of course, I am hugely grateful for all the intervention I received and how much it helped me to live a "normal" life.

As a child, my main goal was to be like my sister and my friends. I did not know anyone else with cerebral palsy, and I resented the appoint-ments that always served to remind me that I was different. What I did not know then, but recognize now, was that I received excellent, timely, and coordinated support that enabled me to attend mainstream school, socialize with my friends, and follow my dreams—going to university, traveling the world, marrying, and becoming a mum.

As an adult, without any integrated care from the authorities, my phys-ical problems increased. I experienced a significant decline in mobility in my late 30s, which led to several surgeries and having to give up work as a speech and language therapist. This came as a big shock to me; having a nonprogressive condition, I didn't anticipate any change in my mobility.

Because cerebral palsy is treated as a childhood condition, not a life-long condition, specialized treatment largely ceases after the age of 18 in the UK, and care becomes reactive rather than proactive. Diagnosis and treatment are often delayed, leaving no room for preventive or long-term maintenance programs.

In my case, when I transitioned from pediatric care, finding the right support for my cerebral palsy proved difficult. My general practitioner referred me back and forth between physiotherapy and other services. I often left my consultations with a prescription for antidepressants, failing to address my increasing hip pain, fatigue, and falls. Hip pain, misdiagnosed as "just CP," worsened due to lack of investigation. Advanced arthritis developed in both hips, and despite needing hip replacements, I was deemed "too young" by surgeons who wanted me to wait until I lost full mobility. Fighting for my surgery, a privilege not accessible to most, allowed me to regain some independence.

My hospitalization after surgery was another hurdle. The orthopedic team lacked understanding of my CP, which made pain management difficult. The complications of developing a grade 4 heel sore and a blood clot added to the struggle. My hospital stay was nearly three weeks instead of the usual five days, and I needed 18 months of intensive rehabilitation afterward to regain my independence.

Five years later, shoulder pain emerged, impacting my arm and my use of crutches. Again, the lack of practitioners with specialist knowledge and understanding of the impact of cerebral palsy as people age left me feeling unsupported. Yet, through physiotherapy and self-advocacy, I found solutions. Splinting, muscle strengthening, and exploring underlying hormonal causes led to trialing hormone replacement therapy, which resulted in significant improvement. Building my upper body strength and balance further reduced my reliance on crutches.

Through all this, I couldn't understand why support for adults with cerebral palsy was so threadbare and uncoordinated. I expressed my frustration in a blog I posted, "From Complainer to Campaigner," in which I started to reach out to the medical and CP communities to set an agenda for change. This led to my starting the charity UP—The Adult Cerebral Palsy Movement to help those in the adult CP community who, like me, were struggling to get the right kind of help and, importantly, to "live well" with the condition. We have worked tirelessly to gain a better understanding of CP as it pertains to adults and to address the lack of coordinated services and trained specialists who understand our unique medical needs. The majority of people with cerebral palsy experience near-normal life expectancies; this means that for many individuals, me included, adult life also comes with challenges in housing, employment, relationships, family life, and overall participation in life.

It is now recognized that there are consequences on the body of living lifelong with cerebral palsy, including the possibility of accelerated aging. It is now also understood that adults with cerebral palsy may be at higher risk for developing secondary conditions such as musculoskeletal deterioration, pain, cardiometabolic diseases, kidney disease, dysphagia, and mental health issues such as depression and anxiety.

I believe that, in light of this new understanding, we have to begin to take a life course perspective when treating and managing adults with cerebral palsy. I live a great life with cerebral palsy, so I do not write this to cause alarm. I believe that knowledge is power and with understanding of some of the consequences of living with cerebral palsy comes opportunity to mitigate risk.

Many people ask me for advice on navigating life with CP. Here are some key principles I've learned from my own journey and from others:

- **Information is key:** Transition from childhood to being an adult is a process, not an event, and children need to be prepared for the change. The research suggests we should be working toward transition from the age of 14. It's important to know and understand what type of cerebral palsy you have so you can learn how to best to manage your condition and grow old with it. Many people I speak with say they regret they were not taught strategies to manage pain, fatigue, and anxiety earlier. To this day, at the age of 47, I am asked about my birth and experience of childhood. Information that was known and relayed by my parents before I was viewed as an adult. As an adult, it is important to know this for sharing with medical professionals in adulthood.
- **Look for the opportunities to build skills:** Research has identified independence, self-advocacy, and decision-making skills as being key to supporting teenagers in their development of independence. In my own family, this is almost an organic process over time—my husband and I slowly giving my son responsibility and opportunity to do things independently. However, when you are parenting an individual with CP who needs more support, these naturally occurring opportunities are more limited. The onus is on parents to create times when a young person can practice making decisions and speaking up for themselves as well as chances to learn how and when to ask for help.
- **Build healthy habits:** As an adult, my focus is on staying healthy, maintaining skills, and being able to participate in all aspects of life. The responsibility to keep myself active is mine, and it is important because it helps me stay mobile, manage my stress, and reduce my pain (which reduces the risk of falls). While I have found a way to stay active, the journey to getting there has been difficult and would have been easier if I had had positive experiences of activity

in my childhood. I now encourage parents to make being active an important part of family life for everyone. Help children try different sports and activities until they find one that they like. In my experience, those adults who found sports that they loved in childhood find it much easier to stay active later in life. Individuals who keep active report they feel less isolated and find it much easier to develop friendships. They find community through a shared love of a sport. Being physically active is also crucial for mental health.

- **Success is being able to participate:** When I grew up, my understanding of the goals of physiotherapy was to help me walk independently. I guarded that success so closely that when it was suggested to me that a walking stick would reduce my pain and keep me safe, I felt like I had failed and refused. But I now know that success is about being able to participate, something I learned after my surgery when I had to use a wheelchair. I discovered that instead of being a symbol of failure, the chair aided my participation. I am no longer embarrassed about using my chair or my crutches because they allow me to be more involved in activities with my children and friends. Using aids sometimes means being in less pain, and that makes my life easier too. We need to teach our children that using aids is okay and better than sitting at home alone.

- **Support is available:** I have always felt quite isolated when it came to trying to manage life events such as starting a relationship, going to university, finding work, or becoming a parent. My peers were going through the same thing, but they didn't have CP. There are a lot of organizations that can help. Some of them are not just for people with CP but for all people with disabilities, and I don't think that matters. It is about knowing that there is support out there and knowing where to look.

- **Connecting and finding role models:** As a child, I always felt different. It would have really helped me to know that I was not alone. Connecting with others with CP helps you discover that there are a lot more people like you. Sharing experiences is powerful, and I have learned so much from other people. I also believe that it is only by seeing other people achieving and succeeding that you can learn what is possible.

Above all, my main message is we need to treat cerebral palsy as a lifelong condition and therefore intervention in childhood and adolescence should also include equipping and preparing them for adulthood.

Justin, an adult, from Oklahoma, US

I am a father, physician, and an individual with hemiplegic CP, and I recently celebrated my 45th year. Over the years, I've thought a lot about how children with CP, particularly those with hemiplegic CP, relate to life.

Throughout the day, I diagnose and treat children with CP and similar conditions. Their parents often fear the unknown and have anxiety about the future for their children—something I can recognize as a parent. Some parents tend to want to hover and protect their children as much as they can. Many are aware that I have CP myself, so ask for my advice. It's important to note that while there are similar patterns within CP, no individual history and experience is the same.

Children with hemiplegia often have higher gait function. They may have varying degrees of hand function and the full spectrum of intellectual and communication abilities. Many children with hemiplegia can "hide in plain sight" from those unfamiliar with the condition. This can be a blessing in many ways, but most of these children are still faced with uncomfortable questions about and frustrations with their body, which they struggle to control. And having impairments that are less obvious can create an identity challenge of sorts. To the outside observer, it may be difficult to understand the challenges of the hand, speech, or overall physical impairment when paired with the ability to walk and talk relatively well.

As kindergarten and first grade come round, children seem more aware of their differences. Both parents and children often fear having to face the inevitable questions: What's that on your leg? (referring to a brace). Why can't you hold that with your hand? Why does your voice sound different?

I advise parents and children of elementary school age to view their peers as they are—curious about everything. Yes, there are circumstances where a child may be excluded because they are different and times when intentionally cruel comments are made. There are more times, though, when interaction is based on underlying curiosity.

I wish I had some of that insight when I was young. Most kids in the classroom or on the playground are preoccupied with their own challenges. It is useful for parents to introduce the idea to their child that every human can teach their community how to relate to them. I advise children to be matter of fact in their responses and not overexplain: "Oh that. Well, that's my brace. It helps me walk."

But I also know that as a physician, my advice isn't always welcome. At an appointment, I may be focused on the form of a leg brace and gait pattern. The teenager I'm seeing may not care about that at all! He may be thinking, What will the girls at school think about this brace? or Will this make it harder to relate to my friends? or I don't want to be different! Once, I was fired by a patient for suggesting that cowboy boots may not be the best option for their shoe wear!

We know that there is a tendency for individuals with CP to isolate themselves when it is more difficult to perform tasks. We know that adults with CP may struggle with social isolation. I advise anyone with CP to seek challenges and to engage in life right from the start. At the same time, it's okay for individuals to take time for themselves in places of peace. That could be something as simple as spending time in a grandfather's barnyard or taking a walk with a dog in a field or forest path.

Patterns we establish when we are young can affect us throughout our lives. It is normal for a child to be angry when they struggle to control their hand. It is normal to feel frustrated that they are the only one not going up the stairs. It is normal for a teenager to believe that they might not be handsome enough to date. It is normal for an adult to fear that someone will not love them because of some of their physical challenges. But I have found, through trial and error, that it is important to acknowledge and challenge these doubts. It is easy to say but harder to live the adage, "more reward, more risk." It is truly better to "have loved and lost than never to have loved at all."

I encourage my patients to consider that every person has their own challenges. It is important to encourage every family to consider compassion and forgiveness. To grow and succeed, we will all require those gifts. When considering these concepts, we need to remember to forgive ourselves.

God and time have taught me these lessons. And having learned them, I remember what I could have done better myself and think of the many blessings I have been given. I have found a woman whom I love and have created a family with. We have two beautiful children who have so much to offer the world. They, too, will have their own challenges in life. I hope to be able to help them as their dad. And as a physician, I hope to watch my terrific patients bring great things to the world.

Chapter 6

Further reading and research

Education is not the filling of a pail,
but the lighting of a fire.
William Butler Yeats

Further reading

For those who would like further reading on this condition, a list of recommended books, websites, and resources has been collated and will be regularly updated. Access to the list is provided in **Useful web resources.**

Research

Research serves as a cornerstone of evidence-based medicine and drives health care advancement. We discussed the importance of evidence-based medicine (or evidence-based practice) in Chapter 3. It is "the conscientious, explicit, and judicious use of current best evidence in making decisions about the care of individual patients." It combines the best available external clinical evidence from research with the clinical expertise of the professional.[170] Family priorities and preferences are also considered.[171]

Evidence is collected by carrying out scientific studies (research studies), the results of which are published as full-length, peer-reviewed research articles (or papers) in scientific journals. "Peer-reviewed" means that experts with relevant content knowledge have reviewed, challenged, and agreed that the scientific method and study conclusions based on the results are sound.

Scientific studies may also be presented in brief at conferences, and conference proceedings are often published. However, conference proceedings present preliminary results and peer review is minimal. *Therefore, full-length published research articles are the most rigorous and sound evidence.*

The above published research outputs are collectively known as scientific literature or, simply, research.

Research may also be discussed on various social media platforms such as X (formerly Twitter), Facebook, LinkedIn, and Instagram. If you consume information this way, it is always important to go back to the original source (i.e., the full-length research article) to ensure the media's portrayal of the study findings is accurate.

You may have familiarity with searching the scientific literature. If not, search engines such as PubMed (ncbi.nlm.nih.gov/pubmed) and Google Scholar (scholar.google.com) are good places to start. They provide a free abstract (a short summary of the article), which can be very useful. In the past, you generally needed to belong to an academic or medical institution to have access to full-length research articles. Many articles are now available online for free. Google Scholar provides links to many full-length articles, and some community libraries allow you to request full-length articles.

You might have heard the phrase, "Just because someone says it, doesn't mean it's true." This is worth remembering in all aspects of life, but it is also relevant to research. While research articles go through a peer review process, you should still read them with a critical eye. Ask yourself, How confident can I be in the results of this research study? Was the sample size big enough to be representative of the larger population? Did the results support the conclusion?

If you aren't a trained scientist, reviewing the quality of the evidence might be more challenging, but you can still make sure the basic methods make sense and the author's conclusions are supported by the data presented. The information below will help you learn about some research study designs and how study design affects how much confidence you can place in a study's conclusions.

Research study design

There are different research study designs, and each has its value. The quality of the evidence, or level of evidence, is graded based on the study design and how well the methods were executed. Research articles sometimes list (often in the abstract) the level of evidence from I to V, with level I being the highest.

The most common research study designs, listed from highest to lowest level of evidence, are:

- Systematic review
- Randomized controlled trial
- Cohort
- Case control
- Cross-sectional
- Case report and case series

Systematic review: A systematic review summarizes the results of several scientific studies on the same topic. They can be qualitative (descriptive) or quantitative (numerical):

- Qualitative: A summary of common themes and findings across studies but without a statistical analysis.
- Quantitative: A statistical analysis carried out that takes a weighted average of the findings across studies to produce one estimate for the effect of a treatment, for example. The quantitative approach is called a "meta-analysis."

The highest level of evidence is a systematic review of randomized controlled trials (described next), although systematic reviews can also include studies that used other types of study designs. Systematic reviews may be published by individual researchers or groups. The Cochrane collaboration is a worldwide association of researchers, health care professionals, patients, and carers that publishes systematic reviews on various topics.

Randomized controlled trial (RCT): An RCT is a study design aimed at identifying cause and effect. The cause is, for example, the treatment, and the effect is the outcome being measured. Strict control of the study method (the "C" in RCT) helps to ensure the treatment of interest is the only factor that could cause the outcome. A treatment group receives the treatment while a nontreatment group (also known as the control group) does not. The participants are randomly assigned (the "R" in RCT) to one of the groups. The random assignment is one of the key strengths of this study design because it takes care of the "unknown unknowns" that may influence the outcome. The treatment effect is found by comparing the outcomes of the treatment and nontreatment groups. RCTs are considered the highest quality study design but are still uncommon in medical literature.

Cohort: A cohort is a group of people who share a common characteristic (e.g., diagnosis, gender). In a cohort study, outcome is measured two or more times. Researchers identify the characteristic of interest and then measure the outcome, looking for associations between the two. A cohort study is a form of longitudinal study ("longitudinal" means that the same outcome is measured on the same participants two or more times over a period of time). You may come across the terms "prospective" and "retrospective" cohort studies.

- In prospective cohort studies, research questions and methods are defined, and a cohort is followed over time, collecting data.
- In retrospective cohort studies, research questions and methods are defined after data has been collected or already exists (e.g., a person's medical record).

Case control: In case control studies, researchers identify the outcome of interest, which defines the groups (e.g., infants with a specific diagnosis and typically developing infants), and then look backward in time at different factors or exposures that might have caused different outcomes. At the beginning of the study, the outcome is known, but the factors or exposures that might have caused that outcome are unknown. This is the opposite of cohort studies. Because the outcome and factors or exposures data already exist, case control studies are always retrospective.

Cross-sectional: Cross-sectional studies take measurements only once from participants. Researchers look for associations between certain factors and exposures, and outcomes.

Case report and case series: A case report (also referred to as a single-subject case study) is an account of a single patient—usually a unique case—and their medical history, status, and outcomes from a treatment, for example. A case series is a group of case reports on patients who were exposed to a similar treatment. These reports are usually retrospective, and data has already been collected by other means (usually as part of routine medical care).

Getting involved in research

There are many opportunities to become involved in research. Together with medical professionals and researchers, people with lived experience can help drive advancement in health care.

a) As a participant

Researchers working in academic and medical settings are always looking for participants for their studies. You might receive an invitation to participate in such a study via an email, letter in the mail, phone call, social media ad, or other method.

Some studies are very easy and may just involve completing one online survey; others may take more time with various measurements being taken on more than one occasion. Just as you are advised to read published research studies with a critical eye, so should you judge new research study opportunities before agreeing to participate. Participating can take time and effort—the expected time commitment will be communicated in the study recruitment material. There is often a small reimbursement offered for time spent in a study.

It's worth noting that you, as the study participant, may not personally benefit from the research study, but the collective population with the condition will likely benefit.

Clinical trials are research studies conducted to evaluate the safety and effectiveness of new medical treatments, including new medications and devices before they can be approved for widespread use. They are often conducted following a randomized controlled trial research study design.

A potential benefit of participating in clinical trials is gaining early access to new medical treatments. Even if you are assigned to the control group (which usually receives standard care), you may have early access to the new treatment once the data collection phase is complete. In addition, standard care is likely to be current best practice.

You can find information about clinical trials through various sources:

- The National Institutes of Health in the US maintains a comprehensive database, ClinicalTrials.gov, where you can learn about clinical trials around the world. You can search this database by specific medical condition, location, or other pertinent criteria to identify relevant clinical trials that may be currently enrolling participants.
- Major academic medical centers, research institutions, and hospitals often conduct clinical trials and can provide information about their ongoing studies.
- Medical professionals may be aware of ongoing clinical trials in their field and can provide guidance to families who are interested in participating.
- Organizations that support particular conditions are another source of information.

Depending on the nature of the treatment in the clinical trial, you may want to, or be required to, consult with your medical professional to help you consider the risks and benefits of participating.

b) As a co-producer

Family engagement in research (FER) plays a crucial role in fostering collaboration and helping improve study design and outcome. When families become involved in research as collaborators on a study rather than simply as participants, researchers gain valuable insights into the lived experiences and perspectives of families. Families participate at every stage of the research process: concept, design, planning, conduct, and reporting of the study findings. These opportunities are still rare but are becoming more common. As an example, a link to the FER program at Gillette Children's is included in **Useful web resources**.

The family engagement in research movement is largely attributed to the similar and earlier patient and public involvement initiative in the UK. Here are some opportunities:

- **CanChild** and the **Kids Brain Health Network** in Canada currently offer The Family Engagement in Research program, a short online training course through McMaster University Continuing Education, to train family members and researchers (including coordinators and assistants) in collaborating on research.
- Online training modules are available at **Patient-Oriented Research Curriculum in Child Health (PORCCH).**
- The **Patient-Centered Outcomes Research Institute (PCORI)** and the **Strategy for Patient-Oriented Research (SPOR)** are two other organizations that encourage family engagement.

USEFUL WEB RESOURCES

Acknowledgments

It takes a village to raise a child
African proverb

And it takes a village to produce a Healthcare Series. Publication of this series began with an idea, then with five titles, and then more titles. These acknowledgments relate to the entire series.

The formula of deep medical information interspersed with lived experience gives readers an appreciation of the childhood-acquired, often lifelong conditions. We thank the many people who contributed to each title: medical professionals at Gillette Children's who willingly came forward to lead each book; Gillette writers who did the research and writing of each, including Michaela Hingtgen who contributed to this book in the early stages; other Gillette team members who contributed from their different specialties; family authors and vignette writers who shared their personal stories; other families who shared photographs; the Gillette editing team who ensured the content and structure worked for the reader; Olwyn Roche who beautifully illustrated each title; advance readers, both professionals and families, whose feedback was invaluable; and Lina Abdennabi who coordinated Gillette Press operations. Behind every book was also a pit team who converted the finished manuscript into the book you now hold. Ruth Wilson led and looked after copyediting and proofreading. Jazmin Welch created the beautiful design and layout. Audrey McClellan indexed each title.

Smoothly creating each title required great teamwork among our villagers.

Staff at Gillette Children's provided continual support to the project and everyone involved. This included the steering committee, in particular Paula Montgomery, Dr. Micah Niermann, and Barbara Joers.

This Healthcare Series is co-published with Mac Keith Press. From the get-go, the journey with Ann-Marie Halligan and Sally Wilkinson was one of great support and collaboration.

Gillette Children's Healthcare Press

Glossary

Grasp the subject, the words will follow.

Cato the Elder

TERM	DEFINITION
Abnormal/atypical	Deviating from the typical expectation.
Achilles tendon	The cord-like structure that attaches the gastrocnemius and soleus muscles (both calf muscles) to the bone at the heel.
Ankle-foot orthosis (AFO)	A type of orthosis (brace or splint) that controls the ankle and foot. See *orthosis*.
Baclofen	A medication used for tone reduction; can be delivered either orally or by using a pump connected to a catheter to deliver the medication to the intrathecal area (the fluid-filled space surrounding the spinal cord). The latter delivery method is called intrathecal baclofen (ITB).
Bilateral CP	A form of cerebral palsy that affects both sides of the body.
Bimanual therapy	A treatment consisting of activities designed to improve the individual's ability to use both arms or hands together (without any restraint placed on the unaffected hand). It involves a high level of repetition.
Botulinum neurotoxin A (BoNT-A)	A medication used for tone reduction. It is delivered by injection directly into the muscle.
Cardiometabolic	Referring to both heart disease and metabolic disorders (such as diabetes).

Casting	The process of stretching a muscle by applying a plaster of paris or a fiberglass cast; for example, a below-knee cast to stretch the tight gastrocnemius and/or soleus muscles (calf muscles) to hold the muscle in a position of maximum stretch.
Centers for Disease Control and Prevention (CDC)	The national public health institute in the US.
Cerebral	Referring to the cerebrum, the front and upper part of the brain, one of the major areas responsible for the control of movement.
Constraint-induced movement therapy	A treatment used for individuals with hemiplegia involving restraint of the unaffected hand and intensive structured therapy.
Contracture	A limitation of the range of motion of a joint. It occurs in the muscle-tendon unit (MTU) and/or capsule of the joint, not just the muscle. See *muscle-tendon unit; range of motion.*
Crouch gait	A persistent flexed-knee gait. The exact degree of knee flexion that constitutes crouch gait varies in the literature but is typically greater than or equal to 20 degrees. This knee flexion is normally also accompanied by persistent hip flexion. The foot position can be variable. See *gait.*
Diplegia	A form of cerebral palsy affecting all limbs, but the lower limbs are much more affected than the upper limbs, which frequently show only fine motor impairment.
Dystonia	A condition characterized by involuntary muscle contractions that cause slow repetitive movements or abnormal postures that can sometimes be painful.
Episode of care (EOC)	A period of therapy (at the appropriate frequency) followed by a therapy break.
Fine motor function	Refers to the smaller movements in the wrists, hands, fingers, and toes. Examples include picking up objects between the thumb and forefinger, and writing. Also called fine motor skills, hand skills, fine motor coordination, or dexterity.

Gait	A person's manner of walking.
Gait analysis	A measurement tool used to evaluate gait. Within gait analysis, multiple variables are evaluated using different measurement tools.
Gross motor function	The ability to make large, general movement of the arms, legs, and other large body parts, such as sitting, crawling, standing, running, jumping, swimming, throwing, catching, and kicking. Also called gross motor skills.
Gross Motor Function Classification System (GMFCS)	A five-level classification system that describes the functional mobilities of children and adolescents with cerebral palsy. Level I has the fewest limitations and level V has the most. It provides an indication of the severity of cerebral palsy.
Hemiplegia	A form of cerebral palsy affecting the upper and lower limbs on one side of the body. The upper limb is usually more affected than the lower limb.
Hypotonia/hypertonia	See *muscle tone*.
International Classification of Functioning, Disability and Health (ICF)	A universal framework for considering any health condition. It helps show the impact of a health condition at different levels and how those levels are interconnected.
Magnetic resonance imaging (MRI)	A noninvasive imaging technology that produces detailed three-dimensional anatomical images without the use of radiation.
Muscle-tendon unit (MTU)	A combination of the muscle, tendon, and other structures.
Muscle tone	The resting tension in a person's muscles. Tone is considered abnormal when it falls outside the range of normal or typical; either too low (hypotonia) or too high (hypertonia). Abnormal muscle tone occurs in all types of cerebral palsy.
Musculoskeletal	Referring to both the muscles and the skeleton; includes muscles, bones, joints, and their related structures (e.g., ligaments, and tendons). The term *neuromusculoskeletal* includes the nervous system.

Neurology	Specialty dealing with disorders of the nervous system.
Neuromusculoskeletal	Referring to the nervous system, muscles, bones, joints, and their related structures.
Neurosurgery	Specialty that involves surgical management of disorders of the nervous system.
Occupational therapy	A type of therapy based on engaging in everyday activities (occupations) to promote health, well-being, and independence.
Orthopedic surgery	Specialty that involves surgical management of disorders affecting the *musculoskeletal* system.
Orthosis	A device designed to hold specific body parts in position to modify their structure and/or function; also called a brace or splint.
Orthotics	The branch of medicine concerned with the design, manufacture, and management of orthoses. See *orthosis*.
Osteoporosis	A medical condition where the bones are weak and brittle, with low density.
Palsy	Paralysis (though paralysis by pure definition is not a feature of cerebral palsy).
Pediatrics	Specialty dealing with children and their conditions.
Percentile	A variable (such as a person's height by age) that divides the distribution of the variable into 100 groups. The 50th percentile is always the median (the midpoint that separates lower and higher values into two groups).
Physiatry	See *physical medicine and rehabilitation*.
Physical medicine and rehabilitation (PM&R)	Specialty that aims to enhance and restore functional ability and quality of life among those with physical disabilities. Also termed *physiatry*.
Physical therapy/ physiotherapy	A type of therapy to develop, maintain, and restore a person's maximum movement and functional ability.
Quadriplegia	A form of cerebral palsy affecting all four limbs and the trunk; also known as tetraplegia.

Range of motion (ROM)	A measure of joint flexibility; the range through which a joint moves, measured in degrees. Also called range of movement.
Selective dorsal rhizotomy (SDR)	Refers to the selective cutting of abnormal sensory nerve rootlets in the spinal cord to reduce spasticity.
Single-event multilevel surgery (SEMLS)	Multiple orthopedic surgical procedures performed during a single operation.
Spasticity	A condition in which there is an abnormal increase in muscle tone or stiffness of muscle that can interfere with movement and speech, and be associated with discomfort or pain.
Speech and language pathology (SLP)	A type of therapy to support those with speech, language, and communication needs as well as feeding and swallowing difficulties. Also called speech and language therapy.
Tendon	The cord-like structure that attaches the muscle to the bone; for example, the *Achilles tendon* attaches both calf muscles to the bone at the heel.
Tone	See *muscle tone*.
Unilateral CP	A form of cerebral palsy that affects one side of the body.
W-sitting	A description of the sitting position often adopted by a child with cerebral palsy where the child's bottom is on the floor while their legs are out to each side; looking from the top, the legs form a "W" shape.

References

1. World Health Organization (2001) *International classification of functioning, disability and health (ICF)*. [online] Available at: <https://www.who.int/standards/classifications/international-classification-of-functioning-disability-and-health> [Accessed February 22 2024].

2. Rosenbaum P, Paneth N, Leviton A, et al. (2007) A report: The definition and classification of cerebral palsy April 2006. *Dev Med Child Neurol Suppl*, 109, 8-14.

3. Graham HK, Rosenbaum P, Paneth N, et al. (2016) Cerebral palsy. *Nat Rev Dis Primers*, 2, 1-24.

4. Smithers-Sheedy H, Waight E, Goldsmith S, McIntyre S (2023) Australian Cerebral Palsy Register report, Available at: <https://cpregister.com/wp-content/uploads/2023/01/2023-ACPR-Report.pdf> [Accessed June 24 2024].

5. McIntyre S, Goldsmith S, Webb A, et al. (2022) Global prevalence of cerebral palsy: A systematic analysis. *Dev Med Child Neurol*, 64, 1494-1506.

6. Centers for Disease Control and Prevention (2024a) *Epidemiology glossary*. [online] Available at: <https://www.cdc.gov/reproductive-health/glossary/> [Accessed June 24 2024].

7. Shepherd E, Salam RA, Middleton P, et al. (2017) Antenatal and intrapartum interventions for preventing cerebral palsy: An overview of Cochrane systematic reviews. *Cochrane Database Syst Rev*, 8, 1-78.

8. Rosenbaum P, Rosenbloom L (2012) *Cerebral palsy: From diagnosis to adult life*. London: Mac Keith Press.

9. National Institute of Neurological Disorders and Stroke (2023a) *Cerebral palsy*. [online] Available at: <https://www.ninds.nih.gov/health-information/disorders/cerebral-palsy> [Accessed June 21 2024].

10. Centers for Disease Control and Prevention (2024b) *Risk factors for cerebral palsy*. [online] Available at: <https://www.cdc.gov/cerebral-palsy/risk-factors/> [Accessed June 18 2024].

11. Centers for Disease Control and Prevention (2017) *Single embryo transfer*. [online] Available at: <https://www.cdc.gov/art/patientresources/transfer.html> [Accessed June 24 2024].

12. National Perinatal Epidemiology and Statistics Unit (2021) IVF success rates have improved in the last decade, especially in older women: Report, Australia, UNSW. Available at: <https://www.unsw.edu.au/newsroom/news/2021/09/ivf-success-rates-have-improved-in-the-last-decade--especially-i> [Accessed January 19 2024].

13. Nelson KB (2008) Causative factors in cerebral palsy. *Clin Obstet Gynecol*, 51, 749-62.

14. Novak I, Morgan C, Fahey M, et al. (2020) State of the evidence traffic lights 2019: Systematic review of interventions for preventing and treating children with cerebral palsy. *Curr Neurol Neurosci Rep*, 20, 1-21.

15. Durkin MS, Benedict RE, Christensen D, et al. (2016) Prevalence of cerebral palsy among 8-year-old children in 2010 and preliminary evidence of trends in its relationship to low birthweight. *Paediatr Perinat Epidemiol*, 30, 496-510.

16. McGuire DO, Tian LH, Yeargin-Allsopp M, Dowling NF, Christensen DL (2019) Prevalence of cerebral palsy, intellectual disability, hearing loss, and blindness, National Health Interview Survey, 2009-2016. *Disabil Health J*, 12, 443-451.

17. Khandaker G, Muhit M, Karim T, et al. (2019) Epidemiology of cerebral palsy in Bangladesh: A population-based surveillance study. *Dev Med Child Neurol*, 61, 601-609.

18. Centers for Disease Control and Prevention (2024c) *Down syndrome*. [online] Available at: <https://www.cdc.gov/ncbddd/birthdefects/downsyndrome.html> [Accessed June 21 2024].

19. National Institutes of Health (2024) *Estimates of funding for various research, condition, and disease categories (RCDC)*. [online] Available at: <https://report.nih.gov/funding/categorical-spending#/> [Accessed June 21 2024].

20. Mathew JL, Kaur N, Dsouza JM (2022) Therapeutic hypothermia in neonatal hypoxic encephalopathy: A systematic review and meta-analysis. *J Glob Health*, 12, 1-22.

21. Novak I, Morgan C, Adde L, et al. (2017) Early, accurate diagnosis and early intervention in cerebral palsy. *JAMA Pediatr*, 171, 1-11.

22. National Institute of Neurological Disorders and Stroke (2024) *Glossary of neurological terms*. [online] Available at: <https://www.ninds.nih.gov/health-information/disorders/glossary-neurological-terms> [Accessed June 14 2024].

23. Byrne R, Noritz G, Maitre NL, N.C.H. Early Developmental Group (2017) Implementation of early diagnosis and intervention guidelines for cerebral palsy in a high-risk infant follow-up clinic. *Pediatr Neurol*, 76, 66-71.

24. Maitre NL, Burton VJ, Duncan AF, et al. (2020) Network implementation of guideline for early detection decreases age at cerebral palsy diagnosis. *Pediatrics*, 145, 1-10.

25. Te Velde A, Tantsis E, Novak I, et al. (2021) Age of diagnosis, fidelity and acceptability of an early diagnosis clinic for cerebral palsy: A single site implementation study. *Brain Sci*, 11, 1-14.

26. King AR, Machipisa C, Finlayson F, et al. (2021) Early detection of cerebral palsy in high-risk infants: Translation of evidence into practice in an Australian hospital. *J Paediatr Child Health*, 57, 246-250.

27. King AR, Al Imam MH, McIntyre S, et al. (2022) Early diagnosis of cerebral palsy in low- and middle-income countries. *Brain Sci*, 12, 1-13.

28. Maitre NL, Damiano D, Byrne R (2023) Implementation of early detection and intervention for cerebral palsy in high-risk infant follow-up programs: U.S. and global considerations. *Clin Perinatol*, 50, 269-279.

29. Maitre NL, Byrne R, Duncan A, et al. (2022) "High-risk for cerebral palsy" designation: A clinical consensus statement. *J Pediatr Rehabil Med*, 15, 165-174.

30. Morgan C, Fetters L, Adde L, et al. (2021) Early intervention for children aged 0 to 2 years with or at high risk of cerebral palsy: International clinical practice guideline based on systematic reviews. *JAMA Pediatr,* 175, 846-858.

31. Ismail FY, Fatemi A, Johnston MV (2017) Cerebral plasticity: Windows of opportunity in the developing brain. *Eur J Paediatr Neurol,* 21, 23-48.

32. Cerebral Palsy Alliance (2019) *Why neuroplasticity is the secret ingredient for kids with special needs.* [online] Available at: <https://cerebralpalsy.org.au/news -stories/why-neuroplasticity-is-the-secret-ingredient-for-kids-with-special-needs/> [Accessed June 14 2024].

33. Kohli-Lynch M, Tann CJ, Ellis ME (2019) Early intervention for children at high risk of developmental disability in low- and middle-income countries: A narrative review. *Int J Environ Res Public Health,* 16, 1-9.

34. McNamara L, Morgan C, Novak I (2023) Interventions for motor disorders in high-risk neonates. *Clin Perinatol,* 50, 121-155.

35. Byrne R, Duncan A, Pickar T, et al. (2019) Comparing parent and provider priorities in discussions of early detection and intervention for infants with and at risk of cerebral palsy. *Child Care Health Dev,* 45, 799-807.

36. Centers for Disease Control and Prevention (2024d) *CDC's developmental milestones.* [online] Available at: <https://www.cdc.gov/ncbddd/actearly/milestones/ index.html> [Accessed June 21 2024].

37. WHO Multicentre Growth Reference Study Group (2006) WHO motor development study: Windows of achievement for six gross motor development milestones. *Acta Paediatr Suppl,* 450, 86-95.

38. Surveillance of Cerebral Palsy in Europe (2000) A collaboration of cerebral palsy surveys and registers. Surveillance of cerebral palsy in Europe (SCPE). *Dev Med Child Neurol,* 42, 816-24.

39. National Institute of Neurological Disorders and Stroke (2021) *Dystonia [pdf].* [online] Available at: <https://catalog.ninds.nih.gov/sites/default/files/publications/ dystonia.pdf> [Accessed January 19 2024].

40. National Institute of Neurological Disorders and Stroke (2023b) *Ataxia and cerebellar or spinocerebellar degeneration.* [online] Available at: <https:// www.ninds.nih.gov/health-information/disorders/ataxia-and-cerebellar-or -spinocerebellar-degeneration> [Accessed January 19 2024].

41. Centers for Disease Control and Prevention (2024e) *About cerebral palsy.* [online] Available at: <https://www.cdc.gov/cerebral-palsy/about/> [Accessed June 21 2024].

42. Australian Cerebral Palsy Register (2023) *Personal communication.*

43. Gorter JW, Rosenbaum PL, Hanna SE, et al. (2004) Limb distribution, motor impairment, and functional classification of cerebral palsy. *Dev Med Child Neurol,* 46, 461-7.

44. Himmelmann K, Beckung E, Hagberg G, Uvebrant P (2006) Gross and fine motor function and accompanying impairments in cerebral palsy. *Dev Med Child Neurol,* 48, 417-23.

45. Shevell MI, Dagenais L, Hall N, Repacq C (2009) The relationship of cerebral palsy subtype and functional motor impairment: A population-based study. *Dev Med Child Neurol,* 51, 872-7.

46. Hidecker MJ, Ho NT, Dodge N, et al. (2012) Inter-relationships of functional status in cerebral palsy: Analyzing gross motor function, manual ability, and communication function classification systems in children. *Dev Med Child Neurol*, 54, 737-42.

47. Aravamuthan BR, Fehlings D, Shetty S, et al. (2021) Variability in cerebral palsy diagnosis. *Pediatrics*, 147, 1-11.

48. Dar H, Stewart K, McIntyre S, Paget S (2023) Multiple motor disorders in cerebral palsy. *Dev Med Child Neurol*, 66, 317-325.

49. Palisano R, Rosenbaum P, Walter S, et al. (1997) Development and reliability of a system to classify gross motor function in children with cerebral palsy. *Dev Med Child Neurol*, 39, 214-23.

50. Palisano RJ, Rosenbaum P, Bartlett D, Livingston MH (2008) Content validity of the expanded and revised Gross Motor Function Classification System. *Dev Med Child Neurol*, 50, 744-50.

51. Alriksson-Schmidt A, Nordmark E, Czuba T, Westbom L (2017) Stability of the Gross Motor Function Classification System in children and adolescents with cerebral palsy: A retrospective cohort registry study. *Dev Med Child Neurol*, 59, 641-646.

52. Huroy M, Behlim T, Andersen J, et al. (2022) Stability of the Gross Motor Function Classification System over time in children with cerebral palsy. *Dev Med Child Neurol*, 64, 1487-1493.

53. McCormick A, Brien M, Plourde J, et al. (2007) Stability of the Gross Motor Function Classification System in adults with cerebral palsy. *Dev Med Child Neurol*, 49, 265-9.

54. Kinsner-Ovaskainen A, Lanzoni M, Martin S, et al. (2017) *Surveillance of cerebral palsy in Europe: Development of the JRC-SCPE central database and public health indicators*, Luxembourg: Publications Office of the European Union.

55. Rosenbaum PL, Walter SD, Hanna SE, et al. (2002) Prognosis for gross motor function in cerebral palsy: Creation of motor development curves. *JAMA*, 288, 1357-63.

56. Hanna SE, Bartlett DJ, Rivard LM, Russell DJ (2008) Reference curves for the gross motor function measure: Percentiles for clinical description and tracking over time among children with cerebral palsy. *Phys Ther*, 88, 596-607.

57. Eliasson AC, Krumlinde-Sundholm L, Rösblad B, et al. (2006) The Manual Ability Classification System (MACS) for children with cerebral palsy: Scale development and evidence of validity and reliability. *Dev Med Child Neurol*, 48, 549-54.

58. Eliasson AC, Ullenhag A, Wahlstrom U, Krumlinde-Sundholm L (2017) Mini-MACS: Development of the Manual Ability Classification System for children younger than 4 years of age with signs of cerebral palsy. *Dev Med Child Neurol*, 59, 72-78.

59. Beckung E, Hagberg G (2002) Neuroimpairments, activity limitations, and participation restrictions in children with cerebral palsy. *Dev Med Child Neurol*, 44, 309-16.

60. Elvrum AK, Andersen GL, Himmelmann K, et al. (2016) Bimanual Fine Motor Function (BFMF) classification in children with cerebral palsy: Aspects of construct and content validity. *Phys Occup Ther Pediatr,* 36, 1-16.

61. Elvrum AG, Beckung E, Saether R, et al. (2017) Bimanual capacity of children with cerebral palsy: Intra- and interrater reliability of a revised edition of the Bimanual Fine Motor Function classification. *Phys Occup Ther Pediatr,* 37, 239-251.

62. Hidecker MJ, Paneth N, Rosenbaum PL, et al. (2011) Developing and validating the Communication Function Classification System for individuals with cerebral palsy. *Dev Med Child Neurol,* 53, 704-10.

63. Pennington L, Mjøen T, Da Graça Andrada M, Murray J (2010) Viking Speech Scale [pdf], EU, European Commission, Available at: <https://eu-rd-platform. jrc.ec.europa.eu/sites/default/files/Viking-Speech-Scale-2011-Copyright_EN.pdf> [Accessed June 18 2024].

64. Pennington L, Virella D, Mjøen T, et al. (2013) Development of the Viking Speech Scale to classify the speech of children with cerebral palsy. *Res Dev Disabil,* 34, 3202-10.

65. Virella D, Pennington L, Andersen GL, et al. (2016) Classification systems of communication for use in epidemiological surveillance of children with cerebral palsy. *Dev Med Child Neurol,* 58, 285-91.

66. Sellers D, Mandy A, Pennington L, Hankins M, Morris C (2014) Development and reliability of a system to classify the eating and drinking ability of people with cerebral palsy. *Dev Med Child Neurol,* 56, 245-51.

67. Sellers D, Pennington L, Bryant E, et al. (2022) Mini-EDACS: Development of the Eating and Drinking Ability Classification System for young children with cerebral palsy. *Dev Med Child Neurol,* 64, 897-906.

68. Baranello G, Signorini S, Tinelli F, et al. (2020) Visual Function Classification System for children with cerebral palsy: Development and validation. *Dev Med Child Neurol,* 62, 104-110.

69. Paulson A, Vargus-Adams J (2017) Overview of four functional classification systems commonly used in cerebral palsy. *Children,* 4, 1-10.

70. Piscitelli D, Ferrarello F, Ugolini A, Verola S, Pellicciari L (2021) Measurement properties of the Gross Motor Function Classification System, Gross Motor Function Classification System-expanded & revised, Manual Ability Classification System, and Communication Function Classification System in cerebral palsy: A systematic review with meta-analysis. *Dev Med Child Neurol,* 63, 1251-1261.

71. Shevell M (2019) Cerebral palsy to cerebral palsy spectrum disorder: Time for a name change? *Neurology,* 92, 233-35.

72. Holsbeeke L, Ketelaar M, Schoemaker MM, Gorter JW (2009) Capacity, capability, and performance: Different constructs or three of a kind? *Arch Phys Med Rehabil,* 90, 849-55.

73. Rosenbaum P, Gorter JW (2012) The 'F-words' in childhood disability: I swear this is how we should think! *Child Care Health Dev,* 38, 457-63.

74. Gage JR (1991) *Gait analysis in cerebral palsy,* London: Mac Keith Press.

75. Howard J, Soo B, Graham HK, et al. (2005) Cerebral palsy in Victoria: Motor types, topography and gross motor function. *J Paediatr Child Health*, 41, 479-83.

76. Carnahan K, Arner M, Hagglund G (2007) Association between gross motor function (GMFCS) and manual ability (MACS) in children with cerebral palsy. A population-based study of 359 children. *BMC Musculoskelet Disord*, 8, 1-7.

77. Rice J, Russo R, Halbert J, Van Essen P, Haan E (2009) Motor function in 5-year-old children with cerebral palsy in the South Australian population. *Dev Med Child Neurol*, 51, 551-6.

78. Unes S, Tuncdemir M, Ozal C, et al. (2022) Relationship among four functional classification systems and parent interpredicted intelligence level in children with different clinical types of cerebral palsy. *Dev Neurorehabil*, 25, 410-416.

79. Delacy MJ, Reid SM, Australian Cerebral Palsy Register Group (2016) Profile of associated impairments at age 5 years in Australia by cerebral palsy subtype and Gross Motor Function Classification System level for birth years 1996 to 2005. *Dev Med Child Neurol*, 58, 50-6.

80. Fehlings D, Krishnan P, Ragguett RM, et al. (2021) Neurodevelopmental profiles of children with unilateral cerebral palsy associated with middle cerebral artery and periventricular venous infarctions. *Dev Med Child Neurol*, 63, 729-735.

81. Keogh J, Sugden DA (1985) *Movement skill development*, London: Macmillan.

82. Day SM, Strauss DJ, Vachon PJ, et al. (2007) Growth patterns in a population of children and adolescents with cerebral palsy. *Dev Med Child Neurol*, 49, 167-71.

83. Brooks J, Day S, Shavelle R, Strauss D (2011) Low weight, morbidity, and mortality in children with cerebral palsy: New clinical growth charts. *Pediatrics*, 128, 299-307.

84. Wright CM, Reynolds L, Ingram E, Cole TJ, Brooks J (2017) Validation of US cerebral palsy growth charts using a UK cohort. *Dev Med Child Neurol*, 59, 933-938.

85. Centers for Disease Control and Prevention (2000a) *2 to 20 years: Girls stature-for-age and weight-for-age percentiles [pdf]*. [online] Available at: <https://www.cdc.gov/growthcharts/data/set2clinical/cj41c072.pdf> [Accessed February 22 2024].

86. Centers for Disease Control and Prevention (2009) *Birth to 24 months: Girls length-for-age and weight-for-age percentiles [pdf]*. [online] Available at: <https://www.cdc.gov/growthcharts/data/who/GrChrt_Girls_24LW_9210.pdf> [Accessed June 19 2024].

87. Centers for Disease Control and Prevention (2000b) *2 to 20 years: Boys stature-for-age and weight-for-age percentiles [pdf]*. [online] Available at: <https://www.cdc.gov/growthcharts/data/set1clinical/cj41l021.pdf> [Accessed February 22 2024].

88. Centers for Disease Control and Prevention (2001) *Birth to 36 months: Boys length-for-age and weight-for-age percentiles [pdf]*. [online] Available at: <https://www.cdc.gov/growthcharts/data/set1clinical/cj41l017.pdf> [Accessed February 22 2024].

89. Park ES, Park CI, Cho SR, Na SI, Cho YS (2004) Colonic transit time and constipation in children with spastic cerebral palsy. *Arch Phys Med Rehabil,* 85, 453-6.

90. Murphy KP, Boutin SA, Ide KR (2012) Cerebral palsy, neurogenic bladder, and outcomes of lifetime care. *Dev Med Child Neurol,* 54, 945-50.

91. Azouz H, Abdelmohsen A, Ghany H, Mamdouh R (2021) Evaluation of autonomic nervous system in children with spastic cerebral palsy: Clinical and electophysiological study. *Egypt Rheumatol Rehabil,* 48, 1-9.

92. Nuckolls GH, Kinnett K, Dayanidhi S, et al. (2020) Conference report on contractures in musculoskeletal and neurological conditions. *Muscle Nerve,* 61, 740-744.

93. Radomski MV, Trombly Latham CA (2014) *Occupational therapy for physical dysfunction,* Philadelphia: Lippincott Williams & Wilkins.

94. Kendall FP, McCreary EK, Provance PG, McIntyre Rodgers M, Romani WA (2005) *Muscles: Testing and function with posture and pain,* Baltimore: Lippincott Williams & Wilkins.

95. Hislop HJ, Montgomery J (1995) *Daniels and Worthingham's muscle testing techniques of manual examination.* Philadelphia: WB Saunders.

96. Gage JR, Schwartz MH (2009a) Normal gait. In: Gage JR, Schwartz MH, Koop SE, Novacheck TF, editors, *The identification and treatment of gait problems in cerebral palsy.* London: Mac Keith Press, pp 31-64.

97. Stout JL (2023) Gait: Development and analysis. In: Palisano R, Orlin M, Schreiber J, editors, *Campbell's physical therapy for children 6th edition.* St. Louis: Elsevier, pp 159-183.

98. Gage JR, Novacheck TF (2001) An update on the treatment of gait problems in cerebral palsy. *J Pediatr Orthop,* 10, 265-74.

99. Gage JR, Schwartz MH (2009b) Consequences of brain injury on musculoskel-etal development. In: Gage JR, Schwartz MH, Koop SE, Novacheck TF, editors, *The identification and treatment of gait problems in cerebral palsy.* London: Mac Keith Press, pp 107-129.

100. Pollock AS, Durward BR, Rowe PJ, Paul JP (2000) What is balance? *Clin Rehabil,* 14, 402-6.

101. Clauser CE, Mcconville JT, Young JW (1969) Weight, volume, and center of mass of segments of the human body [pdf], Available at: <https://ntrs.nasa.gov/api/citations/19700027497/downloads/19700027497.pdf> [Accessed June 19 2024].

102. Peterka RJ (2018) Sensory integration for human balance control. *Handb Clin Neurol,* 159, 27-42.

103. Dewar R, Love S, Johnston LM (2015) Exercise interventions improve postural control in children with cerebral palsy: A systematic review. *Dev Med Child Neurol,* 57, 504-20.

104. Lance JW (1980) Pathophysiology of spasticity and clinical experience with baclofen. In: Feldman RG, Young RR, Koella WP, editors, *Spasticity: Disordered motor control.* Chicago: Year Book Medical, pp 183-203.

105. Bohannon RW, Smith MB (1987) Interrater reliability of a Modified Ashworth Scale of muscle spasticity. *Phys Ther,* 67, 206-7.

106. Numanoglu A, Gunel MK (2012) Intraobserver reliability of Modified Ashworth Scale and Modified Tardieu Scale in the assessment of spasticity in children with cerebral palsy. *Acta Orthop Traumatol Turc,* 46, 196-200.

107. Gracies JM, Burke K, Clegg NJ, et al. (2010) Reliability of the Tardieu Scale for assessing spasticity in children with cerebral palsy. *Arch Phys Med Rehabil,* 91, 421-8.

108. Barry MJ, VanSwearingen JM, Albright AL (1999) Reliability and responsiveness of the Barry-Albright Dystonia Scale. *Dev Med Child Neurol,* 41, 404-11.

109. Jethwa A, Mink J, Macarthur C, et al. (2010) Development of the Hypertonia Assessment Tool (HAT): A discriminative tool for hypertonia in children. *Dev Med Child Neurol,* 52, 83-7.

110. Knights S, Datoo N, Kawamura A, Switzer L, Fehlings D (2014) Further evaluation of the scoring, reliability, and validity of the Hypertonia Assessment Tool (HAT). *J Child Neurol,* 29, 500-4.

111. Wiley ME, Damiano DL (1998) Lower-extremity strength profiles in spastic cerebral palsy. *Dev Med Child Neurol,* 40, 100-7.

112. Dekkers K, Rameckers EAA, Smeets R, et al. (2020) Upper extremity muscle strength in children with unilateral spastic cerebral palsy: A bilateral problem? *Phys Ther,* 100, 2205-2216.

113. Barrett RS, Lichtwark GA (2010) Gross muscle morphology and structure in spastic cerebral palsy: A systematic review. *Dev Med Child Neurol,* 52, 794-804.

114. Modlesky CM, Zhang C (2020) Complicated muscle-bone interactions in children with cerebral palsy. *Curr Osteoporos Rep,* 18, 47-56.

115. Stackhouse SK, Binder-Macleod SA, Lee SC (2005) Voluntary muscle activation, contractile properties, and fatigability in children with and without cerebral palsy. *Muscle Nerve,* 31, 594-601.

116. Theologis T (2013) Lever arm dysfunction in cerebral palsy gait. *J Child Orthop,* 7, 379-82.

117. Kalkman BM, Bar-On L, Cenni F, et al. (2017) Achilles tendon moment arm length is smaller in children with cerebral palsy than in typically developing children. *J Biomech,* 56, 48-54.

118. Bittmann MF, Lenhart RL, Schwartz MH, et al. (2018) How does patellar tendon advancement alter the knee extensor mechanism in children treated for crouch gait? *Gait Posture,* 64, 248-254.

119. Noonan KJ, Farnum CE, Leiferman EM, et al. (2004) Growing pains: Are they due to increased growth during recumbency as documented in a lamb model? *J Pediatr Orthop,* 24, 726-31.

120. Carlon S, Taylor N, Dodd K, Shields N (2013) Differences in habitual physical activity levels of young people with cerebral palsy and their typically developing peers: A systematic review. *Disabil Rehabil,* 35, 647-55.

121. Gough M, Shortland AP (2012) Could muscle deformity in children with spastic cerebral palsy be related to an impairment of muscle growth and altered adaptation? *Dev Med Child Neurol,* 54, 495-9.

122. Nordmark E, Hagglund G, Lauge-Pedersen H, Wagner P, Westbom L (2009) Development of lower limb range of motion from early childhood to adolescence in cerebral palsy: A population-based study. *BMC Med,* 7, 1-11.

123. Smith LR, Chambers HG, Lieber RL (2013) Reduced satellite cell population may lead to contractures in children with cerebral palsy. *Dev Med Child Neurol,* 55, 264-70.

124. Dayanidhi S, Dykstra PB, Lyubasyuk V, et al. (2015) Reduced satellite cell number in situ in muscular contractures from children with cerebral palsy. *J Orthop Res,* 33, 1039-45.

125. Domenighetti AA, Mathewson MA, Pichika R, et al. (2018) Loss of myogenic potential and fusion capacity of muscle stem cells isolated from contractured muscle in children with cerebral palsy. *Am J Physiol Cell Physiol,* 315, 247-257.

126. Barber L, Hastings-Ison T, Baker R, Barrett R, Lichtwark G (2011) Medial gastrocnemius muscle volume and fascicle length in children aged 2 to 5 years with cerebral palsy. *Dev Med Child Neurol,* 53, 543-8.

127. Herskind A, Ritterband-Rosenbaum A, Willerslev-Olsen M, et al. (2016) Muscle growth is reduced in 15-month-old children with cerebral palsy. *Dev Med Child Neurol,* 58, 485-91.

128. Soo B, Howard JJ, Boyd RN, et al. (2006) Hip displacement in cerebral palsy. *J Bone Joint Surg Am,* 88, 121-9.

129. Graham HK, Thomason P, Novacheck TF (2014) Cerebral palsy. In: Weinstein SL, Flynn JM, editors, *Lovell and Winter's pediatric orthopedics, level 1 and 2.* Philadelphia: Lippincott Williams & Wilkins, pp 484-554.

130. Hägglund G, Alriksson-Schmidt A, Lauge-Pedersen H, et al. (2014) Prevention of dislocation of the hip in children with cerebral palsy: 20-year results of a population-based prevention programme. *Bone Joint J,* 96-B, 1546-52.

131. Walker K (2009) Radiographic evaluation of the patient with cerebral palsy. In: Gage JR, Schwartz MH, Koop SE, Novacheck TF, editors, *The identification and treatment of gait problems in cerebral palsy.* London: Mac Keith Press, pp 244-259.

132. Wise CH (2015) *Orthopaedic manual physical therapy: From art to evidence,* Philadelphia: F.A. Davis.

133. Koop SE (2009) Musculoskeletal growth and development. In: Gage JR, Schwartz MH, Koop SE, Novacheck TF, editors, *The identification and treatment of gait problems in cerebral palsy.* London: Mac Keith Press, pp 21-30.

134. Staheli LT, Engel GM (1972) Tibial torsion: A method of assessment and a survey of normal children. *Clin Orthop Relat Res,* 86, 183-6.

135. Inman VT, Ralston HJ, Todd F (1981) *Human walking.* Baltimore: Williams & Wilkins.

136. Hägglund G, Pettersson K, Czuba T, Persson-Bunke M, Rodby-Bousquet E (2018) Incidence of scoliosis in cerebral palsy. *Acta Orthop,* 89, 443-447.

137. Willoughby KL, Ang SG, Thomason P, et al. (2022) Epidemiology of scoliosis in cerebral palsy: A population-based study at skeletal maturity. *J Paediatr Child Health,* 58, 295-301.

138. Saraph V, Zwick EB, Steinwender G, et al. (2006) Leg lengthening as part of gait improvement surgery in cerebral palsy: An evaluation using gait analysis. *Gait Posture,* 23, 83-90.

139. Karaguzel G, Holick MF (2010) Diagnosis and treatment of osteopenia. *Rev Endocr Metab Disord,* 11, 237-51.

140. Finbraten AK, Syversen U, Skranes J, et al. (2015) Bone mineral density and vitamin D status in ambulatory and non-ambulatory children with cerebral palsy. *Osteoporos Int,* 26, 141-50.

141. Van Heest AE, Kozin SH (2022) Spasticity: Cerebral palsy and traumatic brain injury. In: Wolfe SW, Pederson WC, Kozin SH, Cohen MS, editors, *Green's operative hand surgery.* Philadelphia: Elsevier, pp 1243-1264.

142. House JH, Gwathmey FW, Fidler MO (1981) A dynamic approach to the thumb-in palm deformity in cerebral palsy. *J Bone Joint Surg Am,* 63, 216-25.

143. Ottenbacher KJ, Msall ME, Lyon NR, et al. (1997) Interrater agreement and stability of the Functional Independence Measure for Children (WeeFIM): Use in children with developmental disabilities. *Arch Phys Med Rehabil,* 78, 1309-15.

144. Damiano D, Abel M, Romness M, et al. (2006) Comparing functional profiles of children with hemiplegic and diplegic cerebral palsy in GMFCS levels I and II: Are separate classifications needed? *Dev Med Child Neurol,* 48, 797-803.

145. Winters TFJ, Gage JR, Hicks R (1987) Gait patterns in spastic hemiplegia in children and young adults. *J Bone Joint Surg Am,* 69, 437-41.

146. Van Heest AE, House J, Putnam M (1993) Sensibility deficiencies in the hands of children with spastic hemiplegia. *J Hand Surg Am,* 18, 278-81.

147. Svedberg LE, Englund E, Malker H, Stener-Victorin E (2008) Parental perception of cold extremities and other accompanying symptoms in children with cerebral palsy. *Eur J Paediatr Neurol,* 12, 89-96.

148. Collins M (2014) Strabismus in cerebral palsy: When and why to operate. *Am Orthopt J,* 64, 17-20.

149. Huff JS, Murr N (2023) *Seizure.* [e-book] Treasure Island, StatPearls Publishing. Available at: National Library of Medicine <https://www.ncbi.nlm.nih.gov/books/NBK430765/> [Accessed February 9 2024].

150. Vinkel MN, Rackauskaite G, Finnerup NB (2022) Classification of pain in children with cerebral palsy. *Dev Med Child Neurol,* 64, 447-452.

151. Dickinson HO, Parkinson KN, Ravens-Sieberer U, et al. (2007) Self-reported quality of life of 8-12-year-old children with cerebral palsy: A cross-sectional European study. *Lancet,* 369, 2171-2178.

152. Colver A, Rapp M, Eisemann N, et al. (2015) Self-reported quality of life of adolescents with cerebral palsy: A cross-sectional and longitudinal analysis. *Lancet,* 385, 705-16.

153. Baram M, Zuk L, Stattler T, Katz-Leurer M (2023) The prevalence of bladder and bowel dysfunction in children with cerebral palsy and its association with motor, cognitive, and autonomic function. *Dev Neurorehabil,* 26, 155-162.

154. Wiegerink DJ, Roebroeck ME, Van Der Slot WM, et al. (2010) Importance of peers and dating in the development of romantic relationships and sexual activity of young adults with cerebral palsy. *Dev Med Child Neurol,* 52, 576-82.

155. Wiegerink DJ, Roebroeck ME, Bender J, et al. (2011) Sexuality of young adults with cerebral palsy: Experienced limitations and needs. *Sex Disabil,* 29, 119-128.

156. World Health Organization (1995) The World Health Organization Quality of Life Assessment (WHOQOL): Position paper from the World Health Organization. *Soc Sci Med,* 41, 1403-9.

157. World Health Organization (2022) *Mental health.* [online] Available at: <https://www.who.int/news-room/fact-sheets/detail/mental-health-strengthening-our-response> [Accessed February 22 2024].

158. Goodman R, Graham P (1996) Psychiatric problems in children with hemiplegia: Cross sectional epidemiological survey. *BMJ,* 312, 1065-9.

159. Downs J, Blackmore A, Epstein A, et al. (2017) The prevalence of mental health disorders and symptoms in children and adolescents with cerebral palsy: A systematic review and meta-analysis. *Dev Med Child Neurol,* 60, 30-38.

160. Rackauskaite G, Bilenberg N, Uldall P, Bech BH, Ostergaard J (2020) Prevalence of mental disorders in children and adolescents with cerebral palsy: Danish nationwide follow-up study. *Eur J Paediatr Neurol,* 27, 98-103.

161. Lindsay S, McPherson AC (2012a) Experiences of social exclusion and bullying at school among children and youth with cerebral palsy. *Disabil Rehabil,* 34, 101-9.

162. Riad J, Broström E, Langius-Eklöf A (2013) Do movement deviations influence self-esteem and sense of coherence in mild unilateral cerebral palsy? *J Pediatr Orthop,* 33, 298-302.

163. Noritz G, Davidson L, Steingass K, The Council on Children with Disabilities, The American Academy for Cerebral Palsy and Developmental Medicine (2022) Providing a primary care medical home for children and youth with cerebral palsy. *American Academy of Pediatrics,* 150, 1-54.

164. Rosenbaum P, Rosenbloom L, Mayston M (2012) Therapists and therapies in cerebral palsy. In: Rosenbaum P, Rosenbloom L, editors, *Cerebral palsy: From diagnosis to adulthood.* London: Mac Keith Press, pp 124-148.

165. CanChild (2024) *Family-centred service.* [online] Available at: <https://canchild.ca/en/research-in-practice/family-centred-service> [Accessed February 22 2024].

166. Stivers T (2012) Physician-child interaction: When children answer physicians' questions in routine medical encounters. *Patient Educ Couns,* 87, 3-9.

167. Martinek TJ (1996) Fostering hope in youth: A model for explaining learned helplessness in physical activity. *Quest,* 48, 409-421.

168. Jahnsen R, Villien L, Aamodt G, Stanghelle J, Inger H (2003) Physiotherapy and physical activity – experiences of adults with cerebral palsy, with implications for children. *Advances in Physiotherapy,* 5, 21-32.

169. Gillette Children's (2018) *Cerebral palsy road map: What to expect as your child grows [pdf].* [online] Available at: <http://gillettechildrens.org/assets/uploads/care-and-conditions/CP_Roadmap.pdf> [Accessed February 22 2024].

170. Sackett DL, Rosenberg WM, Gray JA, Haynes RB, Richardson WS (1996) Evidence based medicine: What it is and what it isn't. *BMJ,* 312, 71-2.

171. Academy of Pediatric Physical Therapy (2019) Fact sheet: The ABCs of pediatric physical therapy. [pdf], Wisconsin, APTA, Available at: <https://pediatricapta.org/includes/fact-sheets/pdfs/FactSheet_ABCsofPediatricPT_2019.pdf?v=2> [Accessed April 24 2024].

172. Agency for Healthcare Research and Quality (2020) The SHARE approach: A model for shared decisionmaking – fact sheet, Available at: <https://www.ahrq.gov/health-literacy/professional-training/shared-decision/tools/factsheet.html> [Accessed February 18 2024].

173. Palisano RJ (2006) A collaborative model of service delivery for children with movement disorders: A framework for evidence-based decision making. *Phys Ther*, 86, 1295-305.

174. Mayston M (2018) More studies are needed in paediatric neurodisability. *Dev Med Child Neurol*, 60, 966.

175. Morris ZS, Wooding S, Grant J (2011) The answer is 17 years, what is the question: Understanding time lags in translational research. *J R Soc Med*, 104, 510-20.

176. Deville C, McEwen I, Arnold SH, Jones M, Zhao YD (2015) Knowledge translation of the gross motor function classification system among pediatric physical therapists. *Pediatr Phys Ther*, 27, 376-84.

177. Bailes A, Gannotti M, Bellows D, et al. (2018) Caregiver knowledge and preferences for gross motor function information in cerebral palsy. *Dev Med Child Neurol*, 60, 1264-1270.

178. Gross PH, Bailes AF, Horn SD, et al. (2018) Setting a patient-centered research agenda for cerebral palsy: A participatory action research initiative. *Dev Med Child Neurol*, 60, 1278-1284.

179. Wallwiener M, Brucker SY, Wallwiener D, Steering C (2012) Multidisciplinary breast centres in Germany: A review and update of quality assurance through benchmarking and certification. *Arch Gynecol Obstet*, 285, 1671-83.

180. Damiano D, Longo E (2021) Early intervention evidence for infants with or at risk for cerebral palsy: An overview of systematic reviews. *Dev Med Child Neurol*, 63, 771-784.

181. Ogbeiwi O (2018) General concepts of goals and goal-setting in healthcare: A narrative review. *Journal of Management & Organization*, 27, 324-341.

182. Löwing K, Bexelius A, Brogren Carlberg E (2009) Activity focused and goal directed therapy for children with cerebral palsy–do goals make a difference? *Disabil Rehabil*, 31, 1808-16.

183. Phoenix M, Rosenbaum P (2014) Development and implementation of a paediatric rehabilitation care path for hard-to-reach families: A case report. *Child Care Health Dev*, 41, 494-9.

184. Vroland-Nordstrand K, Eliasson AC, Jacobsson H, Johansson U, Krumlinde-Sundholm L (2016) Can children identify and achieve goals for intervention? A randomized trial comparing two goal-setting approaches. *Dev Med Child Neurol*, 58, 589-96.

185. Franki I, De Cat J, Deschepper E, et al. (2014) A clinical decision framework for the identification of main problems and treatment goals for ambulant children with bilateral spastic cerebral palsy. *Res Dev Disabil*, 35, 1160-76.

186. Law M, Baptiste S, Carswell A, et al. (2019) *Canadian Occupational Performance Measure*, Ottawa: COMP Inc.

187. Turner-Stokes L (2009) Goal Attainment Scaling (GAS) in rehabilitation: A practical guide. *Clin Rehabil*, 23, 362-70.

188. Stout JL, Thill M, Munger ME, Walt K, Boyer ER (2024) Reliability of the Gait Outcomes Assessment List questionnaire. *Dev Med Child Neurol*, 66, 61-69.

189. Narayanan U, Davidson B, Weir S (2011) The Gait Outcomes Assessment List (GOAL): A new tool to assess cerebral palsy. *Dev Med Child Neurol*, 53, 79.

190. Thomason P, Tan A, Donnan A, et al. (2018) The Gait Outcomes Assessment List (GOAL): Validation of a new assessment of gait function for children with cerebral palsy. *Dev Med Child Neurol*, 60, 618-623.

191. Boyer E, Palmer M, Walt K, Georgiadis A, Stout J (2022) Validation of the Gait Outcomes Assessment List questionnaire and caregiver priorities for individuals with cerebral palsy. *Dev Med Child Neurol*, 64, 379-386.

192. Elkamil AI, Andersen GL, Hägglund G, et al. (2011) Prevalence of hip dislocation among children with cerebral palsy in regions with and without a surveillance programme: A cross sectional study in Sweden and Norway. *BMC Musculoskelet Disord*, 12, 284.

193. Thomason P, Rodda J, Willoughby K, Graham HK (2014) Lower limb function. In: Dan B, Mayston M, Paneth N, Rosenbloom L, editors, *Cerebral palsy: Science and clinical practice*. London: Mac Keith Press, pp 461-488.

194. Van Heest AE (2023) *Personal communication.*

195. World Confederation for Physical Therapy (2024) *What is physiotherapy?* [online] Available at: <https://world.physio/resources/what-is-physiotherapy> [Accessed February 22 2024].

196. Fowler EG, Ho TW, Nwigwe AI, Dorey FJ (2001) The effect of quadriceps femoris muscle strengthening exercises on spasticity in children with cerebral palsy. *Phys Ther*, 81, 1215-23.

197. Gonzalez A, Garcia L, Kilby J, McNair P (2021) Robotic devices for paediatric rehabilitation: A review of design features. *BioMed Eng OnLine*, 20, 1-33.

198. Pin T, Dyke P, Chan M (2006) The effectiveness of passive stretching in children with cerebral palsy. *Dev Med Child Neurol*, 48, 855-62.

199. American Occupational Therapy Association (2024) *Patients & clients: Learn about occupational therapy.* [online] Available at: <https://www.aota.org/about/what-is-ot> [Accessed February 22 2024].

200. Gilliaux M, Renders A, Dispa D, et al. (2015) Upper limb robot-assisted therapy in cerebral palsy: A single-blind randomized controlled trial. *Neurorehabil Neural Repair*, 29, 183-92.

201. Bailes A, Reder R, Burch C (2008) Development of guidelines for determining frequency of therapy services in a pediatric medical setting. *Pediatr Phys Ther*, 20, 194-8.

202. Gillette Children's (2024) *Episodes of care in childhood and adolescence.* [online] Available at: <https://www.gillettechildrens.org/assets/REHA-006_EOC_English.pdf [Accessed January 19 2024].

203. Novak I, McIntyre S, Morgan C, et al. (2013) A systematic review of interventions for children with cerebral palsy: State of the evidence. *Dev Med Child Neurol*, 55, 885-910.

204. American Council on Exercise (2015) *Physical activity vs. Exercise: What's the difference?* [online] Available at: <https://www.acefitness.org/resources/everyone/blog/5460/physical-activity-vs-exercise-what-s-the-difference/> [Accessed February 22 2024].

205. O'Neil ME, Fragala-Pinkham M, Lennon N, et al. (2016) Reliability and validity of objective measures of physical activity in youth with cerebral palsy who are ambulatory. *Phys Ther*, 96, 37-45.

206. Bjornson K, Fiss A, Avery L, et al. (2019) Longitudinal trajectories of physical activity and walking performance by Gross Motor Function Classification System level for children with cerebral palsy. *Disabil Rehabil,* 42, 1705-1713.

207. Bjornson KF, Zhou C, Stevenson R, Christakis D, Song K (2014) Walking activity patterns in youth with cerebral palsy and youth developing typically. *Disabil Rehabil,* 36, 1279-84.

208. Obeid J, Balemans AC, Noorduyn SG, Gorter JW, Timmons BW (2014) Objectively measured sedentary time in youth with cerebral palsy compared with age, sex, and season-matched youth who are developing typically: An explorative study. *Phys Ther,* 94, 1163-7.

209. Maltais DB, Pierrynowski MR, Galea VA, Bar-Or O (2005) Physical activity level is associated with the O2 cost of walking in cerebral palsy. *Med Sci Sports Exerc,* 37, 347-53.

210. Ryan JM, Hensey O, McLoughlin B, Lyons A, Gormley J (2014) Reduced moderate-to-vigorous physical activity and increased sedentary behavior are associated with elevated blood pressure values in children with cerebral palsy. *Phys Ther,* 94, 1144-53.

211. Slaman J, Roebroeck M, Van Der Slot W, et al. (2014) Can a lifestyle intervention improve physical fitness in adolescents and young adults with spastic cerebral palsy? A randomized controlled trial. *Arch Phys Med Rehabil,* 95, 1646-55.

212. Maher CA, Toohey M, Ferguson M (2016) Physical activity predicts quality of life and happiness in children and adolescents with cerebral palsy. *Disabil Rehabil,* 38, 865-9.

213. Zwinkels M, Verschuren O, Balemans A, et al. (2018) Effects of a school-based sports program on physical fitness, physical activity, and cardiometabolic health in youth with physical disabilities: Data from the sport-2-stay-fit study. *Front Pediatr,* 6, 1-11.

214. Fowler EG, Kolobe TH, Damiano DL, et al. (2007) Promotion of physical fitness and prevention of secondary conditions for children with cerebral palsy: Section on pediatrics research summit proceedings. *Phys Ther,* 87, 1495-510.

215. Verschuren O, Peterson MD, Balemans AC, Hurvitz EA (2016) Exercise and physical activity recommendations for people with cerebral palsy. *Dev Med Child Neurol,* 58, 798-808.

216. World Health Organization (2010) *Global recommendations on physical activity for health.* [online] Available at: <https://www.who.int/publications/i/item/9789241599979> [Accessed February 22 2024].

217. Tipton CM (2014) The history of "exercise is medicine" in ancient civilizations. *Adv Physiol Educ,* 38, 109-17.

218. Adolph KE, Vereijken B, Shrout PE (2003) What changes in infant walking and why. *Child Dev,* 74, 475-97.

219. Loughborough University Peter Harrison Centre for Disability Sport [pdf] (n.d.) *Fit for sport.* [online] Available at: <https://www.lboro.ac.uk/media/media/research/phc/downloads/Cerebral%20Palsy%20guide_Fit_for_Sport.pdf> [Accessed February 22 2024].

220. Loughborough University Peter Harrison Centre for Disability Sport [pdf] (n.d.) *Fit for life.* [online] Available at: <https://www.lboro.ac.uk/media/media/research/phc/downloads/Cerebral%20Palsy%20guide_Fit_for_Life.pdf> [Accessed February 22 2024].

221. World Abilitysport (2024) *World Abilitysport.* [online] Available at: <https://worldabilitysport.org/> [Accessed February 22 2024].

222. O'Sullivan J (2016) *'We all have limits. I am not a disabled athlete, I am a Paralympic athlete.'* [online] Available at: <https://www.irishtimes.com/sport/we-all-have-limits-i-am-not-a-disabled-athlete-i-am-a-paralympic-athlete-1.2787039> [Accessed February 22 2024].

223. Moore J (2016) *Now four Paralympic athletes beat the Olympic gold medal time, perhaps people will stop telling me I can become one too.* [online] Available at: <https://www.independent.co.uk/voices/paralympics-athletes-beat-olympic-gold-medal-time-1500m-race-disability-stop-asking-me-to-become-one-a7245961.html> [Accessed February 22 2024].

224. International Paralympic Committee (2024) *Paralympic sports list.* [online] Available at: <https://www.paralympic.org/sports> [Accessed February 22 2024].

225. World Health Organization (2024a) *Assistive technology.* [online] Available at: <https://www.who.int/news-room/fact-sheets/detail/assistive-technology> [Accessed February 22 2024].

226. Ward M, Johnson C, Klein J, McGeary FJ, Nolin W PM (2021) Orthotics and assistive devices. In: Murphy KP, McMahon MA, Houtrow AJ, editors, *Pediatric rehabilitation principles and practice.* New York: Springer publishing company, pp 196-229.

227. Owen E, Rahlin M, Kane K (2023) Content validity of a collaborative goal-setting pictorial tool for children who wear ankle-foot orthoses: A modified Delphi consensus study. *JPO Journal of Prosthetics and Orthotics,* 32, 89-98.

228. Ward ME (2009) Pharmacologic treatment with oral medications. In: Gage JR, Schwartz MH, Koop SE, Novacheck TF, editors, *The identification and treatment of gait problems in cerebral palsy.* London: Mac Keith Press, pp 349-362.

229. Molenaers G, Desloovere K (2009) Pharmacologic treatment with botulinum toxin. In: Gage JR, Schwartz MH, Koop SE, Novacheck TF, editors, *The identification and treatment of gait problems in cerebral palsy.* London: Mac Keith Press, pp 363-380.

230. Multani I, Manji J, Hastings-Ison T, Khot A, Graham K (2019) Botulinum toxin in the management of children with cerebral palsy. *Paediatr Drugs,* 21, 261-281.

231. Shore BJ, Thomason P, Reid SM, Shrader MW, Graham HK (2021) Cerebral palsy. In: Weinstein S, Flynn J, Crawford H, editors, *Lovell and Winter's pediatric orthopaedics* 8th ed. Philadelphia: Wolters Kluwer, pp 508-589.

232. Williams SA, Elliott C, Valentine J, et al. (2013) Combining strength training and botulinum neurotoxin intervention in children with cerebral palsy: The impact on muscle morphology and strength. *Disabil Rehabil,* 35, 596-605.

233. Love SC, Novak I, Kentish M, et al. (2010) Botulinum toxin assessment, intervention and after-care for lower limb spasticity in children with cerebral palsy: International consensus statement. *Eur J Neurol,* 17, 9-37.

234. Molenaers G, Fagard K, Van Campenhout A, Desloovere K (2013) Botulinum toxin A treatment of the lower extremities in children with cerebral palsy. *J Child Orthop*, 7, 383-7.

235. Fortuna R, Horisberger M, Vaz MA, Herzog W (2013) Do skeletal muscle properties recover following repeat onabotulinum toxin A injections? *J Biomech*, 46, 2426-33.

236. Fortuna R, Vaz MA, Sawatsky A, Hart DA, Herzog W (2015) A clinically relevant BTA-X injection protocol leads to persistent weakness, contractile material loss, and an altered MRNA expression phenotype in rabbit quadriceps muscles. *J Biomech*, 48, 1700-6.

237. Mathevon L, Michel F, Decavel P, et al. (2015) Muscle structure and stiffness assessment after botulinum toxin type A injection. A systematic review. *Ann Phys Rehabil Med*, 58, 343-50.

238. Valentine J, Stannage K, Fabian V, et al. (2016) Muscle histopathology in children with spastic cerebral palsy receiving botulinum toxin type A. *Muscle Nerve*, 53, 407-14.

239. Alexander C, Elliott C, Valentine J, et al. (2018) Muscle volume alterations after first botulinum neurotoxin A treatment in children with cerebral palsy: A 6-month prospective cohort study. *Dev Med Child Neurol*, 60, 1165-1171.

240. Schless SH, Cenni F, Bar-On L, et al. (2019) Medial gastrocnemius volume and echo-intensity after botulinum neurotoxin A interventions in children with spastic cerebral palsy. *Dev Med Child Neurol*, 61, 783-790.

241. Tang MJ, Graham HK, Davidson KE (2021) Botulinum toxin A and osteosarcopenia in experimental animals: A scoping review. *Toxins*, 13, 1-13.

242. Krach LE (2009) Treatment of spasticity with intrathecal baclofen. In: Gage JR, Schwartz MH, Koop SE, Novacheck TF, editors, *The identification and treatment of gait problems in cerebral palsy*. London: Mac Keith Press, pp 383-396.

243. Gillette Children's (2013) *Pediatric spasticity management*. St. Paul: Gillette Children's Hospital. Unpublished.

244. Grunt S, Fieggen AG, Vermeulen RJ, Becher JG, Langerak NG (2014) Selection criteria for selective dorsal rhizotomy in children with spastic cerebral palsy: A systematic review of the literature. *Dev Med Child Neurol*, 56, 302-12.

245. Van Heest AE, House JH, Cariello C (1999) Upper extremity surgical treatment of cerebral palsy. *J Hand Surg Am*, 24, 323-30.

246. Smitherman JA, Davids JR, Tanner S, et al. (2011) Functional outcomes following single-event multilevel surgery of the upper extremity for children with hemiplegic cerebral palsy. *J Bone Joint Surg Am*, 93, 655-61.

247. Van Heest AE, Ramachandran V, Stout J, Wervey R, Garcia L (2008) Quantitative and qualitative functional evaluation of upper extremity tendon transfers in spastic hemiplegia caused by cerebral palsy. *J Pediatr Orthop*, 28, 679-83.

248. Rethlefsen SA, Blumstein G, Kay RM, Dorey F, Wren TA (2017) Prevalence of specific gait abnormalities in children with cerebral palsy revisited: Influence of age, prior surgery, and Gross Motor Function Classification System level. *Dev Med Child Neurol*, 59, 79-88.

249. Rang M (1990) Cerebral palsy. In: Morrissy R, editor, *Pediatric orthopedics.* Philadelphia: Lippincott, pp 465-506.

250. Thomason P, Baker R, Dodd K, et al. (2011) Single-event multilevel surgery in children with spastic diplegia: A pilot randomized controlled trial. *J Bone Joint Surg Am,* 93, 451-60.

251. Vuillermin C, Rodda J, Rutz E, et al. (2011) Severe crouch gait in spastic diplegia can be prevented: A population-based study. *J Bone Joint Surg Br,* 93, 1670-5.

252. McGinley JL, Dobson F, Ganeshalingam R, et al. (2012) Single-event multilevel surgery for children with cerebral palsy: A systematic review. *Dev Med Child Neurol,* 54, 117-28.

253. Van Bommel EEH, Arts MME, Jongerius PH, Ratter J, Rameckers EAA (2019) Physical therapy treatment in children with cerebral palsy after single-event multilevel surgery: A qualitative systematic review. A first step towards a clinical guideline for physical therapy after single-event multilevel surgery. *Ther Adv Chronic Dis,* 10, 1-14.

254. Colvin C, Greve K, Lehn C, et al. (2019) *Evidence-based clinical care guideline for physical therapy management of single event multi-level surgeries (SEMLS) for children, adolescents, and young adults with cerebral palsy or other similar neuromotor conditions [pdf].* [online] Available at: <https://www.cincinnati childrens.org/research/divisions/j/anderson-center/evidence-based-care/ recommendations> [Accessed February 22 2024].

255. Gorton GE, Abel MF, Oeffinger DJ, et al. (2009) A prospective cohort study of the effects of lower extremity orthopaedic surgery on outcome measures in ambulatory children with cerebral palsy. *J Pediatr Orthop,* 29, 903-9.

256. Schranz C, Kruse A, Kraus T, Steinwender G, Svehlik M (2017) Does unilateral single-event multilevel surgery improve gait in children with spastic hemiplegia? A retrospective analysis of a long-term follow-up. *Gait Posture,* 52, 135-139.

257. Amirmudin NA, Lavelle G, Theologis T, Thompson N, Ryan JM (2019) Multilevel surgery for children with cerebral palsy: A meta-analysis. *Pediatrics,* 143, 1-18.

258. Dreher T, Thomason P, Svehlik M, et al. (2018) Long-term development of gait after multilevel surgery in children with cerebral palsy: A multicentre cohort study. *Dev Med Child Neurol,* 60, 88-93.

259. Graham HK, Selber P, Nattrass GR (2005) Comment on: Handelsman JE, Weinberg J, Razi A, Mulley DA, The role of AO external fixation in proximal femoral osteotomies in the pediatric neuromuscular population. *Journal of Pediatric Orthopaedics B,* 14, 307.

260. Lubicky JP (2005) Comment on: Handelsman JE, Weinberg J, Razi A, Mulley DA, The role of AO external fixation in proximal femoral osteotomies in the pediatric neuromuscular population. *Journal of Pediatric Orthopaedics B,* 14, 307.

261. Petersen E, Tomhave W, Agel J, et al. (2016) The effect of treatment on stereognosis in children with hemiplegic cerebral palsy. *J Hand Surg Am,* 41, 91-6.

262. Auld ML, Johnston LM, Russo RN, Moseley GL (2017) A single session of mirror-based tactile and motor training improves tactile dysfunction in children with unilateral cerebral palsy: A replicated randomized controlled case series. *Physiother Res Int,* 22, 1-24.

263. McLean B, Taylor S, Blair E, et al. (2017) Somatosensory discrimination intervention improves body position sense and motor performance in children with hemiplegic cerebral palsy. *Am J Occup Ther,* 71, 1-9.

264. Mus-Peters CTR, Huisstede BMA, Noten S, et al. (2018) Low bone mineral density in ambulatory persons with cerebral palsy? A systematic review. *Disabil Rehabil,* 41, 2392-2402.

265. Mergler S (2018) Bone status in cerebral palsy. In: Panteliadis CP, editor, *Cerebral palsy: A multidisciplinary approach.* Cham: Springer International Publishing, pp 253-257.

266. Gage JR (2009) General issues of recurrence with growth. In: Gage JR, Schwartz MH, Koop SE, Novacheck TF, editor, *The identification and treatment of gait problems in cerebral palsy.* London: Mac Keith Press, pp 546-554.

267. Majnemer A, Shikako-Thomas K, Shevell MI, et al. (2013) Pursuit of complementary and alternative medicine treatments in adolescents with cerebral palsy. *J Child Neurol,* 28, 1443-1447.

268. Graham HK (2014) Cerebral palsy prevention and cure: Vision or mirage? A personal view. *J Paediatr Child Health,* 50, 89-90.

269. King GA, Cathers T, Polgar JM, Mackinnon E, Havens L (2000) Success in life for older adolescents with cerebral palsy. *Qual Health Res,* 10, 734-49.

270. Wehmeyer ML, Palmer S (2003) Adult outcomes for students with cognitive disabilities three-years after high school: The impact of self-determination. *Education and Training in Developmental Disabilities,* 38, 131-144.

271. Damiano DL (2006) Activity, activity, activity: Rethinking our physical therapy approach to cerebral palsy. *Phys Ther,* 86, 1534-40.

272. United Nations (1990) *Convention on the rights of the child.* [online] Available at: <https://www.ohchr.org/en/instruments-mechanisms/instruments/convention-rights-child> [Accessed February 22 2024].

273. United Nations Educational Scientific and Cultural Organization (2017) *School violence and bullying: Global status report.* [online] Available at: <https://unesdoc.unesco.org/ark:/48223/pf0000246970?posInSet=1&queryId=N-EXPLORE-8864b64c-4b12-445e-a56d-b655a1a86afd> [Accessed February 22 2024].

274. Lindsay S, McPherson AC (2012b) Strategies for improving disability awareness and social inclusion of children and young people with cerebral palsy. *Child Care Health Dev,* 38, 809-16.

275. Tindal SR (2017) Students with mild cerebral palsy in the classroom: Information and guidelines for teachers. *Interdisciplinary Journal of Undergraduate Research,* 6, 70-78.

276. Thomason P, Graham HK (2013) Rehabilitation of children with cerebral palsy after single-event multilevel surgery. In: Iansek R, Morris ME, editor, *Rehabilitation in movement disorders.* Cambridge: Cambridge University Press, pp 203-217.

277. Strauss D, Brooks J, Rosenbloom L, Shavelle R (2008) Life expectancy in cerebral palsy: An update. *Dev Med Child Neurol*, 50, 487-93.

278. World Health Organization (2024b) *Adolescent health.* [online] Available at: <https://www.who.int/health-topics/adolescent-health#tab=tab_1> [Accessed February 22 2024].

279. Liptak GS (2008) Health and well being of adults with cerebral palsy. *Curr Opin Neurol*, 21, 136-42.

280. Centers for Disease Control and Prevention (2020) *Disability and health related conditions.* [online] Available at: <https://www.cdc.gov/ncbddd/disabilityand health/relatedconditions.html> [Accessed January 19 2024].

281. Novak I, Walker K, Hunt RW, et al. (2016) Concise review: Stem cell interventions for people with cerebral palsy: Systematic review with meta-analysis. *Stem Cells Transl Med*, 5, 1014-25.

282. Wu YW, Mehravari AS, Numis AL, Gross P (2015) Cerebral palsy research funding from the National Institutes of Health, 2001 to 2013. *Dev Med Child Neurol*, 57, 936-41.

283. Tosi LL, Maher N, Moore DW, Goldstein M, Aisen ML (2009) Adults with cerebral palsy: A workshop to define the challenges of treating and preventing secondary musculoskeletal and neuromuscular complications in this rapidly growing population. *Dev Med Child Neurol*, 51, 2-11.

284. Santilli V, Bernetti A, Mangone M, Paoloni M (2014) Clinical definition of sarcopenia. *Clin Cases Miner Bone Metab*, 11, 177-80.

285. Ni Lochlainn M, Bowyer RCE, Steves CJ (2018) Dietary protein and muscle in aging people: The potential role of the gut microbiome. *Nutrients*, 10, 929.

286. Bauer J, Biolo G, Cederholm T, et al. (2013) Evidence-based recommendations for optimal dietary protein intake in older people: A position paper from the PROT-AGE study group. *J Am Med Dir Assoc*, 14, 542-59.

287. Resnick B, Nahm ES, Zhu S, et al. (2014) The impact of osteoporosis, falls, fear of falling, and efficacy expectations on exercise among community-dwelling older adults. *Orthop Nurs*, 33, 277-88.

288. World Health Organization (2023) *Noncommunicable diseases.* [online] Available at: <https://www.who.int/news-room/fact-sheets/detail/ noncommunicable-diseases> [Accessed February 22 2024].

289. Rauch J (2018) *The happiness curve: Why life gets better after midlife*, London: Bloomsbury Publishing.

290. Sheridan KJ (2009) Osteoporosis in adults with cerebral palsy. *Dev Med Child Neurol*, 51 Suppl 4, 38-51.

291. Ryan JM, Albairami F, Hamilton T, et al. (2023) Prevalence and incidence of chronic conditions among adults with cerebral palsy: A systematic review and meta-analysis. *Dev Med Child Neurol*, 65, 1174-1189.

292. Thomason P, Graham HK (2009) Consequences of interventions. In: Gage JR, Schwartz MH, Koop SE, Novacheck TF, editor, *The identification and treatment of gait problems in cerebral palsy*. London: Mac Keith Press, pp 605-623.

293. Nooijen C, Slaman J, Van Der Slot W, et al. (2014) Health-related physical fitness of ambulatory adolescents and young adults with spastic cerebral palsy. *J Rehabil Med*, 46, 642-7.

294. Gillett JG, Lichtwark GA, Boyd RN, Barber LA (2018) Functional capacity in adults with cerebral palsy: Lower limb muscle strength matters. *Arch Phys Med Rehabil,* 99, 900-906.

295. Cremer N, Hurvitz E, Peterson M (2017) Multimorbidity in middle-aged adults with cerebral palsy. *Am J Med,* 130, 9-15.

296. Peterson MD, Ryan JM, Hurvitz EA, Mahmoudi E (2015) Chronic conditions in adults with cerebral palsy. *JAMA,* 314, 2303-5.

297. O'Connell NE, Smith KJ, Peterson MD, et al. (2019) Incidence of osteoarthritis, osteoporosis and inflammatory musculoskeletal diseases in adults with cerebral palsy: A population-based cohort study. *Bone,* 125, 30-35.

298. Whitney DG, Alford AI, Devlin MJ, et al. (2019) Adults with cerebral palsy have higher prevalence of fracture compared with adults without cerebral palsy independent of osteoporosis and cardiometabolic diseases. *J Bone Miner Res,* 34, 1240-1247.

299. Van Gorp M, Hilberink SR, Noten S, et al. (2020) Epidemiology of cerebral palsy in adulthood: A systematic review and meta-analysis of the most frequently studied outcomes. *Arch Phys Med Rehabil,* 101, 1041-1052.

300. Morgan P, McGinley J (2014) Gait function and decline in adults with cerebral palsy: A systematic review. *Disabil Rehabil,* 36, 1-9.

301. Murphy KP (2010) The adult with cerebral palsy. *Orthop Clin North Am,* 41, 595-605.

302. Thill M, Krach LE, Pederson K, et al. (2023) *Physical and psychosocial consequences of falls in individuals with cerebral palsy [pdf],* [online] Available at: <https://www.medrxiv.org/content/medrxiv/early/2023/08/21/2023.08.16.23294 077.full.pdf> [Accessed June 20 2024].

303. Ryan JM (2023) *Personal communication.*

304. Morgan P, McDonald R, McGinley J (2015) Perceived cause, environmental factors, and consequences of falls in adults with cerebral palsy: A preliminary mixed methods study. *Rehabil Res Pract,* 2015, 1-9.

305. Boyer ER, Patterson A (2018) Gait pathology subtypes are not associated with self-reported fall frequency in children with cerebral palsy. *Gait Posture,* 63, 189-194.

306. Ryan JM, Cameron MH, Liverani S, et al. (2019) Incidence of falls among adults with cerebral palsy: A cohort study using primary care data. *Dev Med Child Neurol,* 62, 477-482.

307. Jahnsen R, Villien L, Aamodt G, Stanghelle JK, Holm I (2004) Musculoskeletal pain in adults with cerebral palsy compared with the general population. *J Rehabil Med,* 36, 78-84.

308. Rodby-Bousquet E, Alriksson-Schmidt A, Jarl J (2021) Prevalence of pain and interference with daily activities and sleep in adults with cerebral palsy. *Dev Med Child Neurol,* 63, 60-67.

309. Whitney DG, Bell S, Whibley D, et al. (2020) Effect of pain on mood affective disorders in adults with cerebral palsy. *Dev Med Child Neurol,* 62, 926-932.

310. Asuman D, Gerdtham UG, Alriksson-Schmidt AI, et al. (2023) Pain and labor outcomes: A longitudinal study of adults with cerebral palsy in Sweden. *Disabil Health J,* 16, 1-8.

311. Jarl J, Alriksson-Schmidt A, Rodby-Bousquet E (2019) Health-related quality of life in adults with cerebral palsy living in Sweden and relation to demographic and disability-specific factors. *Disabil Health J,* 12, 460-466.

312. Vidart D'egurbide Bagazgoitia N, Ehlinger V, Duffaut C, et al. (2021) Quality of life in young adults with cerebral palsy: A longitudinal analysis of the sparcle study. *Front Neurol,* 12, 1-14.

313. Jahnsen R, Villien L, Stanghelle JK, Holm I (2003) Fatigue in adults with cerebral palsy in Norway compared with the general population. *Dev Med Child Neurol,* 45, 296-303.

314. Russchen HA, Slaman J, Stam HJ, et al. (2014) Focus on fatigue amongst young adults with spastic cerebral palsy. *J Neuroeng Rehabil,* 11, 1-7.

315. McPhee PG, Brunton LK, Timmons BW, Bentley T, Gorter JW (2017) Fatigue and its relationship with physical activity, age, and body composition in adults with cerebral palsy. *Dev Med Child Neurol,* 59, 367-373.

316. National Institute of Mental Health (2024a) *Depression.* [online] Available at: <https://www.nimh.nih.gov/health/topics/depression> [Accessed February 22 2024].

317. Smith KJ, Peterson MD, O'Connell NE, et al. (2019) Risk of depression and anxiety in adults with cerebral palsy. *JAMA Neurol,* 76, 294-300.

318. Gannotti ME, Gorton GE, 3rd, Nahorniak MT, Masso PD (2013) Gait and participation outcomes in adults with cerebral palsy: A series of case studies using mixed methods. *Disabil Health J,* 6, 244-52.

319. National Institute of Mental Health (2024b) *Anxiety disorders.* [online] Available at: <https://www.nimh.nih.gov/health/topics/anxiety-disorders> [Accessed February 22 2024].

320. Schmidt AK, Van Gorp M, Van Wely L, et al. (2020) Autonomy in participation in cerebral palsy from childhood to adulthood. *Dev Med Child Neurol,* 62, 363-371.

321. Pettersson K, Rodby-Bousquet E (2021) Living conditions and social outcomes in adults with cerebral palsy. *Front Neurol,* 12, 1-12.

322. Accenture (2018) *Getting to equal: The disability inclusion advantage [pdf].* [online] Available at: <https://www.accenture.com/content/dam/accenture/final/a-com-migration/pdf/pdf-89/accenture-disability-inclusion-research-report.pdf> [Accessed February 22 2024].

323. Hayward K, Chen AY, Forbes E, et al. (2017) Reproductive healthcare experiences of women with cerebral palsy. *Disabil Health J,* 10, 413-418.

324. Van Der Slot WM, Nieuwenhuijsen C, Van Den Berg-Emons RJ, et al. (2010) Participation and health-related quality of life in adults with spastic bilateral cerebral palsy and the role of self-efficacy. *J Rehabil Med,* 42, 528-35.

325. Nieuwenhuijsen C, Van Der Laar Y, Donkervoort M, et al. (2008) Unmet needs and health care utilization in young adults with cerebral palsy. *Disabil Rehabil,* 30, 1254-62.

326. Bagatell N, Chan D, Rauch KK, Thorpe D (2017) "Thrust into adulthood": Transition experiences of young adults with cerebral palsy. *Disabil Health J,* 10, 80-86.

327. Freeman M, Stewart D, Cunningham CE, Gorter JW (2018) "If I had been given that information back then": An interpretive description exploring the information needs of adults with cerebral palsy looking back on their transition to adulthood. *Child Care Health Dev,* 44, 689-696.

328. O'Brien G, Bass A, Rosenbloom L (2009) Cerebral palsy and aging. In: O'Brien G, Rosenbloom L, editor, *Developmental disability and aging.* London: Mac Keith Press, pp 39-52.

329. Hilberink SR, Roebroeck ME, Nieuwstraten W, et al. (2007) Health issues in young adults with cerebral palsy: Towards a life-span perspective. *J Rehabil Med,* 39, 605-11.

330. Ryan JM, Crowley VE, Hensey O, McGahey A, Gormley J (2014) Waist circumference provides an indication of numerous cardiometabolic risk factors in adults with cerebral palsy. *Arch Phys Med Rehabil,* 95, 1540-6.

331. Putz C, Döderlein L, Mertens EM, et al. (2016) Multilevel surgery in adults with cerebral palsy. *Bone Joint J,* 98-b, 282-8.

332. Cassidy C, Campbell N, Madady M, Payne M (2016) Bridging the gap: The role of physiatrists in caring for adults with cerebral palsy. *Disabil Rehabil,* 38, 493-8.

333. Gajdosik CG, Cicirello N (2001) Secondary conditions of the musculoskeletal system in adolescents and adults with cerebral palsy. *Phys Occup Ther Pediatr,* 21, 49-68.

334. Murphy KP (2018) Comment on: Cerebral palsy, non-communicable diseases, and lifespan care. *Dev Med Child Neurol,* 60, 733.

335. Rosenbaum P (2019) Diagnosis in developmental disability: A perennial challenge, and a proposed middle ground. *Dev Med Child Neurol,* 61, 620.

336. Schuh L (2023) *Personal communication.*

337. Imms C, Dodd KJ (2010) What is cerebral palsy? In: Dodd KJ, Imms C, Taylor NF, editor, *Physiotherapy and occupational therapy for people with cerebral palsy: A problem-based approach to assessment and management.* London: Mac Keith Press, pp 7-30.

338. Ryan JM, Allen E, Gormley J, Hurvitz EA, Peterson MD (2018) The risk, burden, and management of non-communicable diseases in cerebral palsy: A scoping review. *Dev Med Child Neurol,* 60, 753-764.

339. Sheridan (2019) *Personal communication.*

340. Louw A, Diener I, Butler DS, Puentedura EJ (2011) The effect of neuroscience education on pain, disability, anxiety, and stress in chronic musculoskeletal pain. *Arch Phys Med Rehabil,* 92, 2041-56.

341. Moseley GL, Butler DS (2015) Fifteen years of explaining pain: The past, present, and future. *J Pain,* 16, 807-13.

342. Gettings J (2019) *Personal communication.*

343. Andraweera ND, Andraweera PH, Lassi ZS, Kochiyil V (2021) Effectiveness of botulinum toxin A injection in managing mobility-related outcomes in adult patients with cerebral palsy: Systematic review. *Am J Phys Med Rehabil,* 100, 851-857.

344. Thomason P, Selber P, Graham HK (2013) Single event multilevel surgery in children with bilateral spastic cerebral palsy: A 5 year prospective cohort study. *Gait Posture*, 37, 23-8.

345. Peterson MD, Gordon PM, Hurvitz EA (2013) Chronic disease risk among adults with cerebral palsy: The role of premature sarcopoenia, obesity and sedentary behaviour. *Obes Rev*, 14, 171-82.

346. Garber CE, Blissmer B, Deschenes MR, et al. (2011) American College of Sports Medicine position stand. Quantity and quality of exercise for developing and maintaining cardiorespiratory, musculoskeletal, and neuromotor fitness in apparently healthy adults: Guidance for prescribing exercise. *Med Sci Sports Exerc*, 43, 1334-59.

Index

Figures and tables indicated by page numbers in italics.

A

abducted forefoot, 116
activities of daily living, 171
acupuncture, 249
adaptive equipment: for daily living, 208–209; for recreation, 210–217
adducted forefoot, 117
aerobic exercise, 188
aging: motor function, 281; musculoskeletal system, 274–276, 279–281, 284, 285, 292–293; nervous system, 292; and pain, 282, 284–285; and physical activity, 184, 281, 298, 299; and spastic hemiplegia, 270–272, 278–289, 291–293; typical, 274–277
alternative treatments, 248–250, *249–250*
ankle-foot orthoses, *203–204*, 205
ankles: flexion, 88, 89; and gait patterns, 129–130; orthoses, 164, 167, 197–198, *202–204. See also* lower limbs
anterior pelvic tilt, 66
arms: external rotation, 87; nonuse, 123; pronated, 65–66; in spastic hemiplegia, 65–66, 86. *See also* upper limbs
art and crafts, adaptive equipment for, 214–215, *215*
arthritis, 280, 284, 285. *See also* osteoarthritis
assistive technology, 196–217. *See also* mobility aids; orthoses
asthma, 285
ataxia, 32, 34–35, 37
autonomy. *See* independence

B

baclofen: intrathecal delivery, 225–226, *226*; oral medication, 221
balance: exercises for, 298; and nervous system, 11; and neuromusculoskeletal system, 90n, 98; service dog, 295; and spastic hemiplegia, 98; and walking, 91–93, 98. *See also* falls
basal ganglia, 12, *13, 34*–35
behavioral health, and CP, 137–138, 246–247
bilateral cerebral palsy, 34
Bimanual Fine Motor Function (BFMF), 46–47, *47*
bimanual therapy, 155, 169–170, *171*
blood pressure, high, 187, 277, 283, 284
body mass index (BMI), 277n, 300
bones: about, 80–82; aging, 274–276, 280–281, 292–293; atypical development, 108–122; density, *120,* 120–121, 245, 292; fractures, 275–276, 281; growth, 108, *108*; health of, 120–121; and muscle growth, 105; and nutrition, 245; orthopedic surgery, 231, 233
botulinum neurotoxin A (BoNT-A) injection, 220, 222–223
brain: injury during development, 4, 6, 15, 23, 75; location of injury, 34–36, *35, 73*–75, *75*; neuroplasticity, 23; structure and functions, 11–13, *12, 13*
bullying, 257–258

C

cancer, 276–277
cardiorespiratory (aerobic) exercise, 188, 298
cardiovascular disease, 276–277, 284
case studies, 336–337
casting, for stretching, 167
cerebellum, 11, *12, 13,* 34–35

cerebral palsy (CP): about, 3–58; and aging, 278–289; causes and risk factors, 14–17; classification, 30–58, *31–32, 33, 34, 35*; definition, 3–4, *4–5*; description, 153; diagnosis, 21–24; early intervention, 23–24; and function, 25–28, 39–52 (*see also* communication function; motor function); and gender, 16, 77–79, *78, 79*; introduction, 3–7; life expectancy, 269; and muscles, 106–107; and non-communicable diseases, 283–285; and physical activity, 187–189, *188–189*; and pregnancy, 288; prevalence, 18–19, 36–37, *37*; prevention, 18; registers, 18; research and funding, 19, 53, 148, 265, 271–272, *272*
cerebrum, 11–12, *12, 13,* 34–35
children, of people with CP, 288
cholesterol, high, 277, 283
choreo-athetosis, 31
chronic diseases. *See* noncommunicable diseases
classification systems: for communication, 48–49; for eating and drinking ability, 49–52; for health and disability, 55–58; for motor functions, 39–47; using, 53; for visual function, 52
clinical trials, 337–338
clonus, 101
clothing, adaptive, 208–209
Cobb angle, 119, *119*
cognition: and aging, 292; definition, 5; and language, 174–175; problems with, 71, 133, 136, 154–155, 246, 257, 270
cohort study, 336
cold extremities, 135
communication function, 25, 48–49, 69, 133, 154–155, 174–175, 243
Communication Function Classification System (CFCS), *48,* 48–49, 68–69, *69*
complementary treatments, 248–250, *249–250*
constipation, 136, 245
constraint-induced movement therapy (CIMT), 155, 169–170, *171*
contractures, 5, 85, 105–106, 197
cranial sacral osteopathy, 249
cross-sectional study, 336
crouch gait, 107–108, 130
cycling, *210,* 210–211

D
data-driven decision-making, 149, 234
degenerative joint disease, 296
depression and anxiety, 286
developmental milestones, 25–27, *27*
diabetes, 276–277, 284, 285
diplegia, 33, 35, 36–37
dogs, as mobility aids, 295
drop foot, 129, 164
dyskinesia, 31, 34–35, 37, 70, 218–219
dystonia, 31, 38, 70, 101–102, 218–219, 228

E
early intervention, 23–24, 27, 150, 154–155
eating ability, 49–52, 69, 133, 175, 209, *209,* 243
Eating and Drinking Ability Classification System (EDACS), 49–52, *50, 51,* 68–69, *69*
education, 256–259
elbow orthosis (EO), *201*
elbows: extension, 87; flexion, 66; orthoses, *201*; in spastic hemiplegia, 66, 86. *See also* upper limbs
electrical stimulation, 164
emphysema, 285
employment, 271, 286–288
epilepsy, 5, 70, 135, 244
episodes of care (EOC) model, 176–178, *178*
equinus gait, 68, 117, 129, 130
evidence-based medicine, 147–148, 333–334
exercise, 186–189, *188–189. See also* physical activity; sports, for individuals with CP
extremities, cold, 135

F
falls, 98, 121, 274, 275–276, 281–282, 295, 298. *See also* balance
family engagement in research, 337–339
family-centered care, 146–147
fatigue, 285
feet: abduction, 67; atypical bone development, 115–117, *116, 117*; dorsiflexion, 89, 205; malalignments, 116, 129; orthoses, *202–204*; in spastic hemiplegia, 67–68, 88. *See also* lower limbs
femoral anteversion, 113–114, *114*
femur, *113,* 113–114, *114*

fine motor function, 26, 69, 125–126. *See also* hand function; manual ability; motor function

fingers: extension, 87; flexion, 66; orthoses, 200; in spastic hemiplegia, 66, 86. *See also* upper limbs

foot orthoses (FO), 202

footdrop, 129, 164

functional electrical stimulation (FES), 164, 205, 206

Functional Independence Measure of Children (WeeFIM), 127, 127

functional mobility, 39–41, 40, 69, 162–163, 281. *See also* motor function

G

gait: and aging, 281; analysis, 234–236; classification system, 128–130, 129–130; computerized motion analysis, 131; crouch gait, 107–108; and foot malalignments, 116, 129; gait training, 162–163; orthopedic surgery, 233–240; and SEMLS, 237–238; and spastic hemiplegia, 128; and tone reduction treatment, 220; typical, 91, 92–93, 93. *See also* walking

games, adaptive equipment for, 216–217

gender: and cerebral palsy, 16; and non-communicable diseases, 283, 284

goal-setting, 150–152, 176–177

gross motor function, 26, 44, 44–45, 69. *See also* motor function

Gross Motor Function Classification System (GMFCS): about, 39–40; associated problems, 132; and bone density, 121; development curves, 44, 44; femoral anteversion, 114; hip displacement, 112; levels, 40, 40, 42–43; recommendations for sports, 190–191; and scoliosis, 120; and self-care, 127, 127; and spastic hemiplegia, 68–69, 69

H

hand finger orthoses (HFO), 200

hand function: about, 90–91; fine motor function, 26; and orthoses, 198; orthoses, 199–201, 200, 205; and sensory problems, 133–134; therapy, 155, 169–170; and tone reduction treatment, 220. *See also* manual ability

health services, for adults, 144, 251, 261, 271, 290–293, 299

hearing problems, 71, 133, 135, 244

heart attacks, 284. *See also* cardiovascular disease

hemiplegia, 33, 35, 36–37

high cholesterol, 277, 283

hiking, 211–212

hips: abduction, 89, 124; adduction, 66, 88, 130; displacement (subluxation and dislocation), 111–112, 112, 156; extension, 89, 129; external rotation, 89; flexion, 67, 88; internal rotation, 66, 88, 130; pelvic obliquity, 123; replacement, 297; in spastic hemiplegia, 66–67, 88; surveillance, 156. *See also* lower limbs

home program: about, 181–182; for adults, 297–298; exercise and physical activity, 186–191, 188–189, 190–191; postural management, 184–186; therapists' homework, 183–184

hydration, 245, 300

hyperactive stretch reflex, 100

hyperbaric oxygen, 249

hypertension, 187, 277, 283, 284, 285

hypertonia, 99

hypotonia, 32, 34–35, 37, 70, 99, 218

I

independence, of individuals with CP, 168, 171, 172, 175, 255, 259–260, 261, 281, 286–287

intelligence. *See* cognition

International Classification of Functioning, Disability and Health (ICF), 55–58, 56, 58

International Clinical Practice Guideline, for early intervention, 154

intrathecal baclofen (ITB), 220, 225–226, 226

J

joints: about, 81; aging, 274, 284, 285; and lower-limb movements, 88–89; and muscles, 84–85, 105–106; and orthoses, 197–198; pain, 284, 285; range of motion (ROM), 83–84, 85, 86–89, 105; replacement, 296; and upper-limb movements, 86–87

jump knee, 130

K
knee immobilizer, 167, *205*
knee orthosis, *205*
knees: extension, 89; flexion, 67, 88, 130;
    hyperextension, 67, 129; orthoses, *205*;
    in spastic hemiplegia, 67, 88. *See also*
    lower limbs

L
learned helplessness, 146
leg length discrepancy, 120, 123, 129,
    240–241
lever-arm dysfunction: about, 108–111;
    excessive femoral anteversion, 113–114;
    hip displacement, 111–112; pes valgus
    or pes varus, 115–118; tibial torsion,
    114–115; upper limb problems, 118
long sitting, 85
lower limbs: orthopedic surgery, 229–230,
    233–241; orthoses, 201–206, *202–205,
    206*; robotics, 163. *See also* ankles; feet;
    hips; knees
lumbar lordosis, 66

M
management and treatment, best practice:
    introduction, 145; principles, 146–152
management and treatment, for adults:
    best practice, 145–152; health services,
    290–293; home program, 297–298;
    mobility, 294–295; orthopedic surgery,
    296–297; overview, 299–300; services,
    144; taking responsibility for health,
    291–292, 299–300; therapies, 293–295;
    tone reduction, 228, 296; transition from
    pediatric, 260–265, *263*
management and treatment, to age 20:
    alternative and complementary treat-
    ments, 248–250, *249–250*; associated
    problems, 243–247; best practice,
    145–152; community integration and
    independence, 251–260; education,
    256–259; home program, 181–191;
    introduction, 143–144; orthopedic
    surgery, 229–241; overall philosophy,
    153–157; taking responsibility for
    health, 146, 151–152, 260, 264;
    therapies, 158–180; tone reduction,
    218–228; transition to adult model,
    260–265, *262, 263*
manual ability, 45–47, 69, 126–127. *See
    also* fine motor function

Manual Ability Classification System
    (MACS), 45–46, *46*, 68–69, *69*
massage, 249
measuring outcomes, 152, 177, 234
mental health, and CP, 137–138, 246–247
metabolic syndrome, 277
mobility aids, 162–163, 207, 294–295
monoplegia, 33
motor function: aging, 281; capacity and
    performance, 57; classification, 39–45,
    40, 42–43, 69; definition, 25; develop-
    ment curves, 44–45; developmental mile-
    stones, 25–27, *27*; early interventions,
    154; lack of control, 97; measuring, 28;
    and spastic hemiplegia, 125–131
motor system. *See* neuromusculoskeletal
    system
multidisciplinary team approach, 147
muscle-tendon unit, 83, 105n, 165
muscles: abnormal tone, 30n, 99–102, *102,*
    155, 218–219; about, 81–82; aging,
    275, 280; atypical growth, 105–108; and
    cerebral palsy, 106–107; contractions,
    types of, 82–83; contractures, 85; and
    joints, 84–85, 105–106; and lower-limb
    movements, *88–89*; orthopedic surgery,
    230, 233; posture, 82–83; strength *vs.*
    power, 83; strengthening, 161, 188;
    stretching, 85, 164–167; tone reduction,
    219–228; and upper-limb movements,
    86–87; weakness, 102. *See also* muscu-
    loskeletal system; neuromusculoskeletal
    system
musculoskeletal system: about, 80–89;
    in adulthood, 270; aging, 274–276,
    279–281, 284, 292–293; atypical bone
    development, 108–122; and balance,
    98; and cerebral palsy, 5; definition, 5;
    and excess weight, 300; and growth,
    77, 105; movement, 111; orthopedic
    surgery, 156–157; overall management,
    155–157; problems arising from spastic
    hemiplegia, 95–96; and selective motor
    control, 97; tone reduction, 219; treating
    problems, 155. *See also* bones; joints;
    muscles; nervous system; neuromusculo-
    skeletal system

N

nerve cells, 10–11, *11*

nervous system: about, 9–13, *10*; aging, 292; and balance, 11, 98; and function, 27; problems arising from brain injury, 95–96

neuromotor exercise, 298

neuromuscular electrical stimulation (NMES), 164

neuromusculoskeletal system, 95–96, 292. *See also* musculoskeletal system; nervous system

neuroplasticity, 23

night splints, 167, *204*

noncommunicable diseases, 276–277, *283*, 283–285, *284, 285*

nutrition, 245, 293, 300

O

obesity, 277, 283, 284, 300

occupational therapy, 168–172, 183–184, 230, 293–295

oral medications, for tone reduction, 220, 221

orthopedic surgery: about, 229–231; for adults, 296–297; bone surgery, 231; leg length discrepancy, 240–241; lower limbs, 233–241; measuring outcomes, 152, 234, 236; minimizing amount needed, 157; rehabilitation, 230, 232, 296–297; soft tissue surgery, 230; and spastic hemiplegia, 156–157; timing, 233; upper limbs, 231–233

orthoses: about, 197–199; for lower extremities, 201–206, *202–205, 206*; in occupational therapy, 169; for stretching, 166–167; for upper extremities, 199–201, *200–201*

osteoarthritis. *See* arthritis

osteopathy, 249

osteopenia, 121, 280

osteoporosis, 120–121, 275–276, 280

P

pain: and aging, 282, 284–285; associated problem, 244–245; and cerebral palsy, 135; and quality of life, 137

Paralympic sports, 194

participation, 56–58, 144, 153, 252, 255, 286–288, *287,* 300

passive stretching, 107, 165

pelvis, 66, 123, 124

periventricular leukomalacia (PVL), 73–74

person-centered care, 146–147

pes valgus, 115–117, *116,* 129

pes varus, 115–117, *117,* 129

phenol injection, 220, 224

physical activity: adaptive equipment, *210,* 210–213, *211, 213*; for adults, 146; and aging, 184, 281, 298, 299; definition, 186; and exercise, 186–188; and individuals with CP, 187–195; limitations, 5, 106; limitations and capability, 56–57; and noncommunicable diseases, 184; recommendations, *188–189*; and spastic hemiplegia, 105; as therapy, 167. *See also* sports, for individuals with CP

physical therapy: about, 159–161; active movement, 167; for adults, 293–295; casting, 167; electrical stimulation, 164; frequency, 176; functional mobility, 162; gait training, 162–163; homework, 183–184; and orthopedic surgery, 230; orthoses, 166–167; positioning, 165–166; strengthening, 161; stretching, 164–165

plantar flexed foot, 68, 88

positioning, for stretching, 165–166

posture: definition, 4; management, 184–186; mechanisms, 82, 83, 90n; and muscles, 107–108; for sitting, standing, sleeping, *185–186*

pregnancy, for individuals with CP, 288

preterm birth, 15, 16, 22n, 36, 75

primary problems: abnormal muscle tone, 99–102, *102*; about, 95–97; lack of selective motor control, 97; muscle weakness, 102; poor balance, 98; sensory problems, 103; treatment, 155

pronated forearm, 66, 86, 118, *118*

pronated midfoot, 116

proprioception, 98, 134

Q

quadriplegia, 33, 35, 36–37

quality of life (QOL), and CP, 137, 245, 282

R

randomized controlled trial, 335–336

range of motion (ROM), 83–84, *85,* 105–107, 219

reading, adaptive equipment for, *215*

reflexology, 250

relationships: intimate or romantic, 136, 286–287; sexual, 136, 246, 288

research: into cerebral palsy, 19, 53, 148, 265, 271–272, 272; and evidence-based medicine, 333–334; funding for, 148; getting involved in, 337–339; types of study design, 334–337
resistance exercise, 188, 298
respiratory disease, 276–277
robot-assisted therapy, 163, 170, 170–171, 171

S
sagittal gait patterns, 128
sarcopenia, 275, 280
scoliosis, 118–120, 119, 156
scooters, 207–208, 208, 295. See also mobility aids
secondary conditions, 270–273
secondary problems: about, 95–96, 104–105; atypical bone development, 108–122; atypical muscle growth, 105–108; definition, 5; orthopedic surgery, 233; treatment, 155
sedentary behavior, 187, 189, 298
selective dorsal rhizotomy (SDR), 220, 227
selective motor control, lack of, 97
self-care, 127, 127
sensory system: and balance, 98; in brain, 74, 75; problems, 103, 133, 243–244; and spastic hemiplegia, 133–135
setting goals, 150–152, 176–177
sexual relationships. See relationships
shared decision-making, 148
shoes: adaptive, 208; for orthoses, 202
shoulders: abduction, 87; adduction, 65, 86; extension, 87; external rotation, 87; flexion, 86; internal rotation, 65, 86; in spastic hemiplegia, 65. See also upper limbs
single-event multilevel surgery (SEMLS): about, 229, 237–238; for adults, 296–297; aftermath, 239–240; bone surgery, 238; and gait analysis, 234–237; goals of, 237–239; for lower limb vs. upper limb, 156–157; rehabilitation, 156, 230, 239–240; soft tissue surgery, 238; upper limbs, 232–233
sleep: importance of, 245, 299; posture, 137; problems, 136, 245–246
SMART goals, 150–151
social connections, 256

spastic hemiplegia: in adulthood, 270–273, 278–300; and aging, 270–272, 278–289, 291–293; alternative and complementary treatments, 248–250, 249–250; areas of unmet need, 288–289; assistive technology, 196–217; associated problems, 70–71, 71, 132–138, 153–154, 243–247; bones, joints, muscles, and movements, 80–89, 86–89; cause, 64; classification, 68–69; co-occurring motor types, 70, 101, 218–219; community integration and independence, 251–260; CP-specific early interventions, 154–155; education, 256–259; and growth, 77–78; having children, 288; home program, 181–191, 297–298; introduction, 63–64; location of brain injury, 73–75, 75; and motor function, 125–131; noncommunicable diseases, 283–285, 284, 285; orthopedic surgery, 229–242, 296–297; and physical activity, 187–189, 188–189; physical features, 64–68, 65–68; primary problems, 95–103; secondary conditions, 270–273; secondary problems, 104–121; tertiary problems, 123–124; therapies, 158–180, 293–295; tone reduction, 218–228, 296; transition from childhood to adulthood, 259–265. See also cerebral palsy (CP); spasticity; management and treatment entries
spasticity: co-occurring motor types, 37–38; definition, 21, 99, 218; description, 31; and dystonia, 38, 70, 101–102; location of brain injury, 34–35; movements affected by, 84–85, 86–89; and muscle tone, 99–102, 218–219; prevalence, 36–37; strengthening muscles, 161; stretching, 165; treatment (see tone reduction)
specialist centers, for CP, 149–150, 228
speech and language pathology, 174–175, 183–184
speech problems, 49, 71, 133, 154–155, 174–175, 243
spine: in nervous system, 9, 10, 12, 12, 13; and spastic hemiplegia, 66, 118–120, 119; surveillance, 156
sports, for individuals with CP, 189–191, 190–191, 194–195, 210, 210–213, 211, 213
stereognosis, 134, 244
strengthening muscles, 161, 169, 188

stretching, 99–100, *100,* 105, 107–108, 164–167, 169, 197–198, 297
strokes, 14, 15, 74, 284, 285
supine midfoot, 117
supramalleolar orthosis (SMO), *202*
systematic review, 335

T
tactile ability, 90, 98, 133–134, 244
technology, adaptive, 213–214, *214*
tendons, 83, 105n, 165, 230, 232, 233, 238
tertiary problems: about, *95–96,* 123–124; correcting, 124
thalamus, 12, *13,* 34–35
therapies: definition, 158; delivery, 176–178, *178;* frequency, 176–177; getting the most from appointment, 179–180; home program, 181–191; occupational therapy, 168–174, 293–295; overall management philosophy, 153–157; physical therapy, 159–167, 293–295; speech and language pathology, 174–175
three-dimensional (3D) computerized motion analysis, 131, 234–236
thumbs: abduction, 87; adduction, 66; extension, 87; flexion, 66; orthoses, *200;* in spastic hemiplegia, 66, 86. *See also* upper limbs
tibial torsion, 114–115, *115*
toe walking, 68, 117, 129
tone reduction: about, 219; for adults, 296; botulinum neurotoxin A (BoNT-A) injection, 222–223; choosing treatment, 228; intrathecal baclofen (ITB), 225–226, *226;* oral medications, 221; phenol injection, 224; selective dorsal rhizotomy (SDR), 227; treatment overview, *220,* 220–221
transition, from childhood to adulthood, 259–265
triplegia, 33
truncal sway, 124

U
unilateral cerebral palsy, 34. *See also* spastic hemiplegia
upper limbs: movements, *86–87;* orthopedic surgery, 229–230, 231–233; orthoses, 199–201, *200–201,* 205; therapy, 155; use of, 125–127, *126. See also* arms; elbows; fingers; hand function; manual ability; shoulders; thumbs; wrists
urinary dysfunction, 135

V
valgus hindfoot, 67, 116, 129. *See also* pes valgus
varus hindfoot, 68, 117, 129. *See also* pes varus
vaulting, 124
ventricles, 12, *13,* 73–74, *75*
Viking Speech Scale, 48–49, *49*
visual function, 52, *52,* 71, 133, 135, 244
Visual Function Classification System (VFCS), 52, *52*

W
W-sitting, 166, *166*
walking: about, 91–93; and aging, 281; developmental milestones, 27; energy conservation, 93, 130–131, 299; and GMFCS, *40, 42–43,* 44; physical therapy, 162–163; and rest, 295, 299; and spastic hemiplegia, 93, 100, 128–131. *See also* gait
wheelchairs, 207–208, 295. *See also* mobility aids
wrist hand finger orthoses (WHFO), *200*
wrist hand orthosis (WHO), *201*
wrists: extension, 87; flexion, 66, 86, 118, *118;* orthoses, *200–201. See also* upper limbs

Y
yoga, 250